AF443581

Cholestatic Liver Diseases:
New Strategies for Prevention and Treatment of Hepatobiliary and Cholestatic Liver Diseases

FALK SYMPOSIUM 75

Cholestatic Liver Diseases:

New Strategies for Prevention and Treatment of Hepatobiliary and Cholestatic Liver Diseases

EDITED BY

G.P. van Berge Henegouwen

Department of Gastroenterology
University Hospital Utrecht
Box 85500
NL-3508 GA Utrecht
The Netherlands

J. De Groote

UZ Gasthuisberg
Hepatologie
Herestraat 49
B-3000 Leuven
Belgium

B. van Hoek

Department of Gastroenterology and
Hepatology
University Hospital Leiden
PO Box 9600
NL-2300 RC Leiden
The Netherlands

S. Matern

III. Medizinische Abteilung
Klinische Anstalten der RWTH
Pauwelsstr.
D-52074 Aachen
Germany

R.W. Stockbrügger

Werkgroep Gastroenterologie/Hepatologie
Interne Geneeskunde
Akademisch Ziekenhuis Maastricht
Postbus 5800
NL-6202 AZ Maastricht
The Netherlands

Proceedings of the 75th Falk Symposium held in Maastricht, The Netherlands, April 22–23, 1994

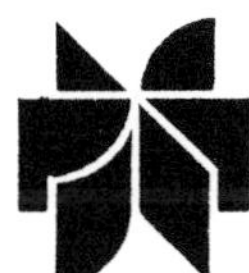

KLUWER ACADEMIC PUBLISHERS
DORDRECHT / BOSTON / LONDON

Distributors

---

for the United States and Canada: Kluwer Academic Publishers, PO Box 358,
Accord Station, Hingham, MA 02018-0358, USA
for all other countries: Kluwer Academic Publishers Group, Distribution
Center, PO Box 322, 3300 AH Dordrecht, The Netherlands

A catalogue record for this book is available from the British Library.

ISBN 0-7923-8867-4

Library of Congress Cataloging-in-Publication Data

Falk Symposium (75th : 1994 : Maastricht, Netherlands)
    Cholestatic liver diseases : new strategies for prevention and treatment of hepatobiliary
and cholestatic liver diseases / edited by G.P. van Berge Henegouwen ... [et al.].
        p.   cm.
    "Proceedings of the 75th Falk Symposium held in Maastricht, The Netherlands, April
22–23, 1994."
    Includes bibliographical references and index.
    ISBN 0-7923-8867-4 (casebound)
    1. Cholestasis—Treatment—Congresses.   2. Cholestasis—Prevention—Congresses.
3. Gallstones—Treatment—Congresses.   4. Gallstones—Prevention—Congresses.
I. Berge Henegouwen, Gerard Pieter van.   II. Title.
    [DNLM: 1. Cholestasis—physiopathology—congresses.   2. Cholestasis—therapy—
congresses.   3. Cholelithiasis—therapy—congresses.   WI 703 F191c 1994]
    RC854.C45F35   1994
    616.3'6—dc20
    DNLM/DLC
    for Library of Congress

94-23373
CIP

Contents

CONTENTS

**SECTION V: GALLBLADDER AND BILE DUCT STONES:
EPIDEMIOLOGY AND TREATMENT**

CONTENTS

List of Principal Authors

IM Arias
Department of Physiology
Tufts University School of Medicine
136 Harrison Ave
Boston, MA 02111
USA

MF Bassendine
Liver Unit
Freeman Hospital
High Heaton
Newcastle Upon Tyne NE7 7DN
UK

GP van Berge Henegouwen
Department of Gastroenterology
University Hospital Utrecht
Box 85500
NL-3508 GA Utrecht
The Netherlands

N Blanckaert
Department of Clinical Pathology
UZ-KUL Medical Center
B-3000 Leuven
Belgium

JL Boyer
Liver Center and Department of
    Medicine
Yale University School of Medicine
333 Cedar Street
New Haven, CT 06510
USA

N Busch
Department of Digestive Diseases
Klinikum der RWTH
Pauwelsstr. 30
D-52057 Aachen
Germany

HR van Buuren
Department of Internal Medicine
    II/Room Ca 326
University Hospital Rotterdam
Dr Molewaterplein 40
NL-3015 GD Rotterdam
The Netherlands

MC Carey
Harvard Medical School
Gastroenterology Division
Brigham & Women's Hospital
75 Francis Street
Boston, MA 02115
USA

RW Chapman
Department of Gastroenterology
John Radcliffe Hospital
Headington
Oxford OX3 9DU
UK

C Colombo
Department of Pediatrics
University of Milano
Via Commenda 9
I-20122 Milano
Italy

PB Cotton
Digestive Disease Center
Medical University of South Carolina
171 Ashley Avenue
Charleston, SC 29425-2220
USA

VJ Desmet
Universitaire Ziekenhuisen Leuven
Dienst Pathologische Ontleedkunde II
Minderbroederstraat 12
B-3000 Leuven
Belgium

RH Dowling
UMDS
Gastroenterology Unit
18th Floor, Guy's Tower
Guy's Hospital
London SE1 9RT
UK

AK Groen
Department of Gastroenterology
Academisch Medisch Centrum
Meibergdreef 9
NL-1105 AZ Amsterdam
The Netherlands

J De Groote
UZ Gasthuisberg
Hepatologie
Herestraat 49
B-3000 Leuven
Belgium

B van Hoek
Department of Gastroenterology and
    Hepatology
Building 1, C4-P
Rijnsburgerweg 10
NL-2333 AA Leiden
The Netherlands

AF Hofmann
Division of Gastroenterology
Department of Medicine (T-013)
University of California, San Diego
La Jolla, CA 92093-0813
USA

RM Janas
Department of Nuclear Medicine
Hormone Laboratory
Child Health Centre
Meml. Hosp., Al. Dzieci Polskich 20
04-736 Warsaw
Poland

F Kuipers
Academic Hospital Groningen
CMC IV, Room Y3137
Oostersingel 59
NL-9713 EZ Groningen
The Netherlands

U Leuschner
Zentrum Innere Medizin
Johann Wolfgang Goethe Universität
Theodor-Stern-Kai 7
D-60596 Frankfurt
Germany

S Matern
Medizinische Klinik III
Klinikum der RWTH Aachen
Pauwelsstr. 30
D-52057 Aachen
Germany

PJ Meier
Abteilung für Klinische Pharmakologie
    und Toxicologie
Medizinische Klinik Universitätsspital
Ramistr. 100
CH-8091 Zurich
Switzerland

TC Northfield
Division of Biochemical Medicine
St George's Hospital Medical School
Cranmer Terrace
London SW17 0RE
UK

R Olsson
Medical Clinic
Sahlgrenska Hospital
Göteborg
Sweden

JB Otte
Department of Pediatric Surgery
Clinique Univeritaires Saint-Luc
Avenue Hippocrate 10
B-1200 Bruxelles
Belgium

G Paumgartner
Department of Medicine II
Klinikum Grosshadern
Marchioninistr. 15
D-81377 München
Germany

P Portincasa
Gastroenterology Department
University Hospital Utrecht
PO Box 85500
NL-3508 GA Utrecht
The Netherlands
and
Istituto di Clinica Medica I
University of Bari Medical School
Policlinico
I-70124 Bari
Italy

LIST OF PRINCIPAL AUTHORS

BC Portmann
Institute of Liver Studies
King's College School of Medicine
Bessemer Road
London SE5 9RS
UK

R Poupon
Unite d'Hepato-Gastroenterologie
Hopital Saint-Antoine
184 rue du Fbg. Saint-Antoine
F-75571 Paris Cedex 12
France

A Radominska
Division of Gastroenterology
Department of Biochemistry
University of Arkansas for Medical
  Sciences
Little Rock, Arkansas
USA

E Roda
Cattedra di Gastroenterologia
Policlinico S. Orsola
Via Massarenti 9
I-40138 Bologna
Italy

KDR Setchell
Division of Clinical Mass
  Spectrometry
Children's Hospital Medical Center
3333 Burnet Ave
Cincinnati, OH 45229
USA

J Sjövall
Department of Medical Biochemistry
  and Biophysics
Karolinska Institutet
S-171 77 Stockholm
Sweden

PB Soeters
University Hospital Maastricht
Department of Surgery
P. Debyelaan 25
NL-6229 HX Maastricht
The Netherlands

W Van Steenbergen
Department of Internal Medicine
Liver Unit
UZ Gasthuisberg
Herestraat 49
B-3000 Leuven
Belgium

B Stieger
Division of Clinical Pharmacology and
  Toxicology
Department of Medicine
University Hospital
CH-8091 Zürich
Switzerland

A Stiehl
Medizinische Universitätsklinik
Bergheimer Str. 58
D-69115 Heidelberg
Germany

RW Stockbrügger
Division of Gastroenterology/
  Hepatology
Department of Internal Medicine
Academic Hospital Maastricht
P. Debyelaan 25
NL-6202 AZ Maastricht
The Netherlands

MFJ Stolk
Department of Gastroenterology
University Hospital Utrecht
Box 85500
NL-3508 GA Utrecht
The Netherlands

OT Terpstra
Department of Surgery
University Hospital Leiden
PO Box 9600
NL-2300 RC Leiden
The Netherlands

RH Wiesner
Gastroenterology Unit
Mayo Clinic and Foundation
200 First Street SW
Rochester, MN 55905
USA

Preface

This book comprises the scientific contributions to Falk Symposium No. 75: 'Cholestatic liver diseases: new strategies for prevention and treatment of hepatobiliary and cholestatic liver diseases'. The focus of this meeting was on cholestasis and gallstone disease.

The liver is the central organ in the metabolism and detoxification of many endogenous and exogenous compounds. Recent studies have led to a better understanding of the pathways of uptake, transport, conjugation and biliary excretion of metabolites. In this book both progress in basic science in this field and the direct application of this knowledge to treatment of hepatobiliary diseases are presented. The emphasis for clinical diseases is on chronic cholestatic conditions, such as primary biliary cirrhosis and primary sclerosing cholangitis, and on gallstone disease. The focus is on the new treatment modalities of these diseases. Recent data on bile acid therapy with the hydrophilic bile salt ursodeoxycholic acid and other new treatment modalities of chronic cholestatic liver diseases are discussed. Furthermore recent developments in the pathogenesis of gallstone disease, such as mechanisms of bile lipid secretion, gallbladder motility and epidemiology, are also presented. Finally, recent strategies for prevention and lithotripsy and endoscopic treatment of gallbladder and bile duct stones are included.

This book should provide both research scientists and clinicians with all the information on cholestatic and hepatobiliary disease currently available. The editors feel that in this symposium a good balance was reached between basic science and clinical applications. In this meeting the new concept of invited oral presentations by selection from the submitted abstracts was tested. The editors feel that this also was a great success. Many investigators were able to present their work by poster or orally, as included in this book. The editors hope that this symposium in the city of Maastricht – like the still partially unfulfilled treaty of Maastricht for the creation of a Europe without borders – will help us also to bring down 'borders of ignorance' in the science of hepatology, and extend cooperation between different research groups.

The editors are grateful to the contributors who made this first Falk Symposium in the Netherlands such a success, with almost 500 participants from many European countries and the USA. They also extend their thanks to Dr Herbert Falk and his staff for the generous support of the meeting, and to Kluwer Academic Publishers for their very helpful cooperation in publishing these proceedings.

Gerard P. van Berge Henegouwen
Jan De Groote
Bart van Hoek
Siegfried Matern
Reinhold W. Stockbrügger (editors)

Section I
Mechanisms of bile formation and cholestasis

1
Histopathology of cholestasis

V. J. DESMET

Liver biopsy is useful in the diagnosis and differential diagnosis of cholestatic syndromes. The histopathological alterations observed in the liver during cholestatic syndromes can be grouped under two general headings: (1) features of cholestasis, common to most – if not all – acute or chronic cholestatic liver disorders; and (2) features which are more or less characteristic for particular entities, and thus are helpful in recognizing individual diseases.

BASIC HISTOLOGICAL FEATURES OF CHOLESTASIS

Parenchymal features

Bilirubinostasis is the most striking histological feature in acute cholestasis, but may be missing for long periods of time in several chronic cholestatic disorders (see below: cholate stasis)[1].

Bilirubinostasis corresponds to the microscopically visible accumulation of bile pigment (bilirubin) in the liver tissue. Bilirubin accumulates in different locations: as smaller or larger inclusions in parenchymal cells (hepatocellular bilirubinostasis), as inclusions in hypertrophic Kupffer cells (Kupffer cell bilirubinostasis); as bile plugs in dilated intercellular canaliculi (canalicular bilirubinostasis), or as inspissated concrements in bile ductules (ductular bilirubinostasis).

Hepatocellular bilirubinostasis in acinar zone 3 is an early change in acute intrahepatic or extrahepatic (obstructive) cholestasis, soon followed by canalicular bilirubinostasis. Retention of bile components results in hepatocellular damage, which leads to Kupffer cell activation; activated and hypertrophic Kupffer cells phagocytose the debris from necrotizing parenchymal cells and the liberated intercellular bile plugs, resulting in Kupffer cell bilirubinostasis. The latter feature thus indicates a cholestatic condition of at least several days duration[2].

Ductular bilirubinostasis represents an intriguing histological change, which is not found in most cholestatic conditions. It is supposed to be caused by an inhibition of the normal secretory function of bile ductular cells. Ductular bilirubinostasis is seen in massive liver cell necrosis[3], in septicaemia and endotoxic shock[4,5], in total parenteral nutrition, during the evolution of extrahepatic bile duct atresia[6], and as sign of 'preservation damage' after liver transplantation[7].

Cholate stasis is a feature of chronic cholestasis. It may be observed together with bilirubinostasis. However, in most diseases characterized by long-standing, incomplete obstruction of intra- or extrahepatic bile ducts, bilirubinostasis may be absent during periods of months or even years. In such cases the histological diagnosis of chronic cholestasis relies heavily on the detection of features of cholate stasis, together with other changes such as feathery degeneration, xanthomatous cells, ductular reaction and periportal fibrosis (see below).

The term cholate stasis refers to a cytological lesion of parenchymal cells in acinar zone 1 (periportal hepatocytes), which is thought to be due to the membrane-damaging effect of retained bile acids with detergent effect[8].

In periportal areas with features of cholate stasis the parenchymal cells appear swollen, pale and coarsely granular. These cells show accumulation of copper and copper-binding protein (metallotheonein), which can be demonstrated by specific stains; e.g. rhodamine staining for copper, and Shikata's orcein stain or Victoria blue for copper-binding protein. With time, Mallory bodies develop in these cells, and eventually bilirubin inclusions[8].

In chronic cholestasis, single hepatocytes or groups of parenchymal cells show *feathery degeneration*; this corresponds to hydropic swelling with variable bilirubin-impregnation of the remaining visible cytoplasm[2].

Xanthomatous cells are a feature of long-standing cholestasis. They correspond to lipid-laden histiocytes with finely vacuolated or foamy cytoplasm, related to the hyperlipidaemia of chronic cholestasis. They usually occur in clusters in portal tracts and in the parenchyma[2].

Cholestatic liver cell rosettes are a very useful feature in the histopathological diagnosis of chronic cholestatic disorders. They correspond to a transformation of the normal, one cell thick parenchymal cell plates into tubular structures. Under the light microscope they appear as glandular structures lined by four or more hepatocytes around a central lumen with variable diameter. The lumen may be empty, or may contain eosinophilic or bilirubin-stained material with variable degree of condensation.

Part or all of the lining hepatocytes may show features of feathery degeneration. These parenchymal tubular structures are in continuity with bile ductular structures[9], and express bile duct-type cytokeratins, indicating a phenotypic shift towards bile duct type cells[10].

Bile infarcts represent a late parenchymal feature in severe cholestasis of long duration, mainly seen in extrahepatic bile duct obstruction. The lesions correspond to necrosis of groups of paraportal hepatocytes, with bilirubin impregnation of the necrotic area; they become gradually replaced by fibrous tissue[2].

Periportal and architectural features

Complete and incomplete blockade in bile secretion, especially when caused by diseases of extra- and intrahepatic bile ducts, is associated with *'ductular reaction'*. This term refers to an increased number of ductular profiles in the periphery of the portal tract, gradually extending into the periportal parenchyma. This increase in number of ductular structures is accompanied by oedema and infiltration by neutrophil polymorphonuclear leucocytes (cholangiolitis) and fibrosis.

The cholangiocytes lining the ductules may show signs of reabsorption of bile constituents, reflected in vacuolization of the cytoplasm, accumulation of lipofuscin and bilirubin inclusions, leading in some instances to formation of inspissated bile concrements in the lumen[8].

The periportal extension of the ductular reaction with its accompanying inflammatory neutrophil infiltrate into the periportal parenchyma showing features of cholate stasis results in an irregular portal–parenchymal interface, which has been termed *'biliary piecemeal necrosis'*.

The progressive wedge-shaped extensions of the periportal ductular reaction eventually result in fibrous linkage of adjacent portal tracts. This stage of *biliary fibrosis*[11,12] is a potentially reversible lesion, since the basic intrahepatic vascular relationships are preserved[13].

With ongoing cholestasis, portal–central septa also develop, accompanied by nodular parenchymal regeneration, resulting in some instances in the final irreversible stage of *biliary cirrhosis*[11,13].

FEATURES CHARACTERIZING SPECIFIC CHOLESTATIC DISEASE

Neonatal cholestatic disorders

Neonatal cholestatic liver diseases are usually associated with parenchymal giant cell transformation, and are often accompanied by extramedullary haematopoiesis[14]. Cryptogenic neonatal cholestasis, often referred to as *'neonatal giant cell hepatitis'*, is characterized by basic features of cholestasis, parenchymal giant cells, extramedullary haematopoiesis, and possibly some degree of parenchymal siderosis and intralobular fibrosis.

In metabolic disorders such as *galactosaemia* and *fructose intolerance*, there is severe bilirubinostasis with bile plugs in pseudoglandular arrangements of hepatocytes and a constant fatty change. The early stage is characterized by ductular proliferation around the portal tracts[15]. In *tyrosinaemia* one finds somewhat similar features, with in addition variable parenchymal siderosis, extramedullary haematopoiesis, and variably sized foci of nodular regeneration[15,16].

α_1-*Antitrypsin deficiency* may be associated with some degree of periportal ductular reaction and parenchymal bilirubinostasis. The diagnostic feature is the presence of PAS-positive, diastase-resistant inclusions in periportal hepatocytes, which react positively on immunostaining with specific antibodies[17]. In a minority of cases, paucity of interlobular bile ducts may also be present[18].

Byler syndrome or *progressive intrahepatic cholestasis* has no pathognomonic histological features. The liver changes include bilirubinostasis in the early stage, giant cell transformation in about half the cases, and bile duct paucity in about three-quarters of patients. Later lesions include periportal and pericentral fibrosis, ductular reaction, and finally cirrhosis of the biliary type[18,19].

Paucity of interlobular bile ducts is recognized by a reduced bile duct-to-portal tract ratio, which normally lies between 0.9 and 1.8[20]. In *syndromic paucity of interlobular bile ducts* (Alagille syndrome), the lesions vary with the ageing of the patient. In early liver biopsies (up to 3 months of age) the number of interlobular ducts may be normal, but the ducts may show signs of duct destruction. The lobular parenchyma reveals parenchymal giant cells and bilirubinostasis. Later changes (in children older than 3 months) include duct paucity of variable degree, often associated with periportal fibrosis, and less parenchymal giant cells[18,21]. The diagnosis of syndromic paucity of interlobular bile ducts relies on the histological demonstration of duct damage and destruction (in early biopsies) or paucity of ducts (in later biopsies), in association with the typical extrahepatic clinical features of Alagille syndrome[18].

Non-syndromic paucity of interlobular bile ducts is characterized by more or less similar histological features, except that bile duct destruction, duct paucity and fibrosis seem to develop earlier and to proceed faster than in the syndromic variety[18]. Non-syndromic paucity of ducts may be associated with a number of other disorders, and is the most frequent diagnosis in infants with conjugated hyperbilirubinaemia in the first month of life. It apparently comprises a heterogeneous group of disorders[18,22].

The histopathology of *extrahepatic bile duct atresia* also evolves with the age of the patient. In the early stage the picture is not diagnostic and resembles that of neonatal giant cell hepatitis. Gradually, portal oedema and ductular reaction set in as sequels of the extrahepatic obstruction. The extending ductular reaction is associated with progressive periductular fibrosis and often ductular bilirubinostasis. Within a few months the lesions evolve into biliary fibrosis and finally biliary cirrhosis.

A further important diagnostic hallmark are the alterations of the interlobular ducts, which show signs of necro-inflammatory destruction to a varying extent. With time the number of interlobular ducts decreases progressively, resulting in a variable degree of ductopenia. The disappearance of interlobular ducts and the ensuing ductopenia suggest that in extrahepatic bile duct atresia the obliterating cholangiopathy is not restricted to some segments of the extrahepatic biliary system, but also involves the intrahepatic ducts[6].

In about one-fifth to one-quarter of cases the interlobular ducts still appear in their primitive embryonic shape, the so-called ductal plate malformation. In this lesion the bile ducts appear as segments of circular profiles, and are also the site of necro-inflammatory epithelial changes as in classical extrahepatic bile duct atresia. Furthermore, one often notes a hypoplasia of the portal vein branches and a more advanced degree of portal and periportal fibrosis[6,23].

Adult cholestatic disorders

Parenchymal diseases

Simple bilirubinostasis – with bilirubin granules in hepatocytes, bile plugs in canaliculi, and bilirubin inclusions in Kupffer cells – is seen in a number of conditions. These include: the very early stage of extrahepatic bile duct obstruction, some forms of drug-induced cholestasis, benign recurrent intrahepatic cholestasis (Summerskill–Tygstrup–De Groote disease), intrahepatic cholestasis of pregnancy, acute fatty liver of pregnancy, and some cases of postoperative cholestasis[24].

Features of parenchymal bilirubinostasis are usually present in *acute alcoholic hepatitis*. The histological picture further comprises a mixed micro- and macrovesicular steatosis, Mallory bodies, satellitosis, possibly central hyaline sclerosis and often paucicellular periportal fibrosis[25,26].

Parenchymal bilirubinostasis of variable degree is part of the histopathological picture of *acute viral hepatitis*. Some forms of acute viral hepatitis A are more cholestatic, and characterized by ductular lesions at the junction between the parenchyma and the intrahepatic biliary tree[27]. Severe acute viral hepatitis with massive parenchymal necrosis may be associated with ductular reaction and ductular bilirubinostasis[3,28].

Parenchymal bilirubinostasis is a frequent component of *drug-induced liver disease*[29]. It may occur as the only lesion, often referred to as 'simple cholestasis' ('Reine Cholestase' of the German literature). The prototype drugs causing this lesion are anabolic steroids and contraceptive drugs. Associated necro-inflammatory parenchymal lesions constitute a picture of 'cholestatic hepatitis', exemplified by chlorpromazine jaundice.

The histopathological diagnosis of drug-induced cholestasis or cholestatic hepatitis is facilitated in cases with marked portal infiltration by eosinophils, or in the presence of smaller or larger epithelioid granulomas, eventually associated with multinucleated giant cells. Examples of drugs preferentially associated with this lesion include diphenylhydantoin, phenylbutazone and sulphonyl urea[29,30].

Acute venous congestion of the liver (e.g. heart decompensation, Budd–Chiari syndrome) may be associated with parenchymal bilirubinostasis, which is often overlooked[31]. The associated features are those of passive venous congestion, with centrolobular sinusoidal dilatation and atrophy, or even necrosis of acinar zone 3 hepatocytes.

Diseases of intrahepatic bile ducts

A number of cholestatic syndromes are characterized by progressive inflammatory destruction of intrahepatic bile ducts of different calibre; they are categorized as 'vanishing bile duct' disorders[32,33]. A detailed description of the histopathology of each of these disorders is beyond the scope of this review. Brief mention is made of the most characteristic features of each disease, but it must be borne in mind that such features are not always sampled in every biopsy specimen, and are not always present in every stage of the disease.

The histological hallmark of *primary biliary cirrhosis* is granulomatous cholangitis[11]. The bile ducts primarily involved are those with a diameter around 80 μm. They show degenerative epithelial changes, lymphocytic infiltration, and finally destruction and disappearance of the duct[1]. The involved portal tracts are the site of dense lymphoplasmocytic infiltration, and epithelioid granulomas often appear close to the affected duct. A similar histological picture is observed in immune cholangitis[34] or autoimmune cholangiopathy[35].

A granulomatous cholangitis associated with intrahepatic bile duct destruction characterizes some cases of *sarcoidosis with intrahepatic cholestasis*[36]. Histological differentiation from primary biliary cirrhosis is difficult, if not impossible.

Primary sclerosing cholangitis has no pathognomonic histological features. The most suggestive lesion is fibro-obliterative cholangitis[11], characterized by concentric periductal fibrosis, followed by progressive atrophy and finally disappearance of the duct. It must be emphasized that similar bile duct changes may also be observed in secondary sclerosing cholangitis, and that the lesion is often missing in needle biopsy specimens from patients with primary sclerosing cholangitis. A diagnostic suggestion has often to be based on periportal ductular reaction, some degree of ductopenia and biliary-type fibrosis, and parenchymal features of chronic cholestasis (e.g. cholate stasis; cholestatic liver cell rosettes).

Idiopathic adulthood ductopenia[37] is characterized by a reduced number of interlobular bile ducts, associated with parenchymal, periportal and often architectural changes of chronic cholestasis. In some cases, necroinflammatory destruction of remaining interlobular ducts may be observed[38]. None of the histological features is pathognomonic. The diagnosis of idiopathic adulthood ductopenia requires exclusion of all other known causes of chronic cholestasis[37,39].

Liver allograft rejection occurs in the settings known as acute, or cellular rejection and chronic, or ductopenic rejection[7,40]. Acute, cellular rejection of the liver transplant is characterized by a triad of lesions: a mixed portal inflammatory infiltrate, including lymphoid blast cells; interlobular bile duct involvement; and endotheliitis of portal and/or central veins[7,41–43]. Parenchymal features include bilirubinostasis and variable degrees of necroinflammatory lesions. Chronic, ductopenic rejection is characterized by absence of interlobular bile ducts; the portal inflammatory infiltrate is usually mild. Obliteration of the lumen of larger branches of the hepatic artery by xanthomatous cells occurs in many cases[7,42,43].

Chronic graft-versus-host disease, occurring after bone marrow transplantation, is diagnosed in liver biopsies on the findings of portal inflammation, bile duct and ductular damage and destruction, possibly endotheliitis of the portal veins, and parenchymal lesions including bilirubinostasis and often reticuloendothelial siderosis and necroinflammatory foci[44].

Damage and destruction of interlobular bile ducts is observed in some forms of *drug-induced cholestatic liver disease*[45,46] and in some patients with *histiocytosis X*[47] and *Hodgkin's lymphoma*[48].

Chronic cholestasis and variable degrees of biliary fibrosis, occasionally resulting in focal biliary cirrhosis, may be a hepatic complication of *mucoviscidosis*[49]. Histopathology reveals increased numbers of ductules with periportal fibrosis; the ductules appear dilated and plugged with dense, PAS-positive, diastase-resistant concrements[50].

Besides the 'vanishing bile duct' disorders briefly enumerated above, other conditions of intrahepatic bile ducts may also predispose to episodes of cholestasis. Examples include Caroli's disease, predisposing to repeated bouts of cholangitis[51] and parasitic infestations of the bile ducts[52].

Extrahepatic bile duct obstruction

A great diversity of lesions may cause obstruction of the extrahepatic bile ducts[53]. Distinction should be made between conditions associated with complete obstruction of the extrahepatic biliary passageways, and those characterized by narrowing only, or incomplete obstruction.

Acute complete obstruction of the extrahepatic bile ducts leads to the full clinical picture of obstructive jaundice. Histologically, the liver is characterized by oedema of the portal tracts and parenchymal bilirubinostasis first restricted to acinar zone 3. After a few days, inflammation occurs in the portal areas, with neutrophil polymorphs predominating around the proliferating ductules in the periportal area (cholangiolitis); the parenchymal bilirubinostasis gradually extends from acinar zone 3 towards the periportal areas.

Chronic complete obstruction of the extrahepatic bile ducts shows all components of the basic features of cholestasis described above: severe panlobular bilirubinostasis, feathery degeneration, cholestatic liver cell rosettes, xanthomatous cells, cholate stasis and paraportal bile infarcts, periportal ductular reaction with periductular fibrosis, development of portal–portal septa, biliary fibrosis and eventually secondary biliary cirrhosis[13].

Chronic incomplete obstruction of the extrahepatic bile ducts is accompanied by some features of chronic cholestasis, such as elevated blood levels of alkaline phosphatase, 5′-nucleotidase and γ-glutamyl transpeptidase, but not necessarily by an increase in the serum levels of conjugated bilirubin. Histologically, the liver biopsy reveals parenchymal and periportal features of chronic cholestasis (compare above), the extent of which varies according to the duration of the condition. However, bilirubinostasis may remain absent for long periods of time. Accordingly, the cholestatic condition needs to be diagnosed in the absence of visible bile pigment accumulation, although the latter represents the most classical histological feature of cholestasis. Examples of chronic incomplete obstruction include narrowing of the common bile duct by strictures, by large duct sclerosing cholangitis, or by annular pancreas. In some chronic alcoholics a sclerosing chronic pancreatitis may be at the origin of the syndrome[54].

A similar constellation of findings may occur in diseases characterized by narrowing and destruction of progressively increasing numbers of *intrahepatic* bile ducts in the presence of an intact extrahepatic biliary system, such as in primary biliary cirrhosis and in small duct primary sclerosing cholangitis.

References

1. Desmet VJ. Chronic cholestasis. In: Hoofnagle JH, Goodman Z, editors. Liver biopsy: interpretation for the 1990s. Thorofare: Slack Inc.; 1991:25–38.
2. Desmet VJ. General pathology. In: McIntyre N, Benhamou J-P, Bircher J, Rizzetto M, Rodes J, editors. Oxford textbook of clinical hepatology, Vol. 1. Oxford: Oxford University Press; 1991:263–9.
3. Schmid M, Cueni B. Portal lesions in viral hepatitis with submassive hepatic necrosis. Hum Pathol. 1972;3:209–16.
4. Lefkowitch JH. Bile ductular cholestasis: an ominous histopathologic sign related to sepsis and 'cholangitis lenta'. Hum Pathol. 1982;13:19–24.
5. Banks JG, Foulis AK, Ledingham IMcA, MacSween RN. Liver function in septic shock. J Clin Pathol. 1982;35:1249–52.
6. Desmet VJ, Callea F. Cholestatic syndromes of infancy and childhood. In: Zakim D, Boyer TD, editors. Hepatology. A textbook of liver disease, Vol. 2, 2nd edn. Philadelphia: Saunders; 1990:1355–95.
7. Demetris AJ. The pathology of liver transplantation. In: Popper H, Schaffner F, editors. Progress in liver diseases, Vol. IX. Philadelphia: Saunders; 1990:687–709.
8. Desmet VJ. Current problems in diagnosis of biliary disease and cholestasis. Semin Liver Dis. 1986;6:233–45.
9. Nagore N, Howe S, Scheuer PJ. The three-dimensional liver. In: Popper H, Schaffner F, editors. Progress in liver diseases, Vol. 9. Philadelphia: Saunders; 1990:1–10.
10. Van Eyken P, Sciot R, Desmet VJ. A cytokeratin immunohistochemical study of cholestatic liver disease: evidence that hepatocytes can express 'bile duct-type' cytokeratins. Histopathology. 1989;15:125–35.
11. Ludwig J. New concepts in biliary cirrhosis. Semin Liver Dis. 1987;7:293–301.
12. Desmet VJ. Modulation of the liver in cholestasis. J Gastroenterol Hepatol. 1992;7:313–23.
13. Desmet VJ. Cirrhosis: aetiology and pathogenesis: cholestasis. In: Boyer JL, Bianchi L, editors. Liver cirrhosis. Falk Symposium 44, Lancaster: MTP Press; 1987:101–18.
14. Desmet VJ. Pathology of paediatric cholestasis. In: Lentze M, Reichen J, editors. Paediatric cholestasis: novel approaches to treatment. Dordrecht: Kluwer; 1992:55–73.
15. Ishak KG, Sharp HL. Metabolic errors and liver disease. In: MacSween RNM, Anthony PP, Scheuer PJ, editors. Pathology of the liver, 2nd edn. Edinburgh: Churchill Livingstone; 1987:99–180.
16. Ishak KG. Pathology of inherited metabolic disorders. In: Balistreri WF, Stocker JT, editors. Pediatric hepatology. New York: Hemisphere; 1990:77–158.
17. Callea F, Brisigotti M, Faa G, Lucini L, Eriksson S. Identification of PiZ gene products in liver tissue by a monoclonal antibody specific for the Z mutant of alpha-1-antitrypsin. J Hepatol. 1991;12:372–6.
18. Kahn E. Paucity of interlobular bile ducts. Arteriohepatic dysplasia and nonsyndromic duct paucity. In: Abramowsky CR, Bernstein J, Rosenberg HS, editors. Perspectives in pediatric pathology. Transplantation pathology – hepatic morphogenesis. Basel: Karger: 1991:168–215.
19. Whitington PF, Freese DK, Alonso EM, Fishbein MH, Emond JC. Progressive familial intrahepatic cholestasis (Byler's disease). In: Lentze M, Reichen J, editors. Paediatric cholestasis. Novel approaches to treatment. Dordrecht: Kluwer; 1992:165–180.
20. Alagille D. Intrahepatic biliary atresia (hepatic ductular hypoplasia). In: Berenberg SR, editor. Liver disease in infancy and childhood. Baltimore: Williams & Wilkins; 1976: 129–42.
21. Hashida Y, Yunis EJ. Syndromatic paucity of interlobular bile ducts: hepatic histopathology of the early and endstage liver. Pediatr Pathol. 1988;8:1–15.
22. Watkins JB. Neonatal cholestasis: developmental aspects and current concepts. Semin Liver

Dis. 1993;13:276–88.

23. Desmet VJ. Congenital diseases of intrahepatic bile ducts: variations on the theme 'ductal plate malformation'. Hepatology. 1992;16:1069–83.

24. Desmet V. Morphologic aspects of intrahepatic cholestasis. In: Gentilini P, Teodori U, Gorini S, Popper H, editors. Intrahepatic cholestasis. New York: Raven Press; 1975:7–23.

25. Desmet VJ. Alcoholic liver disease. Histological features and evolution. Acta Med Scand Suppl. 1985;703:111–26.

26. Sciot R, Desmet VJ. Alcoholic liver disease: histopathology. In: Watson RR, editor. Alcohol and cancer. Boca Raton: CRC Press; 1992:203–33.

27. Sciot R, Van Damme B, Desmet VJ. Cholestatic features in hepatitis A. J Hepatol. 1986;3:172–81.

28. Desmet V, De Groote J, Van Damme B. Acute hepatocellular failure. A study of 17 cases treated with exchange transfusion. Hum Pathol. 1972;167–82.

29. Desmet VJ. Drug-induced liver disease: pathogenetic mechanisms and histopathological lesions. Eur J Med. 1993;2:36–47.

30. Zimmerman HJ. Hepatotoxicity. The adverse effects of drugs and other chemicals on the liver. New York: Appleton Century Crofts; 1978.

31. Nolte D. Ikterus der Leber bei chronischer Herzinsuffizienz. Virchows Arch A. 1966;341: 37–42.

32. Desmet VJ. Vanishing bile duct disorders. In: Boyer JL, Ockner RK, editors. Progress in liver diseases, Vol. X. Philadelphia: Saunders; 1992:89–121.

33. Woolf GH, Vierling JM. Disappearing intrahepatic bile ducts: the syndromes and their mechanisms. Semin Liver Dis. 1993;13:261–75.

34. Brunner G, Klinge O. Ein der chronisch-destruierenden nicht-eitrigen Cholangitis ähnliches Krankheitsbild mit antinukleären Antikörpern. Dtsch Med Wochenschr. 1987;112: 1454–58.

35. Ben-Ari Z, Dhillon AP, Sherlock S. Autoimmune cholangiopathy: part of the spectrum of autoimmune chronic active hepatitis. Hepatology. 1993;18:10–15.

36. Rudzki C, Ishak KG, Zimmerman HJ. Chronic intrahepatic cholestasis of sarcoidosis. Am J Med. 1975;59:373–87.

37. Ludwig J, Wiesner RH, La Russo NF. Idiopathic adulthood ductopenia. A cause of chronic cholestatic liver disease and biliary cirrhosis. J Hepatol. 1988;7:193–9.

38. Faa G, Van Eyken P, Demelia L, Vallebona E, Costa V, Desmet VJ. Idiopathic adulthood ductopenia presenting with chronic recurrent cholestasis. A case report. J Hepatol. 1991;12:14–20.

39. Zafrani ES, Metreau J-M, Douvin C et al. Idiopathic biliary ductopenia in adults: a report of five cases. Gastroenterology. 1990;99:1823–8.

40. Ludwig J. Terminology of hepatic allograft rejection (Glossary). Semin Liver Dis. 1992;12: 89–92.

41. Snover DC, Freese DK, Sharp HL, Bloomer JR, Najarian JS, Ascher NL. Liver allograft rejection. Analysis of the use of biopsy in determining outcome of rejection. Am J Surg Pathol. 1987;11:1–10.

42. Ludwig J. Histopathology of the liver following transplantation. In: Maddrey WC, editor. Transplantation of the liver. New York: Elsevier; 1988:191–218.

43. Wight DGD, Portmann B. Pathology of liver transplantation. In: Calne R, editor. Liver transplantation, 2nd edn. London: Grune & Stratton; 1987:385–435.

44. Snover DC. Biopsy diagnosis of liver disease. Baltimore: Williams & Wilkins; 1992:218–31.

45. Bianchi L. Intrahepatic bile duct damage in various forms of liver diseases. In: Brunner H, Thaler H, editors. Hepatology, a festschrift for Hans Popper. New York: Raven Press; 1985:295–310.

46. Degott C, Feldmann G, Larrey D et al. Drug-induced prolonged cholestasis in adults: a histological semiquantitative study demonstrating progressive ductopenia. Hepatology. 1992;15:244–51.

47. Leblanc A, Hadchouel M, Jehan P, Odievre M, Alagille D. Obstructive jaundice in children with histiocytosis X. Gastroenterology. 1981;80:134–9.

48. Hubscher SG, Lumley MA, Elias E. Vanishing bile duct syndrome: a possible mechanism for intrahepatic cholestasis in Hodgkin's lymphoma. Hepatology. 1993;17:70–7.

49. Park RW, Grand RJ. Gastrointestinal manifestations of cystic fibrosis: a review. Gastroenter-

    ology. 1981;81:1143–61.
50. International Group. Histopathology of the intrahepatic biliary tree. Liver. 1983;3:161–75.
51. Summerfield JA, Nagafuchi Y, Sherlock S, Cadafalch J, Scheuer PJ. Hepatobiliary fibropolycystic disease: a clinical and histological review of 51 patients. J Hepatol. 1986;2:141–56.
52. Ishak KG. New developments in diagnostic liver pathology. In: Farber E, Phillips J, Kaufman N, editors. Pathogenesis of liver diseases. Baltimore: Williams & Wilkins; 1987:223–373.
53. Desmet VJ. Cholestasis: extrahepatic obstruction and secondary biliary cirrhosis. In: MacSween RNM, Anthony PP, Scheuer PJ, editors. Pathology of the liver, 2nd edn. Edinburgh: Churchill Livingstone; 1987:364–423.
54. Afroudakis A, Kaplowitz N. Liver histopathology in chronic common bile duct stenosis due to chronic alcoholic pancreatitis. Hepatology. 1981;1:65–72.

2
Mechanisms of bile formation

J. L. BOYER

INTRODUCTION

Bile formation is the process by which the liver generates a complex secretion of water, electrolytes and many different organic solutes for delivery to the intestine. It begins with formation of a primary secretion at the hepatocyte, known as canalicular bile, by both bile salt-dependent and -independent mechanisms, followed by modifications at more distal sites along the length of the bile ductular epithelium[1,2]. This review briefly summarizes present concepts of the mechanism of bile formation, emphasizing more recent concepts which have provided insights at the cellular and molecular level.

CANALICULAR BILE

Canalicular bile is formed by a process of osmotic filtration in response to osmotic gradients created within the lumen of the bile canaliculus between adjacent hepatocytes. These osmotic gradients are formed by sinusoidal and canalicular membrane transport systems that generate the bile acid-dependent and bile acid-independent components of canalicular bile flow[2]. An additional component of bile is elaborated by the *bile duct epithelium*, which generates a bicarbonate-enriched secretion in response to the hormone, secretin.

BILE ACID-DEPENDENT BILE FLOW (BADF)

Bile acid excretion is a major determinant of canalicular bile flow and is dependent on a series of membrane transport systems on hepatocyte membranes. Bile acids are first transported from sinusoidal blood into the liver by highly specific high-affinity carriers that remove the majority of bile acid from the circulation in a single pass. These transport carriers are both sodium-dependent and sodium-independent. The sodium-dependent co-transporter has been cloned from rat (ntcp) and more recently from human liver (NTCP)[3,4]. The rat cDNA encodes for a 362 amino acid polypeptide with five membrane-spanning domains. The human protein also has five membrane-spanning domains but is slightly smaller, consisting of 349 amino acids of which 77% are identical to the rat. When the rat transporter is expressed in either oocytes or COS-7 cells[3,5], kinetic studies reveal a K_m of approximately 30 μmol/l, essentially identical to the kinetic properties in isolated hepatocyte preparations. Substrate inhibition studies in transfected cell lines (Meier *et al.*, personal communication) suggest that this carrier is specific for conjugated and unconjugated bile acids and sulphated oestrogen. Both the rat and human co-transporters have an obligate requirement for sodium ions which provide the driving force for transport into the hepatocyte against 10-fold concentration gradient. These transporters are secondary active transport systems, since the inwardly directed sodium gradients which sustain hepatic bile acid uptake are maintained by Na^+,K^+-ATPase, a basolateral membrane ion transporter that exchanges three Na^+ ions for two K^+ ions. The intracellular negative electrical potential also facilitates hepatic bile acid uptake[6,7]. The electrical driving force is regulated by the outward conductance of K^+ via K^+ channels in the basolateral membrane[8,9].

There is no known homology with other sodium-coupled transport systems with the exception of the recently cloned hamster ileal bile acid transport system, which is 63% identical to the rat liver protein and thus represent a unique gene family[10]. Moreover, these polypeptides do not contain a previously described consensus sequence for sodium binding found in other sodium-coupled transporters, such as the ileal D-glucose transporter among others[10]. Antibodies prepared against fusion proteins and peptides from the C-terminus have localized the rat sodium-coupled bile acid transport to the basolateral domain of the hepatocyte throughout the lobular gradient[11,12]. Thus all hepatocytes appear to express this mechanism for bile acid uptake. The expression of this transporter is highly regulated, however, at both transcriptional and post-transcriptional levels, and the peptide is no longer expressed in animals following bile duct ligation[13]. The rat bile acid co-transporter is transcribed only in mammalian liver, as its messenger RNA is not expressed in lower vertebrates[14]. During development the message is first detected immediately prior to birth, reaching adult levels of expression within a week or two after parturition[14].

A high-affinity basolateral sodium-*independent* transporter for bile acids has also been cloned from both rat and human liver, although the driving forces for this transport system are not yet known[15]. The rat cDNA encoding for this transporter demonstrates specificity for a variety of other organic anions, including bilirubin and BSP, as well as unconjugated and conjugated bile acids. This transporter has a requirement for Cl^- ions. Multispecific organic anion transporters have also been demonstrated in lower vertebrates and expressed in *Xenopus* oocytes, but it is not yet known if they are part of a larger gene family or are distinct gene products[14,16].

Following transport into the hepatocyte, bile acids accumulate in the cytosol in concentrations approximately 10-fold those obtained in the sinusoidal circulation, and bind to cytosolic bile acid-binding proteins which may facilitate intracellular movement to the canalicular domain[17]. The most specific is the 3α-hydroxysteroid dehydrogenase, a member of the oxidoreductase superfamily, a 37 kDa protein consisting of 322 amino acids with a high affinity for bile acids[18] (K_m, 1–2 μmol/l).

Recent evidence suggests that bile acids may also be transported into intracellular vesicular compartments within the microsomal membrane system of the liver. Here an epoxide hydrolase has been identified with a high capacity for bile acid transport which is both sodium-independent and electrogenic[19]. The precise role of this transporter (which has also been found at the sinusoidal membrane[20]) in intrahepatic bile acid transport is not clear, but this system may be of more importance when bile acid levels increase in the hepatocyte during cholestatic liver injury. Transcytotic microtubule-dependent vesicular transport may also be involved in movement of bile acids from the sinusoidal domain to the canalicular membrane. Apically located proteins appear to be directed to the basolateral domain after synthesis prior to being targeted in vesicles to their canalicular membrane residence[21,22]. Thus the bile acid transporters should be present in transcytotic vesicles *en route* to the bile canaliculus. It is therefore of interest that recent studies show that inhibition of microtubule function inhibits the accumulation of fluorescent bile acids within the canalicular lumen in isolated hepatocyte couplets in association with a reduction in canalicular membrane surface and reduced targeting of canalicular domain proteins[23]. These findings support the view that canalicular excretory function may be regulated by the movement of vesicles into and out of the canalicular domain.

Distinct transport systems exist on the canalicular domain for the movement of bile acids across the canalicular membrane into bile, where they are further concentrated and result in the osmotic stimulation of BADF[24,25]. These transporters consist of an ATP-dependent bile acid transporter identified in isolated canalicular membrane vesicles[26,27], a potential-driven transport system[28–30], and an ecto-ATPase[31,32]. The membrane potential is an important driving force for canalicular excretion of bile acids in the intact hepatocyte couplet or perfused rat liver; however, the size of this potential can account for the excretion of no more than 50% of the transported solute, so that the more recently described ATP-dependent bile acid transport system appears to play an important physiological role[33]. Whether the ATP-dependent and potential-dependent functions reside on the same transporter is not clear, and must await efforts to clone the(se) proteins. However, recent experiments have separated these functions into two populations of vesicles using free-flow electrophoresis techniques[34]. These studies suggest that the ATP-dependent system is found on both canalicular and intracellular vesicles, whereas the potential-driven system is present only on the intracellular membranes. As yet it is not clear how an intracellular location could account for the *in-vivo* effects of the membrane potential on canalicular bile acid excretion[30,33].

Controversy also exists concerning the role of a canalicular ecto-ATPase in bile acid excretion. This approximately 100–110 kDa protein is a Ca^{2+},Mg^{2+}-ATPase which has been cloned and is part of the immunoglobulin superfamily. When its cDNA is transiently transfected into COS-1 cells, bile acid translocating properties are conferred on the COS cells which normally do not excrete bile acids[31]. This transport function is distinct from the protein's

ATPase activity and is dependent on the C-terminal portion of the construct[32]. This highly glycosylated protein (the cDNA encodes for only a 57 kDa polypeptide) has only a single membrane-spanning domain and ATP must bind from the luminal side. Thus a physiological role in bile acid excretion has not yet been accepted.

As previously mentioned, bile acid transport is a highly regulated process, influenced by both transcriptional and post-transcriptional modifications. However, the specific factors that influence this regulation remain to be determined. For example how do protein kinase A agonists stimulate the uptake and excretion of bile acids, as recently demonstrated[35]? Another intriguing observation is the effect of bile acids on cell volume and the bile acid transport maximum, presumably a function of transporters on the canalicular domain. Infusions of bile acids, both taurocholate and tauroursodeoxycholate, in the isolated perfused liver increase cell volume[36,37]. Other studies indicate that factors which increase hepatocyte swelling result in the fusion of pericanalicular vesicles with the canalicular domain, stimulating bile flow by exocytosis and increasing the transport maximum of the liver for bile acid transport[38,39]. This phenomenon is blocked by microtubule inhibitors. Tauroursodeoxycholate appears to stimulate vesicular exocytosis in the perfused rat liver by mobilizing extracellular calcium[40]. These observations suggest that bile acids may autoregulate the capacity for canalicular bile acid transport through osmotically or calcium-activated canalicular fusion of transporters on pericanalicular vesicles.

BILE ACID-INDEPENDENT BILE FLOW (BAIF)

A significant fraction of canalicular bile formation, although variable in different mammalian species, is independent of the secretion of bile acids. In general, BAIF forms a major portion of secretion from pericentral hepatocytes, whereas periportal parenchymal cells are thought to be the major sites of bile acid-dependent secretion.

While the mechanisms which generate BAIF are not fully understood, there is accumulating indirect evidence that a significant component is stimulated by the canalicular excretion of glutathione and glutathione ligands[41,42]. In the rat, concentrations of glutathione reach levels comparable to the intermicellar concentrations of bile acids[43]. However, the relationship between bile flow and the osmotic activity of glutathione is complicated by the intraluminal hydrolysis of this peptide into its constituent amino acids, which are also reabsorbed from the canaliculus and the bile duct lumen[43-45]. Canalicular membrane transport for GSH is driven by the membrane potential[46], and the cDNA for this transporter has recently been cloned from rat liver[47].

An additional component of BAIF appears to be generated by the secretion of bicarbonate, and is generated by the activity of a canalicular Cl^-/HCO_3^- exchanger which also resides on the canalicular domain[48,49]. This exchanger is the major acid-loading mechanism in hepatocytes and is activated when intracellular pH is increased above the normal set point[50]. Interestingly, recent studies suggest that the activity of this exchanger is higher in cells derived from pericentral regions of the lobule where BAIF is believed to be more prominent[51]. Recent studies in the isolated perfused rat liver indicate that bile flow and bicarbonate excretion are stimulated in parallel by manoeuvres that result in acute intracellular alkalinization[52]. This phenomenon, which is also inhibited by DIDS, is consistent with activation of the Cl^-/HCO_3^- exchanger. Activation of this exchanger also appears to be associated with the movement of pericanalicular vesicles to the canalicular domain, since inhibitors of microtubules block activation of the exchanger in isolated hepatocytes[53] as well as the stimulation of bile flow and the biliary excretion of horseradish peroxidase (markers of vesicular transport) in the isolated perfused rat liver following stimulation by intracellular alkalinization or administration of DBcAMP[52]. Thus both BAIF and BADF appear to be regulated by vesicle insertion of transporters into the apical domain.

It is likely that other canalicular transport systems may also contribute to BAIF. A tertiary active transporter, HCO_3^-/SO_4^{2-} exchange resides in the canalicular domain and has recently been cloned from rat liver[54,55]; however, its function remains to be established.

BILE DUCT EPITHELIUM

An understanding of the role of the bile duct epithelium in the process of bile formation at the cellular and molecular level has lagged behind the accumulation of information about canalicular bile. However, it is clear that primary canalicular bile can be modified by both secretory and absorptive processes as it passes along the biliary epithelium. Following the discovery of secretin, it was learned that this hormone could stimulate bicarbonate secretion in most species, and that the source of this secretion was the biliary epithelium[56]. Now the cellular mechanisms for this effect are beginning to be understood, as techniques have been developed to isolate bile duct epithelial cells and bile duct units[57-60]. Ion transporters have been identified in isolated bile duct epithelial cells from the rat that regulate intracellular pH, including a Na^+/H^+ exchanger, Na^+/HCO_3^- symport, and Cl^-/HCO_3^- exchanger[58,59]. While the non-polarized nature of these isolated cell preparations precludes assignment of domain localization, the physiology argues for placement of the Cl^-/HCO_3^- exchanger on the luminal domain of the bile duct cell, a conclusion supported by recent studies in isolated polarized bile duct segments where forskolin, a stimulator of adenylcyclase, increases luminal pH in the presence but not the absence of bicarbonate[60]. Additional electrophysiological studies in isolated cells have demonstrated a chloride channel[59,61] and the CFTR gene product (thought to represent the chloride channel in secretory epithelia) has been immunolocalized to the apical or luminal membrane of duct cells in both human and rat, the predominant site of CFTR mRNA expression in the liver[62,63]. Furthermore, secretin receptors have been identified in bile duct epithelium[64] and secretin increases cAMP levels[65,66], opens chloride channels[59], and stimulates Cl^-/HCO_3^-

exchange activity in isolated rat bile duct cells[59].

Based on these findings the following model for secretin stimulation of a HCO_3^--rich secretion is proposed. Secretin stimulates increases in cAMP, activating luminal chloride channels, which result in chloride leaving the duct cell by conduction. This loss of negative charge depolarizes the cell, resulting in electrogenic stimulation of Na^+/HCO_3^- symport, presumably at the basolateral domain, leading to increased entry of HCO_3^- anions and activation of the Cl^-/HCO_3^- exchanger on the luminal membrane[59,62]. As long as the chloride channel, which is closed in the resting state[62], remains open, the secretion of HCO_3^- should continue with chloride recycling across the apical membrane. Secretin also stimulates vesicle exocytosis in the rat[67] and pig[68,69], and studies in the pig suggest that acid is secreted at the basolateral domain, possibly secondary to insertion of H^+-ATPases since the process is inhibited by baflomycin, a specific inhibitor of vacuolar H^+-ATPases[70]. Whether this latter phenomenon is generalizable or species-specific remains to be determined. There is also accumulating evidence that the bile duct epithelium is heterogeneous with respect to transport function, and that secretin receptors may reside only on medium-sized and larger bile ducts in the rat[71]. This phenomenon may explain why some but not all isolated bile duct epithelial cell preparations respond to secretin with activation of the Cl^-/HCO_3^- exchanger.

Constituents of bile are also reabsorbed by the biliary epithelium, including fluid, a process that is stimulated by somatostatin[72]. Other solutes excreted in canalicular bile may also be reabsorbed from the canalicular lumen and across bile duct epithelium including glucose[73] (the GLUT-1 gene product for glucose transport is localized to bile duct epithelium[74]), and amino acid products of glutathione hydrolysis, glutamic acid[75], glycine[76], and cysteine, as well as the dipeptide, glycyl-cysteine[45].

Thus bile, the final 'exocrine' product of the liver, is the net result of a highly complex process, beginning with the osmotic filtration of water and electrolytes at the bile canaliculus, to which products of canalicular exocytosis are added and constituents further modified by secretory and reabsorptive transport functions along the length of the canalicular conduits within the lobule and the bile duct epithelium. Rapid progress is being made to unravel the complexity of this process at the cellular and molecular level.

References

1. Nathanson MH, Boyer JL. Mechanisms and regulation of bile secretion. Hepatology. 1991;14:551–66.
2. Boyer JL, Graf J, Meier PJ. Hepatic transport systems regulating pHi, cell volume, and bile secretion. Annu Rev Physiol. 1992;54:415–38.
3. Hagenbuch B, Stieger B, Foguet M, Lubbert H, Meier PJ. Functional expression cloning and characterization of the hepatocyte Na^+/bile acid cotransport system. Proc Natl Acad Sci USA. 1991;88:10629–33.
4. Hagenbuch B, Meier PJ. Molecular cloning, chromosomal localization, and functional characterization of a human liver Na^+/bile acid cotransporter. J Clin Invest. 1994;93: 1326–31.
5. Boyer JL, Ng OC, Ananthanarayanan M et al. Expression and characterization of a

functional rat liver Na$^+$ bile acid cotransport system in COS-7 cells. Am J Physiol. 1994;266:G382–7.

6. Lidofsky SD, Fitz JG, Weisiger RA, Scharschmidt BF. Hepatic taurocholate uptake is electrogenic and influenced by transmembrane potential difference. Am J Physiol. 1993;264:G478–85.

7. Weinman SA, Weeks RP. Electrogenicity of Na-coupled bile salt transport in isolated rat hepatocytes. Am J Physiol. 1993;265:G73–80.

8. Henderson RM, Graf J, Boyer JL. Inward-rectifying potassium channels in rat hepatocytes. Am J Physiol. 1989;256:G1028–35.

9. Graf J, Henderson RM, Krumpholz B, Boyer JL. Cell membrane and transepithelial voltages and resistances in isolated rat hepatocyte couplets. J Membr Biol. 1987;95:241–54.

10. Wong MH, Oelkers P, Craddock AL, Dawson PA. Expression cloning and characterization of the hamster ileal sodium-dependent bile acid transporter. J Biol Chem. 1994;269:1340–7.

11. Ananthanarayanan M, Ng OC, Boyer JL, Suchy FJ. Characterization of the cloned rat liver sodium–bile acid cotransporter using C-terminal peptide and fusion protein antibodies. Am J Physiol. 1994 (in press).

12. Stieger B, Hagenbuch B, Cornacchia L, Schroeder A, Landmann L, Meier PJ. Molecular properties of the Na$^+$-dependent taurocholate cotransporting polypeptide (ntcp) of rat liver. Hepatology. 1993;18:143A.

13. Gartung C, Ananthanarayanan M, Rahman MA, Stolz A, Suchy FJ, Boyer JL. Cholestasis induces down-regulation of the sodium dependent bile acid (BA) cotransporter and cytosolic binding proteins following bile duct ligation (BDL) in the rat. Hepatology. 1993;18:139A.

14. Boyer JL, Hagenbuch B, Ananthanarayanan M, Suchy F, Stieger B, Meier PJ. Phylogenic and ontogenic expression of hepatocellular bile acid transport. Proc Natl Acad Sci USA. 1993;90:435–8.

15. Jacquemin E, Hagenbuch B, Stieger B, Wolkoff AW, Meier PJ. Expression cloning of a rat liver Na$^+$-independent organic anion transporter. Proc Natl Acad Sci USA. 1994;91:133–7.

16. Jacquemin E, Hagenbuch B, Wolkoff AW, Meier PJ, Boyer JL. Expression of sodium-independent organic anion uptake systems of skate liver in *Xenopus luevis* oocytes. Am J Physiol. 1994 (in press).

17. Stolz A, Takikawa H, Ookhtens M, Kaplowitz N. The role of cytoplasmic proteins in hepatic bile acid transport. Annu Rev Physiol. 1989;51:161–76.

18. Stolz A, Hammond L, Lou H, Takikawa H, Ronk M, Shively JE. cDNA cloning and expression of the human hepatic bile acid-binding protein – a member of the monomeric reductase gene family. J Biol Chem. 1993;268:10448–57.

19. Alves C, von Dippe P, Amoui M, Levy D. Bile acid transport into hepatocyte smooth endoplasmic reticulum vesicles is mediated by microsomal epoxide hydrolase, a membrane protein exhibiting two distinct topological orientations. J Biol Chem. 1993;268:20148–55.

20. von Dippe P, Amoui M, Alves C, Levy D. Na$^+$-dependent bile acid transport by hepatocytes is mediated by a protein similar to microsomal epoxide hydrolase. Am J Physiol. 1993;264:G528–34.

21. Bartles JR, Feracci HM, Stieger B, Hubbard AL. Biogenesis of the rat hepatocyte plasma membrane in vivo: comparison of the pathways taken by apical and basolateral proteins using sub-cellular fractionation. J Cell Biol. 1987;105:1241–51.

22. Schell MJ, Maurice M, Stieger B, Hubbard AL. 5′ Nucleotidase is sorted to the apical domain of hepatocytes via an indirect route. J Cell Biol. 1992;119:1173–82.

23. Boyer JL, McGrath JW, Ng OC. Microtubule dependent targeting of transporters to the apical membrane determines the canalicular excretion of bile acids in hepatocyte couplets. Hepatology. 1993;18(4):107A.

24. Arias IM, Che MX, Gatmaitan Z, Leveille C, Nishida T, St Pierre M. The biology of the bile canaliculus. Hepatology. 1993;17:318–29.

25. Meier PJ. Transport processes at the canalicular surface of rat hepatocytes. In: Reutter W, editor. Modulation of liver cell expression (Falk Symposium No. 43). Boston: MTP; 1986:127–41.

26. Muller M, Ishikawa T, Berger U et al. ATP-dependent transport of taurocholate across the hepatocyte canalicular membrane mediated by a 110-kDa glycoprotein binding ATP

and bile salt. J Biol Chem. 1991;266:18920–6.

27. Nishida T, Gatmaitan Z, Che MX, Arias IM. Rat liver canalicular membrane vesicles containing an ATP-dependent bile acid transport system. Proc Natl Acad Sci USA. 1991;88:6590.

28. Inoue M, Kinne R, Tran T, Arias IM. Taurocholate transport by rat liver canalicular membrane vesicles. J Clin Invest. 1984;73:659–63.

29. Meier PJ, Meier-Abt AS, Barrett C, Boyer JL. Mechanisms of taurocholate transport in canalicular and basolateral rat liver plasma membrane vesicles. J Biol Chem. 1984;259:10614–22.

30. Weinman SA, Graf J, Boyer JL. Voltage-driven, taurocholate-dependent secretion in isolated hepatocyte couplets. Am J Physiol. 1989;256:G826–32.

31. Sippel CJ, Suchy FJ, Ananthanarayanan M, Perlmutter DH. The rat liver ecto-ATPase is also a canalicular bile acid transport protein. J Biol Chem. 1993;268:2083–91.

32. Sippel CJ, McCollum MJ, Perlmutter DH. Bile acid transport by the rat liver canalicular bile acid transport ecto-ATPase protein is dependent on ATP but not on its own ecto-ATPase activity. J Biol Chem. 1994;269:2800–26.

33. Weinman SA, Graf J, Veith C, Boyer JL. Electroneutral uptake and electrogenic secretion of a fluorescent bile salt by rat hepatocyte couplets. Am J Physiol. 1993;264:G220–30.

34. Kast C, Stieger B, Winterhalter KH, Meier PJ. Hepatocellular transport of bile acids – evidence for distinct subcellular localizations of electrogenic and ATP-dependent taurocholate transport in rat hepatocytes. J Biol Chem. 1994;269:5179–86.

35. Grune S, Engelking LR, Anwer MS. Role of intracellular calcium and protein kinases in the activation of hepatic Na^+/taurocholate cotransport by cyclic AMP. J Biol Chem. 1993;268:17734–41.

36. Hallbrucker C, Lang F, Gerok W, Haussinger D. Cell swelling increases bile flow and taurocholate excretion into bile in isolated perfused rat liver. Biochem J. 1992;281:593–6.

37. Haussinger D, Hallbrucker C, Saha N, Lang F, Gerok W. Cell volume and bile acid excretion. Biochem J. 1992;288:681–90.

38. Bruck R, Haddad P, Graf J, Boyer JL. Regulatory volume decrease stimulates bile flow, bile acid excretion, and exocytosis in isolated perfused rat liver. Am J Physiol. 1992;262:G806–12.

39. Haussinger D, Saha N, Hallbrucker C, Lang F, Gerok W. Involvement of microtubules in the swelling-induced stimulation of transcellular taurocholate transport in perfused rat liver. Biochem J. 1993;291:355–60.

40. Beuers U, Nathanson MH, Isales CM, Boyer JL. Tauroursodeoxycholic acid stimulates hepatocellular exocytosis and mobilizes extracellular Ca^{++} mechanisms defective in cholestasis. J Clin Invest. 1993;92:2984–93.

41. Ballatori N, Truong AT. Relation between biliary glutathione excretion and bile acid-independent bile flow. Am J Physiol. 1989;2560:G22–30.

42. Ballatori N, Truong AT. Glutathione as a primary osmotic driving force in hepatic bile formation. Am J Physiol. 1992;263:G617–24.

43. Ballatori N, Truong AT, Ma AK, Boyer JL. Determinants of glutathione efflux and biliary GSH/GSSG ratio in perfused rat liver. Am J Physiol (Gastrointest Liver Physiol). 1989;256:G482–90.

44. Ballatori N, Jacob R, Boyer JL. Intrabiliary glutathione hydrolysis. J Biol Chem. 1986;261:7860–5.

45. Abbott WA, Meister A. Intrahepatic transport and utilization of biliary glutathione and its metabolism. Proc Natl Acad Sci USA. 1986;83:1246–50.

46. Fernandez-Checa JC, Ookhtens M, Kaplowitz N. Selective induction by phenobarbital of the electrogenic transport of glutathione and organic anions in rat liver canalicular membrane vesicles. J Biol Chem. 1993;268(15):10836–41.

47. Yi J, Lu S, Knezic Z, Erhart N, Fernandez-Checa J, Kaplowitz N. cDNA cloning and initial characterization of the canalicular GSH transporter of rat liver. Hepatology. 1993;18:107A.

48. Hardison WGM, Wood GA. Importance of bicarbonate in bile salt independent fraction of bile flow. Am J Physiol (Endocrinol Metab Gastrointest Physiol 4). 1978;235:E158–64.

49. Meier PJ, Knickelbein RG, Moseley RH, Dobbins JW, Boyer JL. Evidence for carrier-mediated chloride/bicarbonate exchange in canalicular rat liver plasma membrane vesicles. J Clin Invest. 1985;75:1256–63.

50. Benedetti A, Strazzabosco M, Corasanti JG, Haddad P, Graf J, Boyer JL. Cl^- HCO_3 exchanger in isolated rat hepatocytes: role in regulation of intracellular pH. Am J Physiol. 1991;261:G512–22.

51. Benedetti A, Baroni GS, Marucci L, Mancini R, Jezequel AM, Orlandi F. Regulation of intracellular pH in isolated periportal and perivenular rat hepatocytes. Gastroenterology. 1993;105:1797–805.

52. Bruck R, Benedetti A, Strazzabosco M, Boyer JL. Intracellular alkalinization stimulates bile flow and vesicular-mediated exocytosis in IPRL. Am J Physiol. 1993;265(2):G347–53.

53. Benedetti A, Strazzabosco M, Ng OC, Boyer JL. Regulation of activity and apical targeting of the Cl^-/HCO_3^- exchanger in rat hepatocytes. Proc Natl Acad Sci USA. 1994;91:792–6.

54. Meier PJ, Valantinas J, Hugentobler G, Rahm I. Bicarbonate sulfate exchange in canalicular rat liver plasma membrane vesicles. Am J Physiol. 1987;253:G461–8.

55. Bissig M, Hagenbuch B, Stieger B, Koller T, Meier PJ. Functional expression cloning of the canalicular sulfate transport system of rat hepatocytes. J Biol Chem. 1994;269:3017–21.

56. Boyer JL. Mechanisms of bile secretion and hepatic transport. In: Andreoli TE, Hoffman JF, Fanestil DD, Schultz SG, editors. Physiology of membrane disorders. New York: Plenum; 1986;609–36.

57. Mathis GH, Walls SA, Sirica AE. Biochemical characteristics of hyperplastic rat bile ductular epithelial cells cultured 'on top' and 'inside' different extracellular matrix substitutes. Cancer Res. 1988;48:6145–53.

58. Strazzabosco M, Mennone A, Boyer JL. Intracellular pH regulation in isolated rat bile duct epithelial cells. J Clin Invest. 1991;87:1503–12.

59. Alvaro D, Cho WK, Mennone A, Boyer JL. Effect of secretin on intracellular pH regulation in isolated rat bile duct epithelial cells. J Clin Invest. 1993;92:1314–25.

60. Roberts SK, Kuntz SM, Gores GJ, LaRusso NF. Regulation of bicarbonate-dependent ductular bile secretion assessed by lumenal micropuncture of isolated rodent intrahepatic bile ducts. Proc Natl Acad Sci USA. 1993;90:9080–4.

61. Fitz JG, Basavappa S, McGill J, Melhus O, Cohn JA. Regulation of membrane chloride currents in rat bile duct epithelial cells. J Clin Invest. 1993;91:319–28.

62. Fitz JG, Basavappa S, McGill J, Melhus O, Cohn JA. Regulation of membrane chloride currents in rat bile duct epithelial cells. J Clin Invest. 1993;91:319–28.

63. Cohn JA, Strong TV, Picciotto MR, Nairn AC, Collins FS, Fitz JG. Localization of the cystic fibrosis transmembrane conductance regulator in human bile duct epithelial cells. Gastroenterology. 1993;105:1857–64.

64. Farouk M, Vigna S, McVey DC, Meyers WC. Localization and characterization of secretin binding sites expressed by rat bile duct epithelium. Gastroenterology. 1992;102:963–8.

65. Lenzen R, Alpini G, Tavoloni N. Secretin stimulates bile ductular secretory activity through the cAMP system. Hepatology. 1990;12:891 (abstr.).

66. Lenzen R, Alpini G, Tavoloni N. Secretin stimulates bile ductular secretory activity through the cAMP system. Am J Physiol. 1992;263:G527–32.

67. Kato A, Gores GJ, LaRusso NF. Secretin stimulates exocytosis in isolated bile duct epithelial cells by a cyclic AMP-mediated mechanism. J Biol Chem. 1992;267:227–34.

68. Veel T, Buanes T, Grotmol T, Engeland E, Raeder MG. Colchicine blocks the effects of secretin on bile duct cell tubulovesicles and plasma membrane geometry and impairs ductular HCO_3^--secretion in the pig. Acta Physiol Scand. 1990;139:603–7.

69. Buanes T, Grotmol T, Landsverk T, Raeder MG. Secretin empties bile duct cell cytoplasm of vesicles when it initiates ductular HCO_3^- secretion in the pig. Gastroenterology. 1988;95:417–24.

70. Villanger O, Veel T, Raeder MG. Secretin causes H^+ secretion from intrahepatic bile ductules by vacuolar-type H^+-ATPase. Am J Physiol. 1993;28:G719–24.

71. Alpini G, Phillips JO, Kuntz SM et al. Morphologic and functional heterogeneity of intrahepatic bile duct epithelial cells from normal rat liver. Hepatology. 1993;18:109A.

72. Kaminski DL, Dehpande YG. Effect of somatostatin and bombesin on secretin-stimulated ductular bile flow. Gastroenterology. 1983;85:1239–47.

73. Guzelian P, Boyer JL. Glucose reabsorption from bile: evidence for a biliohepatic circulation. J Clin Invest. 1974;53:526–35.

74. Bilir BM, Gong TWL, Kwasiborski V et al. Novel control of the position-dependent expression of genes in hepatocytes. J Biol Chem. 1993;268:19776–84.

75. Ballatori N, Moseley RH, Boyer JL. Sodium gradient-dependent L-glutamate transport is localized to the canalicular domain of liver plasma membranes. J Biol Chem. 1986;261: 6216–21.
76. Mosley RH, Ballatori N, Murphy SM. Na$^+$-glycine co-transport in canalicular liver plasma membrane vesicles. Am J Physiol. 1988;255:G253–9.

3
Enterohepatic circulation of bile acids in mammals

A. F. HOFMANN

INTRODUCTION

Molecules are considered to undergo an enterohepatic circulation (EHC) when they are secreted into bile, efficiently absorbed from the intestine, and resecreted into bile. Cellular transport – that is, secretion by the hepatocyte and absorption by the enterocyte – is mediated by apical and basolateral membrane transporters for organic anions. Movement along the intestine is mediated by intestinal motility and may be termed 'flow'. A similar 'flow' is involved in the movement of molecules from the intestine to the liver in portal venous blood. Molecules may be biotransformed during hepatocyte or enterocyte transport; and if a steady state is to be maintained, loss in faeces and urine must be balanced by input, either *de-novo* synthesis or dietary ingestion or both. Thus, to describe the EHC of molecules, it is necessary to consider: (1) cellular transport; (2) flow in blood, bile, and intestinal content; and (3) biotransformation during transport and flow. In the steady state, input is equivalent to loss. The mass of circulating molecules is termed a 'pool', since it is commonly measured by isotope dilution and is defined as the mass of material with which a tracer exchanges.

As a result of enterohepatic cycling, hepatic secretion greatly exceeds input. The 'gain' in the system may be described by a simple fraction:

$$\text{Gain} = \frac{\text{Hepatic secretion}}{\text{Input}} \qquad (1)$$

When molecules are absorbed from the intestine and are resecreted in bile, this value exceeds 1 and the molecule undergoes an EHC, by definition. For bile acids (in humans), this ranges from 20 to 100.

Hepatic secretion varies diurnally, increasing with eating and decreasing during fasting. The EHC has a rhythm which is largely determined by the eating pattern. For bile acids, secretion depends on the return from the intestine, since uptake by the hepatocyte is efficient, intracellular storage is small, and canalicular secretion is rapid and complete. Efficient hepatic uptake keeps the bile acid content in the systemic circulation low; the small amount of bile acids entering the glomerular filtrate is efficiently reabsorbed by the renal tubules.

Return from the intestine is determined in part by the rate of secretion into the intestine which, in those species possessing gallbladders, is determined by gallbladder evacuation. This in turn is determined by neurohormonal signals, which cause the gallbladder to empty with meals and refill between meals. Thus the daily rhythm of the EHC is determined by the eating pattern. This differs greatly between grazing herbivores, who eat constantly, and hunting carnivores, who eat intermittently. In hunting carnivores the EHC also has an annual rhythm, increasing when the animal is active during the warmer months and decreasing during winter hibernation.

This chapter will summarize briefly current views on the chemistry and biology of the EHC of bile acids in mammals. Both the hepatobiliary and intestinal components of the EHC have been discussed in more detail elsewhere[1–5]. Space does not permit a consideration of the perturbations of the EHC of bile acids that can be induced by drugs, or that occur in genetic or acquired disease[6,7].

CONSTITUENTS

Patterns of nuclear and side-chain hydroxylation

All mammals except for the most ancient ones have predominantly C_{24} bile acids in their EHC. The four most ancient mammals – manatee, elephant, hyrax, and rhinoceros – have solely C_{27} bile alcohols (conjugated with sulphate). The horse, also an ancient mammal, has a mixture of C_{27} bile alcohols and C_{24} bile acids[8].

Bile acids that are formed in the liver from cholesterol are termed *primary bile acids*, and most mammals have not more than three primary bile acids as their major bile acids. Because cholesterol has a 3-hydroxy group, and cholesterol 7-hydroxylase is the rate-limiting bile acid, the simplest primary bile acid is chenodeoxycholic acid (CDCA), which has a 3(α) and a 7(α) hydroxy group. CDCA may be considered 'the mother of all C_{24} bile acids'. In general, it is common for vertebrate hepatocytes to add a hydroxyl group during bile acid biosynthesis. In most mammals, this 'third' site of hydroxylation is at C-12, and the resultant bile acid is cholic acid. (Cholic acid was the first acid isolated from bile – hence its simple name.) In pigs there is 6α-hydroxylation to form hyocholic acid. In rodents, there is 6β-hydroxylation to form β-muricholic acid. Thus, in most mammals, the site of additional hydroxylation of CDCA is at C-6 or C-12.

In bears and the nutria the 7α-hydroxy group undergoes epimerization during biosynthesis, resulting in the formation of a 3α,7β-dihydroxy acid, termed ursodeoxycholic acid (UDCA)[9]. UDCA does not undergo additional hydroxylation, and the 12α-hydroxy derivative of UDCA has not been reported to occur in mammals. In mice and rats, in addition to 6-epimerization, there may also be subsequent epimerization at the 7-position.

The recommended semi-systematic nomenclature of the 3,6,7-trihydroxy bile acids has changed during the past few years[10]. The configuration of the 6-hydroxy group indicates the name of the compound; the configuration of the 7-hydroxy group indicates a given epimer (Table 1).

In Australian marsupials, additional hydroxylation of CDCA occurs at uncommon sites. For example, in the Australian opossum, α-hydroxylation occurs at the 1-carbon[11]. In the wombat, hydroxylation occurs at the 15-position (J. Pyrek, personal communication).

The foregoing discussion indicates that there should be some nine common primary bile acids. These include the common primary bile acids – CDCA, cholic acid, the two epimers of MCA (myocholic acid), and the two epimers of HCA (hyocholic acid). In addition there is UDCA, and the uncommon trihydroxy bile acids of the Australian marsupials.

Side-chain hydroxylation also occurs. The only site identified in mammals having C_{24} bile acids occurs at C-23 (the α-carbon), and such hydroxy bile acids are common in marine mammals. These considerations indicate that, at least in principle, there should be a total of 18 primary bile acids – nine with the common unsubstituted C_5 side-chain and nine with an α-hydroxy group. However, to date, only two α-hydroxy bile acids have been identified in biliary bile acids.

The composition of the circulating bile acids becomes more complex in animals with caeca[12]. Here, anaerobic bacteria remove the 7-hydroxy group to form 7-deoxy bile acids. Such bile acids are termed *secondary bile acids*, the term being used for bile acids whose nuclear substituents have been altered by bacterial enzymes. (Bacterial enzymes can oxidize (dehydrogenate) or epimerize any of the nuclear hydroxy groups, but 7-dehydroxylation is considered the most important bacterial biotransformation.)

In principle then, six new secondary bile acids could be formed by 7-dehydroxylation. To date, only 23-hydroxy deoxycholic acid (DCA), the 7-deoxy derivative of 23-hydroxy cholic acid, has been identified, perhaps because 7-dehydroxylation involves the formation of a coenzyme A derivative. Esterification with coenzyme A occurs more slowly with α-hydroxy bile acids, probably because of their lower pK_a values. Conjugation with taurine or glycine is incomplete, and α-oxidation may occur[13,14]. Thus four major secondary bile acids should occur in principle in mammals. These include lithocholic acid (LCA; 3α-OH) that is formed from CDCA and DCA (3α-OH, 7α-OH) that is formed from cholic acid. The 7-dehydroxylation of the two HCA epimers results in the formation of $3\alpha,6\alpha$-dihydroxy hyodeoxycholic acid (HDCA). The 7-dehydroxylation of the two MCA epimers results in the formation of $3\alpha,6\beta$-dihydroxy murideoxycholic acid (MDCA). In principle the two novel trihydroxy bile acids occurring in Australian mammals could also undergo 7-dehydroxylation, but this has not been examined.

In most mammals, bile is a mixture of primary and secondary bile acids. The pool of a given primary bile acid depends on its biosynthesis and the efficiency of its intestinal conservation. In the steady state:

$$\text{Pool size (mass)} = \frac{\text{Biosynthesis (mass per day)}}{[1 - \text{fraction conserved (per day)}]} \qquad (2)$$

Table 1 Names and structures of common C_{24} bile acids (5β-cholanoic acids) in mammalian bile[a,b]

Name	Position and orientation of substituents: nucleus					Comment
	$3(R_1)$	$6(R_2)$	$7(R_3)$	$12(R_4)$	Other	
I. C_{24} bile acids (5β-cholanoates) with an unsubstituted side-chain						
Chenodeoxycholic acid group[c]						
1. Chenodeoxycholic	α-OH		α-OH			Simplest and common primary bile acid
2. Ursodeoxycholic	α-OH		β-OH			Primary bile acid in bear and nutria; 'BP' in other species
3. 7-Oxolithocholic	α-OH		$=0$			Primary BA in koala and guinea pig
4. Lithocholic	α-OH					B7-DP of 1 and 2
Cholic acid group[c]						
5. Cholic	α-OH		α-OH	α-OH		Common primary bile acid
6. 7-Epicholic	α-OH		β-OH	α-OH		Can be primary bile acid in human
7. 7-Oxodeoxycholic	α-OH		$=0$	α-OH		Can be primary bile acid in human
8. Deoxycholic	α-OH			α-OH		B7-DP of 4
Hyocholic group						
9. α-Hyocholic	α-OH	α-OH	α-OH			Primary bile acid in pigs
10. β-Hyocholic	α-OH	α-OH	β-OH			'BP' in rat; also termed α-muricholic
11. Hyodeoxycholic	α-OH	α-OH				HHP of 3; also B7-DP of 9 and 10
Muricholic group						
12. α-Muricholic	α-OH	β-OH	α-OH			Primary bile acid in rodent
13. β-Muricholic	α-OH	β-OH	β-OH			Primary bile acid in rodent
14. Murideoxycholic	α-OH	β-OH				HHP of 3; also B7-DP of 12 and 13
Other trihydroxy bile acids[d]						
15. 1α-Hydroxy-chenodeoxycholic	α-OH		α-OH		1α-OH	Primary bile acid in Australian marsupials
16. 15α-Hydroxy-chenodeoxycholic					15-OH	Primary bile acid in Australian marsupials

Continued

26

Table 1 *Continued*

Name	Position and orientation of substituents: nucleus					Comment
	$3(R_1)$	$6(R_2)$	$7(R_3)$	$12(R_4)$	Other	
II. C$_{24}$ bile acids (5β) with a 23R-hydroxy group in the side chain						
23R-Hydroxy-cholic acid group						
17. 23R-Hydroxy-cholic	α-OH		α-OH	α-OH		Primary bile acid in marine mammals
18. 23R-Hydroxy-deoxycholic	α-OH			α-OH		B7-DP of 14; unidentified in mammalian bile
23R-Hydroxy-chenodeoxycholic acid group						
19. 23R-Hydroxy-chenodeoxycholic[d]	α-OH		α-OH			Primary bile acid in marine mammals

[a]Abbreviations: BA, bile acid; BP, bacterial product; B7-DP, bacterial 7-dehydroxylation product; HHP, hepatic hydroxylation product. The term 'BP' means that bacteria may form the index compound or generate a precursor that is further metabolized to the index compound by hepatic enzymes.
[b]Nomenclature follows recommendations of a recent consensus statement[17]
[c]5α-(allo) isomers of these bile acids have been identified in some species.
[d]Whether B7-DP of these bile acids is formed *in vivo* is not known.

The fraction conserved per day is the resultant of multiple intestinal transport processes, as will be discussed. The denominator of equation (2) is equivalent to the daily fractional turnover rate. To determine pool size and biosynthesis, an isotope dilution technique is used[15]. In humans the pool of cholic acid, CDCA, or DCA behaves as a single well-mixed pool, and is thus described adequately by first-order kinetics.

For secondary bile acids the term biosynthesis is replaced by 'input', which denotes the flux of newly formed secondary bile acid into the exchangeable pool of that bile acid. In some species (but not in humans), 7-rehydroxylation occurs. This decreases the input of secondary bile acids into the exchangeable bile acid pool and alters the denominator, denoting efficiency of conservation.

The relative proportions of primary and secondary bile acids in bile depend on the relative pool sizes of each of the individual bile acids. One cannot infer relative rates of input from biliary bile acid composition, because the pool size of any bile acid is always influenced by input and conservation.

To determine the extent of bacterial 7-dehydroxylation, faecal bile acids must be analysed. To determine the input of secondary bile acids into the exchangeable bile acid pool, isotope dilution studies must be performed. It is useful to define a fraction, $f_{\text{dehydroxy}}$, which is the input of a secondary bile acid divided by the synthesis rate of its (primary) bile acid precursor[16].

The majority of bile acids in the biliary bile acids of most mammals are primary bile acids. This is probably because there is inefficient absorption of 7-deoxy bile acids from the colon, and because, in some species, efficient 7-rehydroxylation occurs. An exception to the principle that primary bile acids predominate in bile is the rabbit, in which DCA constitutes 90% of biliary bile acids. In certain non-human primates and sperm whales the proportion of DCA exceeds 50%[8].

Patterns of bile acid conjugation

After biosynthesis, bile acids are conjugated efficiently with taurine or glyine before secretion into bile. Such conjugates are termed N-acyl amidates or aminoacyl amidates and are resistant to hydrolysis by pancreatic carboxypeptidases. Conjugation converts a relatively weak acid ($pK_a = 5$) to a stronger acid, since the pK_a of taurine-conjugated bile acids is < 1 and that of glycine-conjugated bile acids[17] is about 3.9. Conjugation improves solubility at acidic pH and prevents precipitation by Ca^{2+} ions[18]. It also decreases passive absorption in the biliary tract and small intestine. In non-mammalian species, conjugation with taurine is the rule, with only a rare exception[8].

A considerable fraction of secreted conjugated bile acids are deconjugated in the distal intestine. The liberated, unconjugated moiety is absorbed in part, and is reconjugated during hepatocyte transport[1]. Such reconjugation is likely to occur in periportal cells, whereas de-novo bile acid biosynthesis is considered to occur predominantly in pericentral cells[19].

Conjugation with taurine (or glycine) involves formation of the coenzyme A ester, followed by transfer to the amino acid. The resulting conjugated bile acids are secreted across the canalicular membrane without further

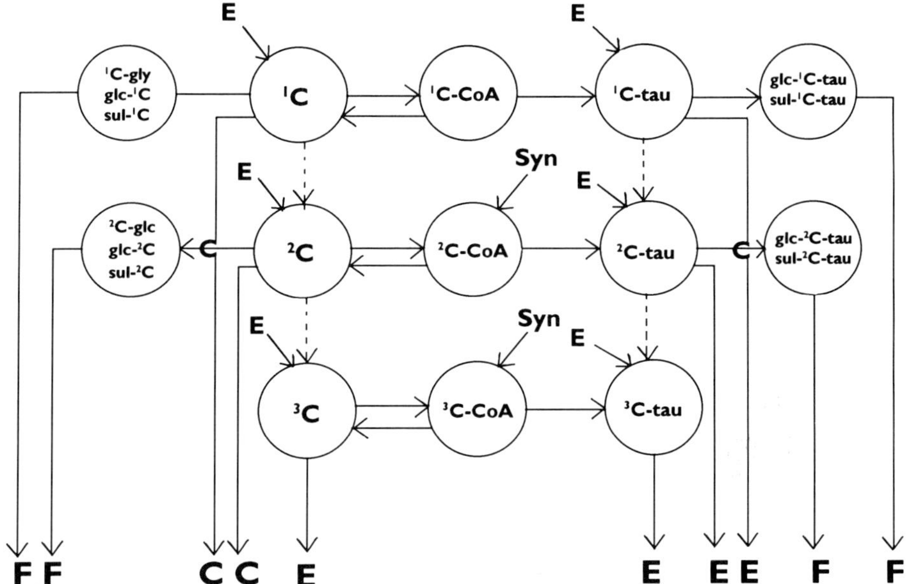

Fig. 1 Overall pattern of bile acid metabolism in mammals. Only taurine conjugation is shown, for simplicity, but glycine conjugation is preferred in many mammals. The superscript denotes the number of nuclear hydroxyl groups. CDCA (²C) and its 6- or 12-hydroxylation product(s) (³C) are synthesized (syn) in the form of their CoA derivatives from cholesterol. They are conjugated with taurine (tau) (or glycine), excreted in bile, and undergo an enterohepatic circulation (E). In severe cholestasis, CDC-taurine undergoes an additional conjugation step: sulphation at the 3-position (sul-²C-tau); this is eliminated in urine (not shown). In humans, hyodeoxycholic acid (3α,6α-dihydroxy) undergoes hydroxylation at the 6-position (glc-²C-tau), which is eliminated in faeces (F) as well as urine (not shown). Unconjugated dihydroxy bile acids (²C) are returned from the intestine (E), are esterified with CoA (²C-CoA), and are then conjugated with taurine (or glycine). When unconjugated bile acids are given intravenously in high doses, they may enter the hepatocyte at a rate exceeding the conjugation capacity. Under these circumstances the molecule may partition into the endoplasmic reticulum and undergo ethereal glucuronidation (glc-²C), sulphation (sul-²C), or ester glucuronidation (²C-glc). These atypical conjugates are secreted in bile, and excreted in the faeces (F). If the dihydroxy compound is secreted in unconjugated form in bile, it undergoes cholehepatic shunting (C). Deoxycholic acid (also shown as ²C) is absorbed from the colon; in the liver it may be hydroxylated to form a trihydroxy bile acid before or after conjugation, as indicated by the dashed vertical lines. (Rehydroxylation of DCA does not occur in humans.) Lithocholic acid, a monohydroxy bile acid (¹C), undergoes a similar metabolism, except that in some species it is hydroxylated extensively (dashed vertical line). In humans it is efficiently sulphated (sul-¹C-tau) and excreted rapidly in faeces (F), with the result that it does not accumulate in bile even during ingestion of chenodeoxycholic acid or ursodeoxycholic acid

biotransformation.

There are some exceptions to this general rule, as shown in Fig. 1. In humans the taurine and glycine *N*-acyl amidates of LCA undergo sulphation at the 3-position. In some animals, deoxycholyl *N*-acyl amidates undergo additional hydroxylation at C-12 to form cholyl conjugates. In humans, HDCA, after *N*-acyl amidation, is transported into the smooth endoplasmic reticulum, and undergoes (ethereal) glucuronidation at the 6-position[20]. The resultant double-conjugates are eliminated in both bile and urine. In patients ingesting UDCA for therapeutic purposes, a small proportion of UDCA *N*-acyl amidates undergoes conjugation with *N*-acetylglucosamine at the 7-position, again to form a 'double' conjugate[21].

All conjugation with taurine or glycine involves formation of the CoA derivative as the initial step. If the side-chain of the bile acid is shortened by a single methylene group, as in *nor* bile acids, CoA formation is inefficient[22]. Dihydroxy bile acids are sufficiently hydrophobic to partition into the SER, where they undergo glucuronidation on the side-chain (ester glucuronidation) or on the 3-hydroxy group (ethereal glucuronidation)[23–26]. A similar pattern of hepatic metabolism has been observed for 23-methyl bile acids[27]. Extremely hydrophilic bile acids, for example epimers of cholic acid, do not partition into the SER, and are secreted largely unchanged into bile[28].

A small proportion of *nor* dihydroxy bile acids escapes partitioning into the SER and is secreted as such across the canalicular membrane. The unconjugated dihydroxy bile acids are sufficiently hydrophobic to undergo passive absorption across the biliary ductular epithelial cells. Here they may be conjugated with taurine or glycine in part. These conjugates, as well as the fraction that escapes conjugation, are transported across the basolateral membranes of the cholangiocytes. The bile acids return to the sinusoids via the periductular capillary plexus, and are once again taken up and secreted into the canaliculus by the hepatocyte. Such intrahepatic cycling is termed cholehepatic circulation, and is evidenced by a bicarbonate-enriched bile acid-depleted bile flow termed 'hypercholeresis'[23,29].

In mammals either glycine or taurine is used for conjugation; no other amino acids are used. The anti-cancer drug, 5-fluorouracil, is metabolized to a compound (2-fluoro-β-alanine) that is similar in structure and physico-chemical properties to taurine; it is used for bile acid conjugation in rodents and humans[30].

BILE ACID TRANSPORT IN THE EHC

Vectorial transport of bile acids occurs in the hepatocyte, in the renal tubular cell, and in enterocytes. Hepatocyte uptake proteins in the basolateral (sinusoidal) membrane are responsible for efficient extraction of bile acids from sinusoidal blood (50–90%, depending on the bile acid). One or more canalicular transport proteins are responsible for the uphill transport of bile acid molecules into the canaliculus. Such secretion induces bile flow and biliary lipid secretion, as discussed elsewhere in this volume.

Bile acid transport by the renal tubular cell and by enterocytes may be considered 'salvage', since they return bile acids to the liver, decreasing faecal loss. Intestinal conservation of bile acids leads to the accumulation of a recycling bile acid pool. Only intestinal transport mechanisms will be considered here.

The bile acids that are secreted into the small intestine are largely conjugated bile acids. Conjugated bile acids are absorbed actively from the jejunum and the ileum, and are also absorbed to a limited extent passively

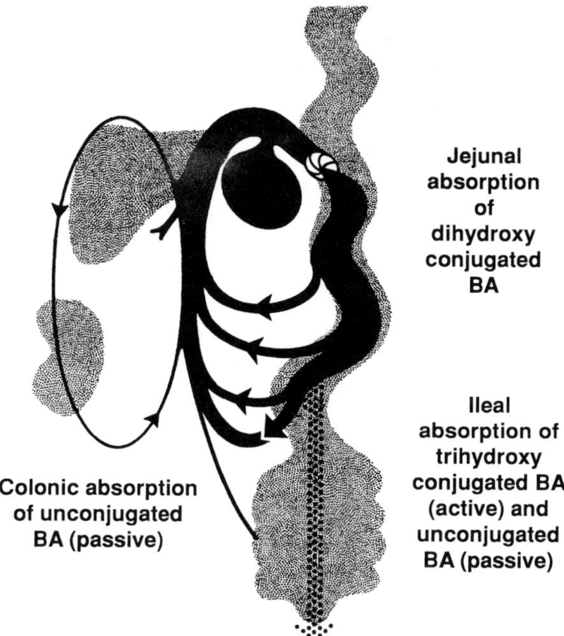

Fig. 2 Enterohepatic circulation of bile acids in mammals. Jejunal absorption is likely to be active, at least in some species, with the transporter preferring dihydroxy conjugates. In species possessing dihydroxy glycine-conjugated bile acids, passive absorption can occur during moments when intraluminal pH is acidic. Ileal absorption involves active transport of all conjugates, as well as passive absorption of newly formed unconjugated bile acids. Unconjugated bile acids may undergo 7-dehydroxylation in the colon, forming secondary bile acids which are absorbed passively. The spillover of bile acids into the systemic circulation is shown. Bile acids not bound to plasma proteins enter the glomerular filtrate, but are absorbed by the renal tubular epithelial cells and are thus conserved. In the steady state, hepatic synthesis is balanced by faecal loss

from the jejunum. In the distal small intestine and colon, bile acids are deconjugated. The resulting unconjugated bile acids are absorbed passively from both ileum and colon; for a given aqueous phase concentration the more hydrophobic the bile acid, the more rapid its absorption (Figure 2).

Jejunal absorption

Jejunal pH is slightly acidic (pH 6–7), but there are occasional dips of intraluminal pH to pH 4–5. Glycine dihydroxy bile acids have a pK_a of 3.9; and when the pH is sufficiently low to protonate an appreciable fraction, passive absorption occurs, as has been shown in experimental animals[31]. The amide bond of conjugated bile acids has the approximate polarity of a hydroxy group, so that glycine-conjugated dihydroxy bile acids, when protonated, have the hydrophobicity of unconjugated cholic acid, which is known to be absorbed passively across membranes, albeit slowly[32].

Recent work from our laboratory indicates that a carrier mechanism for taurine-conjugated dihydroxy bile acids is present in the jejunum, at least in guinea pigs[31]. Whether this carrier is present in other mammals has not yet been determined, but there is ample evidence for a jejunal absorption of dihydroxy-conjugated bile acids in humans[16,33]. Bile acids are likely to be too large to undergo appreciable paracellular absorption.

In the distal ileum there is a powerful Na^+/conjugated bile acid transport system that has recently been cloned[34]. This system is likely to have a far higher V_{max} for conjugated bile acid transport than the jejunal transporter, although its expression may occur over a much smaller segment of intestine than the jejunal transporter.

As noted, in the distal ileum, bile acid deconjugation occurs. The unconjugated bile acids that are formed are absorbed passively. Unconjugated dihydroxy bile acids are absorbed much more rapidly than unconjugated trihydroxy bile acids because their rate of transmembrane 'flipflop' is much more rapid[35].

In the large intestine some passive absorption of unconjugated bile acids occurs, as evidenced by the presence of DCA and LCA in bile. The surface area of bacteria is likely to be far greater than that of the colonic epithelium, and absorption is rather inefficient. Estimates of the efficiency of DCA absorption suggest that 20–50% of newly formed DCA is absorbed[16]; the few available experimental observations suggest that the percentage of newly formed LCA which is absorbed is considerably lower[36]. The extremely low aqueous solubility of LCA (0.05 μmol/l) is likely to contribute to its limited colonic absorption[17].

The overall efficiency of intestinal conservation is high – about 90%/meal or 70%/day for the major conjugated bile acids. In humans, conservation is more efficient for the dihydroxy-bile acids (CDCA and DCA) than for cholic acid[1]. Sulphated amidates of bile acids, such as are formed by LCA during hepatic transport, are much less efficiently conserved from the small intestine[36]. As a consequence, LCA has a rapid turnover rate in humans.

REGULATION OF THE EHC

The EHC of bile acids may be considered to be regulated at two levels. The first is input, that is, biosynthesis in the hepatocyte of new molecules from cholesterol. The second is intestinal transport, that is conservation of secreted bile acids. There may also be homeostatic regulation at a third site, that is, at the level of the gallbladder, since gallbladder emptying is the determinant of delivery of bile acids to the small intestine.

Feedback control of bile acid biosynthesis is under active investigation at the present time. The rate-limiting enzyme appears to be cholesterol 7α-hydroxylase, and considerable evidence indicates that the activity of the enzyme is determined in part at a transcriptional level, directly or indirectly, by the intracellular concentration of bile acids in the hepatocyte[37]. Cloning of the hydroxylase and elucidation of its promoters and enhancers[38] will certainly provide more insight into this problem. Other areas of active investigation involve regulation at the message stability level. Irrespective of the biochemical mechanisms of feedback inhibition of synthesis, it has been amply demonstrated that interruption of the EHC causes a marked increase in bile acid biosynthesis that ranges from two-fold in some species to up to 20-fold in others[39].

Increased bile acid biosynthesis is invariably accompanied by increased cholesterol biosynthesis and up-regulation of low-density lipoprotein (LDL) receptors. Recent work from the Vlahcevic group has described provocative experiments suggesting that an intestinal factor mediates the feedback inhibition of bile acid biosynthesis caused by increased return of bile acids to the liver[40].

Regulation of intestinal conservation is also under active investigation at the present time. In the adult guinea pig, bile acid administration down-regulates ileal transport, and cholestyramine administration up-regulates ileal transport[41]. In the dog[42] and rhesus monkey[43], circumstantial evidence also supports negative feedback of transport. Nonetheless in the rat, creation of a biliary fistula causes striking down-regulation of ileal transport[44]. Such results suggest that ileal transport responds to substrate load; that is, there is positive feedback rather than negative feedback. The explanation for these divergent results is not clear. Nor is it known whether jejunal and ileal transport in humans exhibits negative or positive feedback. The point is not inconsequential since up-regulation, if it were to occur in cholestatic liver disease because of decreased intraluminal bile acids, would exacerbate parenchymal cell injury.

The final level of control of the EHC is delivery to the intestine with meals and storage of the bile acid pool in the gallbladder between meals. Gallbladder emptying is under vagal control, with cholecystokinin considered to act on the vagus nerve and enhance gallbladder emptying together with relaxation of the sphincter of Oddi[45]. Bile acids appear to cause somatostatin release from the small intestine during digestion[46], and somatostatin is a potent inhibitor of CCK-mediated gallbladder contraction[47]. Consequently, gallbladder contraction during meals is likely to be determined by the balance between the agonistic effects of CCK and the antagonistic effects of somatostatin. During meals there may also be secretion by the gallbladder, which enhances emptying of its contents.

Between meals the gallbladder receives about half of the hepatic bile that is secreted[48]. The remainder of secreted bile acids bypass the cystic duct and enter the small intestine, presumably whenever the sphincter of Oddi relaxes in association with the interdigestive motility complex. However, motilin, which is released in association with the interdigestive motility complex, appears to decrease bile flow through the sphincter of Oddi[49]. The secreted bile acids are absorbed from the jejunum and to a lesser extent from the ileum. They return to the liver, are secreted in bile, and once again about half enter the gallbladder. As a consequence the mass (and concentration) of bile acids in the gallbladder continues to increase, although bile remains isotonic.

FUNCTIONS OF THE EHC

The EHC results in a large flux of molecules that traverse the liver, biliary tract and intestine. Because of the rapid portal venous blood flow in relation to the rate of intestinal absorption, the concentration of bile acids in portal venous blood is less than 200 μmol/l in every species that has been examined. Estimates of the concentration of unbound bile acids in the hepatocyte[50] are in the range of $<2\,\mu$mol/l. In contrast, concentrations of bile acids in hepatic bile[51] are 30–50 mmol/l, are still higher in the gallbladder, and are in the range 5–20 mmol/l in the small intestine[1]. In the biliary tract and small intestinal lumen, bile acids are present in the physical form of mixed micelles.

In the hepatocyte, bile acids induce bile acid-dependent canalicular bile flow by their osmotic effects[52]. In addition, bile acids induce phospholipid and cholesterol secretion. The mechanism is currently considered to involve desorption of the outer hemi-leaflet of the lipid bilayer of the canalicular membrane[53]. Recent work from Kitani and his colleagues suggests that the flux of bile acids through the hepatocyte may modulate the activity of some enzymes involved in xenobiotic conjugation such as glutathione *S*-transferase[54].

In the biliary tract, bile acids solubilize lipid vesicles into mixed micelles. Such solubilization involves conversion of a lamellar phase into a hexagonal phase[55].

In the small intestine, bile acids solubilize the fatty acids and monoglycerides that are formed at the oil/water interface by the action of pancreatic lipase (and colipase). Other key dietary lipids, such as fat-soluble vitamins, are also solubilized. In the small intestine, bile acids may also evoke somatostatin release, may modulate intestinal motility, may disperse surface mucus, and may act as bacteriostatic agents.

In the large intestine the concentration of bile acids decreases markedly for a number of reasons. First, all bile acids undergo deconjugation–dehydroxylation, and the resultant monohydroxy and dihydroxy bile acids are less water-soluble for a given pH than their dihydroxy- and trihydroxy-precursors[18]. In addition, the intraluminal pH becomes much more acidic because of organic acid production. Finally, the mass of membranes increases markedly because of the bacteria-rich contents, and bile acids must adsorb to their lipid domains. Since the amount of bile acids entering the colon is increased only modestly because of enterohepatic cycling, the functions of the EHC can be considered to be limited to the liver, biliary tract and small intestine.

EPILOGUE

The EHC in the human, the pig, the hamster and the rat is rather well characterized. Little is known about the EHC in the several thousand other mammalian species, and still less is known about the EHC in the thousands of other vertebrate species. An adequate description of the EHC in a given species requires assessment of cellular transport, flow and biotransformations, and thus is an interdisciplinary study involving the three disciplines of cell biology, physiology and biochemistry. Let us hope that progress in this rather traditional biology will continue, and prove to be almost as interesting as the new frontiers of molecular biology and structure biochemistry. It should be as fascinating to study the interaction of gene products as it is to study only the genes responsible for these products.

Acknowledgements

The author's work is supported in part by a grant from the National Institutes of Health (DK 21506) as well as grants-in-aid from the Falk Foundation e.V., Germany; the Burroughs Wellcome Co.; and Ciba-Geigy, Inc.

References

1. Hofmann AF. Enterohepatic circulation of bile acids. In: Schultz SG, editor. Handbook of physiology. The gastrointestinal system, Vol. III: Salivary, gastric, pancreatic, and hepatobiliary secretion. Bethesda: American Physiological Society; 1989:567–96.
2. Hofmann AF, Molino G, Milanese M, Belforte G. Description and simulation of a physiological pharmacokinetic model for the metabolism and enterohepatic circulation of bile acids in man. Cholic acid in healthy man. J Clin Invest. 1983;71:1003–22.
3. Hofmann AF. Biliary secretion and excretion: the hepatobiliary component of the enterohepatic circulation of bile acids. In: Johnson LR, Alpers DH, Christensen J, Jacobson ED, Walsh JH, editors. Physiology of the gastrointestinal tract. New York: Raven Press; 1994:1555–76.
4. Hofmann AF. Intestinal absorption of bile acids and biliary constituents: the intestinal component of the enterohepatic circulation and the integrated system. In: Johnson LR, Alpers DH, Christensen J, Jacobson ED, Walsh JH, editors. Physiology of the gastrointestinal tract. New York: Raven Press; 1994:1845–65.
5. Carey MC, Duane WC. Enterohepatic circulation. In: Arias IM, Boyer JC, Fausto N, Jacoby WB, Schachter D, Shafritz DA, editors. The liver: biology and pathobiology, 3rd edn. New York: Raven Press; 1994:719–68.
6. Hofmann AF. Bile acids. In: Arias IM, Jakoby WB, Popper H, Schachter D, Shafritz DA, editors. The liver: biology and pathobiology. New York: Raven Press; 1988:553–72.
7. Hofmann AF. The enterohepatic circulation of bile acids in health and disease. In: Sleisenger MH, Fordtran JS, editors. Gastrointestinal disease: pathology, diagnosis, management, 5th edn. Philadelphia: Saunders; 1993:127–50.
8. Hagey LR. Bile acid biodiversity in vertebrates: chemistry and evolutionary implications. San Diego, CA: University of California, San Diego; 1992.
9. Hagey LR, Crombie DL, Espinosa E, Carey MC, Igimi H, Hofmann AF. Ursodeoxycholic acid in the Ursidae: biliary bile acids of bears, pandas, and related carnivores. J Lipid Res. 1993;34:1911–17.
10. Hofmann AF, Sjövall J, Kurz G et al. A proposed nomenclature for bile acids. J Lipid Res. 1992;33:599–604.
11. St Pyrek J, Lee SP, Thomsen L, Tasman-Jones C, Leydon B. Bile acids of marsupials. 2. Hepatic formation of vulpecholic acid ($1\alpha,3\alpha,7\alpha$-trihydroxy-5β-cholan-24-oic acid) from chenodeoxycholic acid in a marsupial, *Trichosurus vulpecula* (Lesson). J Lipid Res. 1992;32:1417–27.
12. Macdonald IA, Bokkenheuser VD, Winter J, McLernon AM, Mosbach EH. Degradation of steroids in the human gut. J Lipid Res. 1983;24:675–700.
13. Roda A, Grigolo B, Minutello A, Pellicciari R, Natalini B. Physicochemical and biological properties of natural and synthetic C-22 and C-23 hydroxylated bile acids. J Lipid Res.

1990;31:289–98.

14. Merrill JR, Peng Y, Schteingart CD *et al.* Ecological and metabolic properties of phocaecholic acid, a natural α-hydroxy bile acid present in wading birds. Gastroenterology. 1991;100:A835 (abstr.).

15. Hofmann AF, Hoffman NE. Measurement of bile acid kinetics by isotope dilution in man. Gastroenterology. 1974;67:314–23.

16. Hofmann AF, Cravetto C, Molino G, Belforte G, Bona B. Simulation of the metabolism and enterohepatic circulation of endogenous deoxycholic acid in man using a physiological pharmacokinetic model for bile acid metabolism. Gastroenterology. 1987;93:693–709.

17. Roda A, Grigolo B, Pellicciari R, Natalini B. Structure–activity relationship studies on natural and synthetic bile acid analogs. Dig Dis Sci. 1989;34:24S–35S.

18. Hofmann AF, Mysels KJ. Bile acid solubility and precipitation *in vitro* and *in vivo*: the role of conjugation, pH and Ca^{2+} ions. J Lipid Res. 1992;33:617–26.

19. Ugele B, Kempen HJM, Gebhardt R, Meijer P, Burger H-J, Princen HMG. Heterogeneity of rat liver parenchyma in cholesterol 7α-hydroxylase and bile acid synthesis. Biochem J. 1991;276:73–7.

20. Parquet M, Pessah M, Sacquet E, Salvat C, Raizman A, Infante R. Glucuronidation of bile acids in human liver, intestine and kidney. An *in vitro* study on hyodeoxycholic acid. FEBS Lett. 1985;189:183–7.

21. Marschall H-U, Griffiths WJ, Gotze U *et al.* The major metabolites of ursodeoxycholic acid in human urine are conjugated with *N*-acetylglucosamine. Hepatology. 1994 (In press).

22. Kirkpatrick RB, Green MD, Hagey LR, Hofmann AF, Tephly TR. Effect of side chain length on bile acid conjugation: glucuronidation, sulfation, and CoA formation of *nor*-bile acids and their natural C_{24} homologues by human rat liver fractions. Hepatology. 1988;8:353–7.

23. Yoon YB, Hagey LR, Hofmann AF, Gurantz D, Michelotti EL, Steinbach JH. Effect of side-chain shortening on the physiological properties of bile acids: hepatic transport and effect on biliary secretion of 23-*nor*-ursodeoxycholate in rodents. Gastroenterology. 1986;90:837–52.

24. Clayton LM, Gurantz D, Hofmann AF, Hagey LR, Schteingart CD. The role of bile acid conjugation in hepatic transport of dihydroxy bile acids. J Pharmacol Exp Ther. 1989;248:1130–7.

25. Oude Elferink RPJ, de Haan J, Lambert KJ, Hagey LR, Hofmann AF, Jansen PLM. Selective hepatobiliary transport of nordeoxycholate side chain conjugates in mutant rats with a canalicular transport defect. Hepatology. 1989;9:861–5.

26. Zakko S, Lira M, Clerici C *et al.* Novel metabolism and hypercholeretic effect of *nor*-ursodeoxycholic acid in man. Gastroenterology. 1987;92:1792 (abstr.).

27. Roda A, Aldini R, Grigolo B *et al.* 23-Methyl-3α,7β-dihydroxy-5β-cholan-24-oic acid: dose–response study of biliary secretion in rat. Hepatology. 1988;8:1571–6.

28. Borgström B, Barrowman J, Krabisch L, Lindstrom M, Lillienau J. Effects of cholic acid, 7β-hydroxy- and 12β-hydroxy-isocholic acid on bile flow, lipid secretion and bile acid synthesis in the rat. Scand J Clin Lab Invest. 1986;46:167–75.

29. Hofmann AF. The cholehepatic circulation of unconjugated bile acids: an update. In: Paumgartner G, Stiehl A, Gerok W, editors. Bile acids and the hepatobiliary system. Boston: Kluwer; 1993:143–60.

30. Sweeny DJ, Barnes S, Diasio RB. Formation of conjugates of 2-fluoro-β-alanine and bile acids during the metabolism of 5-fluorouracil and 5-fluoro-2-deoxyuridine in the isolated perfused rat liver. Cancer Res. 1988;48:2010–14.

31. Amelsberg A, Boyapalli RR, Schteingart CD, Hofmann AF. Carrier mediated transport of conjugated bile acids in the guinea pig jejunum: a new mechanism for conjugated bile acid absorption. Gastroenterology. 1994;106:A219 (abstr.).

32. Dupas J-L, Hofmann AF. Passive jejunal absorption of bile acids *in vivo*: structure-activity relationships and rate limiting steps. Gastroenterology. 1984;86:1067 (abstr.).

33. Molino G, Hofmann AF, Cravetto C, Belforte G, Bona B. Simulation of the metabolism and enterohepatic circulation of endogenous chenodeoxycholic acid in man using a physiological pharmacokinetic model. Eur J Clin Invest. 1986;16:397–414.

34. Wong MH, Oelkers P, Craddock AL, Dawson PA. Expression cloning and characterization of the hamster ileal sodium-dependent bile acid transporter. J Biol Chem. 1994;269:1–8.

35. Cabral DJ, Small DM, Lilly HS, Hamilton JA. Transbilayer movement of bile acids in model membranes. Biochemistry. 1987;26:1801–4.
36. Allan RN, Thistle JL, Hofmann AF. Lithocholate metabolism during chenotherapy for gallstone dissolution. II. Absorption and sulphation. Gut. 1976;17:413–19.
37. Stravitz RT, Hylemon PB, Heuman DM et al. Transcriptional regulation of cholesterol 7α-hydroxylase mRNA by conjugated bile acids in primary cultures of rat hepatocytes. J Biol Chem. 1993;268:13987–93.
38. Crestani M, Galli G, Chiang HY. Genomic cloning, sequencing, and analysis of the hamster cholesterol 7α-hydroxylase gene (CYP7). Arch Biochem Biophys. 1993;306:451–60.
39. Vlahcevic ZR, Heuman DM, Hylemon PB. Regulation of bile acid synthesis. Hepatology. 1991;13:590–600.
40. Pandak WM, Vlahcevic ZR, Heuman DM, Chiang JYL, Hylemon PB. Intraduodenal (ID), but not intravenous (IV) infusion of taurocholate (TCA) down-regulates HMG-CoA reductase (HMG-CoA-R) and cholesterol 7α-hydroxylase (C7αH). Gastroenterology. 1994;106:A958 (abstr.).
41. Lillienau J, Munoz J, Longmire-Cook SJ, Hagey LR, Crombie DL, Hofmann AF. Negative feedback regulation of the ileal bile acid transport system in rodents. Gastroenterology. 1993;104:38–46.
42. Berman AL, Snapp E, Ivy AC, Atkinson AJ. On the regulation or homeostasis of the cholic acid output in biliary-duodenal fistula dogs. Am J Physiol. 1941;131:776–82.
43. Redinger RN. The economy of the enterohepatic circulation of bile acids in the baboon. 2. Regulation of bile acid synthesis by enterohepatic circulation of bile acids. J Lipid Res. 1984;25:437–47.
44. Higgins JV, Paul JM, Dumaswala R, Heubi JE. Down-regulation of taurocholate transport by the ileum and liver in biliary diverted rats. Am J Physiol. 1994 (In press).
45. Li Y, Owyang C. Vagal afferent pathway mediates physiological action of cholecystokinin on pancreatic enzyme secretion. J Clin Invest. 1993;92:418–24.
46. Riepl RL, Fiedler F, Teufel J, Lehnert P. Effect of intraduodenal bile and taurodeoxycholate on exocrine pancreatic secretion and on plasma levels of vasoactive intestinal polypeptide and somatostatin in man. Pancreas. 1994;9:109–16.
47. Fisher RS, Rock E, Levin G, Malmud L. Effects of somatostatin on gallbladder emptying. Gastroenterology. 1987;92:885–90.
48. van Berge Henegouwen GP, Hofmann AF. Nocturnal gallbladder storage and emptying in gallstone patients and healthy subjects. Gastroenterology. 1978;75:879–85.
49. Saccone GT, Liu YF, Thune A, Harvey JR, Baker RA, Toouli J. Erythromycin and motilin stimulate sphincter of Oddi motility and inhibit trans-sphincteric flow in the Australian possum. Naunyn-Schmiedebergs Arch Pharmacol. 1992;346:701–6.
50. Weinman SA, Maglova L, Hofmann AF, Schteingart CD. Measurement of free cytoplasmic concentrations of fluorescent bile salts and organic anions in rat hepatocytes. Hepatology. 1992;16:144A.
51. Shiffman ML, Sugerman HJ, Kellum JM, Moore EW. Changes in gallbladder bile composition following gallstone formation and weight reduction. Gastroenterology. 1992;103:214–21.
52. Boyer JL. New concepts of mechanisms of hepatocyte bile formation. Physiol Rev. 1980;60:303–20.
53. Verkade HJ, Havinga R, Gerding A, Vonk RJ, Kuipers F. Mechanism of bile acid-induced biliary lipid secretion in the rat: effect of conjugated bilirubin. Am J Physiol. 1993;264:G462–9.
54. Kitani K, Kanai S, Sato Y. Primary bile acids can also increase the hepatic glutathion S-transferase (GST) activities in mice. Hepatology. 1994;19:82I (abstr.).
55. Hjelm RP Jr, Thiyagarajan P, Alkan-Onyuksel H. Organization of phosphatidylcholine and bile salt in rodlike mixed micelles. J Physiol Chem. 1992;96:8653–61.

4
Relationship between hepatobiliary transport and cholestatic properties of lithocholic acid conjugates in rats

F. KUIPERS, R. HAVINGA, R. VAN DER MEER, N. R. KOOPEN and R. J. VONK

INTRODUCTION

Lithocholic acid (LCA = 3α-hydroxy-5β-cholanoic acid) is a normal, but minor, component of the human bile acid pool and a well-known cholestatic agent of endogenous origin. LCA is formed mainly by bacterial 7α-dehydroxylation of chenodeoxycholic acid in the intestine, but can also be formed as an intermediate in an alternative route of bile acid synthesis involving initial 26-hydroxylation of cholesterol. The significance of this latter pathway in humans is still a matter of debate; it is clear, however, that it is of importance during the fetal/neonatal period, as well as in children and adults with cholestatic liver disease[1,2]. The cholestatic properties of LCA, a very hydrophobic monohydroxy bile acid, and of its glycine and taurine conjugates, were established in experimental animals more than three decades ago by the pioneering studies of Javitt and Emerman[3,4]. Characteristic ultrastructural alterations caused by LCA and its taurine conjugate (TLCA) include dilatation of bile canaliculi, loss of canalicular microvilli and lamellar transformation of the canalicular membrane[5]. As reviewed extensively (e.g. refs 6 and 7) multiple mechanisms have been proposed to explain LCA-induced cholestasis: (1) accumulation of cholesterol and LCA in the bile canalicular membrane leading to impaired transport function; (2) reduction of bile acid-independent bile flow associated to impaired Na^+,K^+-ATPase activity, which, however, is disputed by other studies; (3) alteration of intracellular Ca^{2+} metabolism; and (4) as proposed initially by Javitt and Emerman[4], obstruction of the bile canaliculus by insoluble LCA precipitates. The involvement of protein synthesis in LCA-induced cholestasis is suggested by its (until now unexplained) prevention by cycloheximide administration[8]. It should be emphasized that multiple actions may contribute to the overall effect of LCA administration, i.e. the decrease of bile flow. In addition, it should be realized that multiple metabolites of LCA, possibly with opposing effects on bile formation, may be involved, as it is well established that LCA is rapidly metabolized in the liver of experimental animals and humans. As studied extensively by Zimniak *et al.*[9], rat liver is capable of efficient hydroxylation of LCA, yielding a variety of polyhydroxylated bile acid species, known to be less cholestatic than the mother compound or even choleretic. In addition, as much as one-third of LCA which is administered to rats is secreted in the form of its 3-*O*-glucuronide[10]. This is of importance, since this derivative itself is three or four times more potent as a cholestatic agent than the parent compound. Also, rat liver contains the enzymic machinery to form LCA sulphates, a pathway of bile acid metabolism first described by Palmer[11]. Sulphation preceded by amino acid conjugation appears to represent the main route of metabolism for LCA in humans[12]; because of the predominance of glycine over taurine conjugation in humans, sulphated glycolithocholic acid (SGLCA) is the major LCA metabolite found in human bile (e.g. ref. 13). This product of phase II biotransformation still has a high cholestatic potency when administered in milligram amounts to experimental animals. In contrast, its taurine-conjugated counterpart (STLCA) is not cholestatic[14,15]. In a series of studies[16-20], we have investigated the mechanisms of hepatobiliary transport of sulphated LCA conjugates and of SGLCA-induced cholestasis in rats, making use of (mutant) bile fistula rats and of *in-vitro* systems; in this respect it is important to realize that the sulphated compounds are not metabolized by rat liver and that, in contrast to the generally accepted view, they are virtually exclusively removed from the body via the bile[18].

HEPATOBILIARY TRANSPORT OF SULPHATED BILE ACIDS

During the past 3–4 years our knowledge of transport systems in the bile canalicular membrane involved in hepatobiliary secretion of anionic cholephils has greatly expanded; the work of many groups has established firmly that these processes are, in part, due to primary, ATP-dependent active transport (see ref. 21 for review). Primary ATP-dependent bile acid transport has been identified in canalicular membrane vesicles from rat[22,23] and human[24] liver. The presence of such a system provides a mechanism for the concentrative secretion of bile acids, unexplained by the previously identified membrane potential-dependent transport activity[25]. Likewise, hepatobiliary transport of non-bile acid organic anions, exemplified by the model substrate *S*-(dinitrophenyl)glutathione (DNP-SG) and the natural substrate bilirubin diglucuronide, appears to comprise an electrogenic component and an ATP-dependent component. The availability of transport-impaired rat mutants lacking ATP-dependent organic anion transport has clearly established that the latter system is distinct from the ATP-dependent bile acid transporter. These mutant rats, designated Groningen Yellow (GY)[18], TR$^-$ [26] and EHBR[27], respectively (probably all three sharing the same genetic defect), have been of great help in defining substrate specificity of the organic anion-ATPase and in elucidating the localization of the (patho)physiological effects of certain organic anions (see below). A detailed discussion of mechanisms of hepatobiliary transport is beyond the scope of this chapter; it should be realized, however, that in view of the multiplicity of the transporters, their probably overlapping patterns of substrate specificity and their complex kinetic properties and interactions, a clear-cut definition of the physiological roles of the above-mentioned transporters awaits their biochemical separation, purification and molecular characterization. Nevertheless, making use of our mutant GY rats and of *in-vivo* and *in-vitro* competition studies, we were able to demonstrate that sulphated (and 3-*O*-glucuronidated) bile acids are secreted into bile (predominantly) via the so-called multispecific organic anion transporter (cMOAT) and not via the bile acid transporter, probably due to the introduction of an additional negative charge to the molecules. Thus, after intravenous injection of tracer amounts of radiolabelled sulphated bile acids, their bile secretion, but not their hepatic uptake, was impaired in mutant GY rats in the order SGLCA > STLCA > sulphated taurochenodeoxycholic acid > sulphated taurocholic acid[18]. Secretion of the unsulphated counterparts was not impaired in GY rats when compared to control Wistar rats. In addition, biliary output of SGLCA, but not that of taurocholic acid, was significantly delayed in control rats by preinjection of the model organic anion dibromosulphthalein (DBSP)[18]. Under no condition was appreciable secretion of sulphated compounds into urine observed. In collaboration with Oude Elferink and co-workers[28], it was found that cMOAT-mediated efflux of the model substrate DNP-SG from isolated rat hepatocytes was significantly inhibited by preincubation of the cells with SGLCA and STLCA. The unsulphated parent compounds, GLCA and TLCA, respectively, as well as a variety of cationic and neutral cholephils, had no effect. Finally, in collaboration with Zimniak and colleagues[29], it was observed that the sulphated and glucuronidated dianionic LC conjugates catalyse ATP hydrolysis by a protein isolated from rat liver plasma membranes by affinity chromatography using DNP-SG Sepharose, providing additional evidence that these compounds are transported by cMOAT.

BILE SECRETION OF SGLC IS REQUIRED FOR ITS CHOLESTATIC ACTION IN RATS

As described in the introduction, SGLCA is highly cholestatic when administered to experimental animals in milligram amounts. Its taurine-conjugated analogue STLCA, on the other hand, is not cholestatic. We have recently provided evidence that the difference in cholestatic potential between SGLCA and STLCA is attributable to their differential interactions with calcium[19]. We found that:

1. *In vitro,* SGLCA is readily precipitated by calcium in physiological concentrations (< 5 mmol/l); SGLCA and calcium coprecipitate with a stoichiometry of 1, implying that the two negative charges of SGLCA are neutralized by calcium. In contrast, STLCA precipitates under these conditions only at high, unphysiological calcium concentrations (see Fig. 1).

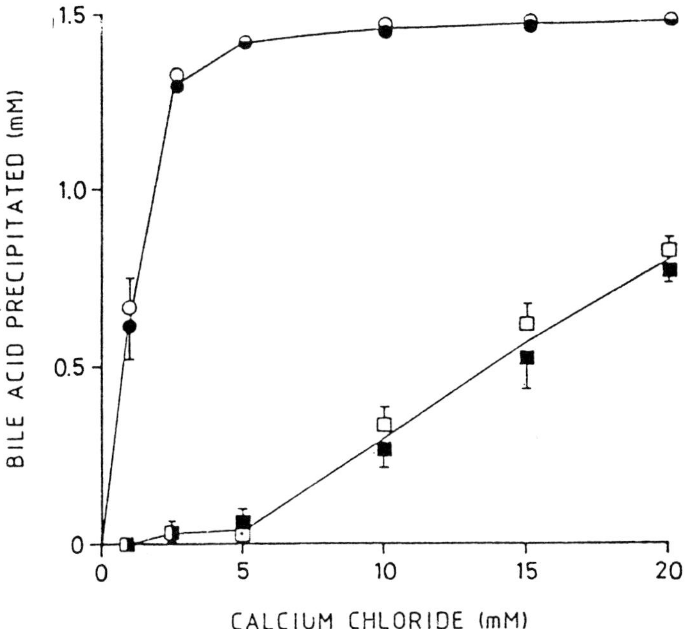

Fig. 1 Precipitation of SGLCA (circles) and STLCA (squares) by calcium chloride at pH 7 (closed symbols) and pH 8.4 (open symbols). Total bile acid concentration is 1.5 mmol/l. Means of three different experiments are shown; SDs are either smaller than size of symbols or indicated by bars. From ref. 19, with permission

2. The onset of SGLCA-induced cholestasis in rats is preceded by the appearance of SGLCA-calcium precipitates in the bile. Based on these findings it was proposed that occlusion of the small bile channels due to a time-dependent accumulation of SGLCA-calcium precipitates is the cause of SGLCA-induced cholestasis in the rat or, in other words, that it represents a form of intrahepatic bile duct obstruction.

In a subsequent study[20], we have used mutant GY rats to test this hypothesis, reasoning that if cholestasis is caused by occlusion, a process that obviously requires secretion of the compound into the bile, these animals should be less vulnerable to the cholestatic action of SGLCA. If, on the other hand, the mechanism of cholestasis is localized intracellularly, the cholestatic effects of SGLCA should be at least similar in GY and control rats. Figure 2 shows that intravenous injection of a low dose (0.6 μmol/100 g body weight) of [^{14}C]SGLCA did not induce cholestasis in GY or control Wistar rats. However, as expected, secretion of the compound was markedly impaired in the mutants. Injection of a 10-fold higher dose (6.0 μmol/100 g body weight), on the other hand, caused an almost complete cessation of bile formation in controls within 3 h. This effect did not occur in GY rats. As expected, cholestasis in control rats was preceded by coprecipitation of [^{14}C]SGLCA

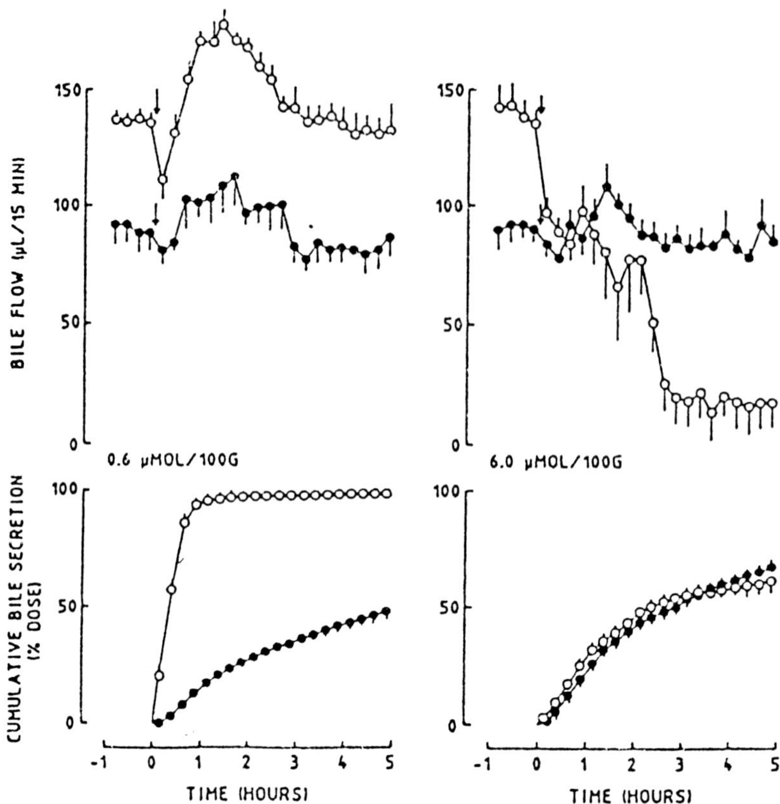

Fig. 2 Bile flow (top panels) and biliary secretion of radioactivity (bottom panels) after i.v. administration of 0.6 or 6.0 μmol/100 g body weight of SGLCA to control rats (open symbols) or GY rats (closed symbols) with permanent biliary drainage. Arrows indicate time of injection. Data are means ± SE of four or five rats per group. From ref. 20, with permission

and calcium in bile and incomplete biliary recovery of radioactivity. The hepatic content at 15 min after injection of $[^{14}C]$SGLCA was similar in control and GY rats, 51% and 49% of the dose, respectively. To test whether the low recovery of $[^{14}C]$SGLCA in bile of control rats was due to exceeding the maximal capacity of its hepatobiliary transport system, we injected control rats with the same dose of $[^{14}C]$STLCA. In contrast to SGLCA, this amount of STLCA was rapidly and virtually completely secreted into the bile within 1 h after injection in control rats.

The resistance of GY rats to SGLCA-induced cholestasis is not due to a general and aspecific feature related to the genetic defect, as it was found that a variety of other cholestatic agents, including LCA, GLCA and ethinyloestradiol, act as potently in GY as in control Wistar rats. On the other hand, it was also found that the mutants in comparison to controls are resistant to cholestasis induced by LCA-3-*O*-glucuronide[30], oestradiol-17β-glucuronide and indocyanine green (unpublished results), compounds of which secretion is impaired in these animals. This indicates that efficient hepatobiliary secretion is also required for the induction of cholestasis by these agents.

In conclusion, our studies have clearly established that SGLCA causes cholestasis in rats by an extracellular, obstructive mechanism, in which the compound forms an insoluble complex with calcium after its secretion into the bile. Because the onset of SGLCA-cholestasis requires relatively high bile concentrations of the bile acid, a direct role in the development of cholestatic phenomena in humans seems less likely. A (patho)physiological role for SGLCA in the human situation, e.g. in benign recurrent intrahepatic cholestasis[31], may be related more to potential interactions with hepatobiliary transport of endogenous organic anions, such as conjugated bilirubin, and/or its very strong inhibitory effect on biliary lipid secretion, which occurs even at low biliary concentrations[32].

Acknowledgement

This work was supported by NWO-GMW grant 900-523-133.

References

1. Setchell KDR, Dumaswala R, Colombo C, Ronchi M. Hepatic bile acid metabolism during early development revealed from the analysis of human fetal gallbladder bile. J Biol Chem. 1988;263:16637–44.
2. Bremmelgaard A, Sjovall J. Bile acid profiles in urine of patients with liver diseases. Eur J Clin Invest. 1979;9:341–8.
3. Javitt NB. Cholestasis in rats induced by taurolithocholate. Nature. 1966;210:1262.
4. Javitt NB, Emerman S. Effect of sodium taurolithocholate on bile flow and bile acid excretion. J Clin Invest. 1968;47:1002–14.
5. Miyai K, Richardson AL, Mayr W, Javitt NB. Subcellular pathology of rat liver in cholestasis and choleresis induced by bile salts. 1. Effects of lithocholic, 3β-hydroxy-5-cholenoic, cholic, and dehydrocholic acids. Lab Invest. 1977;36:249–58.
6. Oelberg DG, Lester R. Cellular mechanisms of cholestasis. Annu Rev Med. 1986;37:297–317.
7. Tuchweber B, Weber A, Roy CC, Yousef IM. Mechanisms of experimentally induced intrahepatic cholestasis. In: Popper H, Shaffner F, editors. Progress in liver disease. New York: Grune & Stratton; 1986:161–78.
8. Yousef IM, Tuchweber B, Weber A. Prevention of lithocholate-induced cholestasis by cycloheximide, an inhibitor of protein synthesis. Life Sci. 1983;33:103–10.
9. Zimniak P, Holsztynska EJ, Lester R, Waxman DJ, Radominska A. Detoxification of lithocholic acid. Elucidation of the pathways of oxidative metabolism in rat liver microsomes. J Lipid Res. 1989;30:907–18.
10. Little JM, Zimniak P, Shattuck KE, Lester R, Radominska A. Metabolism of lithocholic acid in the rat: formation of lithocholic acid 3-*O*-glucuronide *in vivo*. J Lipid Res. 1990;31:615–22.
11. Palmer RH. The formation of bile acid sulfates; a new pathway of bile acid metabolism in humans. Proc Natl Acad Sci USA. 1967;58:1047–50.
12. Cowen AE, Korman MG, Hofmann AF, Cass OW. Metabolism of lithocholate in healthy man. I. Biotransformation and biliary excretion of intravenously administered lithocholate, lithocholylglycine, and their sulfates. Gastroenterology. 1975;69:59–66.
13. Hay DW, Cahalane MJ, Timofeyeva N, Carey MC. Molecular species of lecithins in human gallbladder bile. J Lipid Res. 1993;34;759–68.

14. Yoursef IM, Tuchweber B, Vonk RJ, Masse D, Audet M, Roy CC. Lithocholate cholestasis-sulfated glycolithocholate-induced intrahepatic cholestasis in rats. Gastroenterology. 1981;80:233–41.
15. Dorvil NP, Yousef IM, Tuchweber B, Roy CC. Taurine prevents cholestasis induced by lithocholic acid sulfate in guinea pigs. Am J Clin Nutr. 1983;37:221–32.
16. Kuipers F, Havinga R, Vonk RJ. Cholestasis induced by sulphated glycolithocholic acid in the rat: protection by endogenous bile acids. Clin Sci. 1985;68:127–34.
17. Kuipers F, Heslinga H, Havinga R, Vonk RJ. Intestinal absorption of lithocholic acid sulfates in the rat: inhibitory effects of calcium. Am J Physiol. 1986;251:G189–94.
18. Kuipers F, Enserink M, Havinga R *et al.* Separate transport systems for biliary secretion of sulfated and unsulfated bile acids in the rat. J Clin Invest. 1988;81:1593–9.
19. van der Meer R, Vonk RJ, Kuipers F. Cholestasis and the interactions of sulfated glyco- and taurolithocholate with calcium. Am J Physiol. 1988;254:G644–9.
20. Kuipers F, Hardonk MJ, Vonk RJ, van der Meer R. Bile secretion of sulfated glycolithocholic acid is required for its cholestatic action in rats. Am J Physiol. 1992;262:G267–73.
21. Zimniak P, Awasthi YC. ATP-dependent transport systems for organic anions. Hepatology. 1993;17:330–9.
22. Muller M, Ishikawa T, Berger U *et al.* ATP-dependent transport of taurocholate across the hepatocyte canalicular membrane is mediated by a 100-kDa glycoprotein binding ATP and bile salt. J Biol Chem. 1991;266:18920–6.
23. Nishida M, Gatmaitan Z, Che M, Arias IM. Rat liver canalicular membrane vesicles contain an ATP-dependent bile acid transport system. Proc Natl Acad Sci USA. 1991;88:6590–4.
24. Wolters H, Kuipers F, Slooff MJH, Vonk RJ. ATP-dependent taurocholate transport in human liver plasma membranes. J Clin Invest. 1992;90:2321–6.
25. Inoue M, Kinne R, Tran T, Arias IM. Taurocholate transport by rat liver canalicular membrane vesicles: evidence for the presence of a Na^+-independent transport system. J Clin Invest. 1984;73:659–63.
26. Jansen PLM, Peters WH, Lamers WH. Hereditary chronic conjugated hyperbilirubinemia in mutant rats caused by defective hepatic anion transport. Hepatology. 1985;5:573–9.
27. Takikawa H, Sano H, Narita T *et al.* Biliary excretion of bile acid conjugates in a hyperbilirubinemic mutant Sprague-Dawley rat. Hepatology. 1991;14:352–60.
28. Oude Elferink RPJ, Ottenhoff R, Radominska A, Hofmann AF, Kuipers F, Jansen PLM. Inhibition of glutathioneconjugate secretion from isolated hepatocytes by dipolar bile acids and other organic anions. Biochem J. 1991;274:281–6.
29. Zimniak P, Ziller SA, Panfil A *et al.* Identification of an anion-transport ATPase that catalyzes glutathione conjugate-dependent ATP hydrolysis in canalicular membranes from normal rats and rats with conjugated hyperbilirubinemia (GY mutant). Arch Biochem Biophys. 1992;292:534–8.
30. Kuipers F, Radominska A, Zimniak P *et al.* Defective biliary secretion of bile acid-3-*O*-glucuronides in rats with hereditary conjugated hyperbilirubinemia. J Lipid Res. 1989;30:1835–45.
31. Kuipers F, Bijleveld CMA, Kneepkens CMF, van Zanten A, Fernandes J, Vonk RJ. Sulphated lithocholic acid conjugates in serum from children with hepatic and intestinal diseases. Scand J Gastroenterol. 1985;20:1255–61.
32. Kuipers F, Derksen JTP, Gerding A, Scherphof GL, Vonk RJ. Biliary lipid secretion in the rat; the uncoupling of biliary cholesterol and phospholipid secretion from bile acid secretion by sulfated glycolithocholic acid. Biochem Biophys Acta. 1987;922:136–44.

5
Profiles of steroids and bile acids in plasma of patients with intrahepatic cholestasis of pregnancy – effect of ursodeoxycholic acid therapy

L. J. MENG, H. REYES, J. PALMA, I. HERNANDEZ, J. RIBALTA and J. SJÖVALL

INTRODUCTION

The daily synthesis of progesterone in late pregnancy is approximately 250–300 mg/24 h[1]. The hepatic metabolism of progesterone involves 5α- and 5β-reduction of the 4,5-double bond and reduction of the 3- and 20-oxo groups to yield a number of isomeric pregnanolones and pregnanediols. While the 5β-isomers are in part glucuronidated, all isomers undergo sulphation[2–4]. The monosulphates may be hydroxylated in the 16α- or 21-positions[3,4]. The sulphated pregnanolones, pregnanediols and 5α-pregnane-3α,20α,21-triol are present in micromolar concentrations in plasma, and the concentrations increase with time of gestation. Women with intrahepatic cholestasis of pregnancy (ICP) have markedly elevated levels of sulphated pregnanediols and 5α-pregnane-3α,20α,21-triol[5]. Whether this is a reflection of a primary defect in progesterone metabolism or is secondary to the cholestasis has not been established. Oral administration of ursodeoxycholic acid (UDCA) reduces itching, decreases cholestasis and improves liver function tests in patients with ICP[6]. It was therefore of interest to study whether plasma steroid levels and patterns were affected by this treatment.

MATERIALS AND METHODS

Patients

Three patients were hospitalized for routine care of ICP that had appeared between the 21st and 32nd week of pregnancy. Physical examinations were normal, and the patients did not have other concomitant diseases. UDCA

(Ursofalk, Dr Falk Pharma GmbH, Freiburg, Germany) was given orally, 1 g/day, divided into three doses. The mean daily dosage was 14 mg/kg body weight (range 12–17). All patients remained hospitalized until they delivered the babies. No other drugs were used to relieve pruritus or improve liver function tests. Two patients received the UDCA for a period of 20 days; they delivered 1–8 days afterwards. Another patient with a disease of earlier onset received two periods of treatment, each lasting 20 days, separated by a 14-day interval free of the drug. Blood samples were collected before and after 20 days of treatment. Serum was frozen at $-20°C$ until analysed.

Analytical procedure

Metabolic profiles of steroids and bile acids were analysed by gas–liquid chromatography (GLC) and gas chromatography–mass spectrometry (GC/MS) following a group fractionation of the conjugates. A flow scheme of the analytical method is shown in Fig. 1. Identifications were based upon retention indices and mass spectra. Quantities were estimated by comparing the GLC peak areas given by the compounds from serum with that of the internal standard. Recoveries of added radioactive steroids and bile acids were about 80–95% except for steroid disulphates, the recovery of which was about 60%.

RESULTS

The steroid sulphates found in the serum of women with ICP were the same as those previously identified in normal pregnancy[2,5] both before and during administration of UDCA. The bile acids were also the same as in normal pregnancy except for the presence of UDCA which constituted 66%, 11% and 64% of the conjugated bile acids in serum in the three patients during treatment. The levels of total bile acids before UDCA were 6–50 times higher than in normal pregnancy and decreased by an average of 64% during UDCA (UDCA not included).

In agreement with previous studies, the concentrations of sulphated 5α-pregnane-3α,20α-diol and 5β-pregnane-3α,20α-diol in serum were several times higher than in healthy pregnant women at the same gestational time[5]. The pregnanolones were less different from normal; this is exemplified in Fig. 2. Upon treatment with UDCA the levels of monosulphated pregnanediols decreased by 49%, 70% and 62%, respectively, in the three patients. The corresponding values for the disulphates were 79%, 85% and 52%. In healthy pregnancy, 5α-pregnane-3β,20α-diol is usually the predominant disulphate[2]. It was less elevated in the patients (see ref. 5) but decreased during UDCA in all patients (Fig. 2) to become the major disulphated steroid in two of the patients. The concentration of 5α-pregnane-3α,20α,21-triol sulphates was also markedly increased, and decreased by an average of 76% during UDCA.

In contrast to the steroid sulphates, the steroid glucuronides in serum

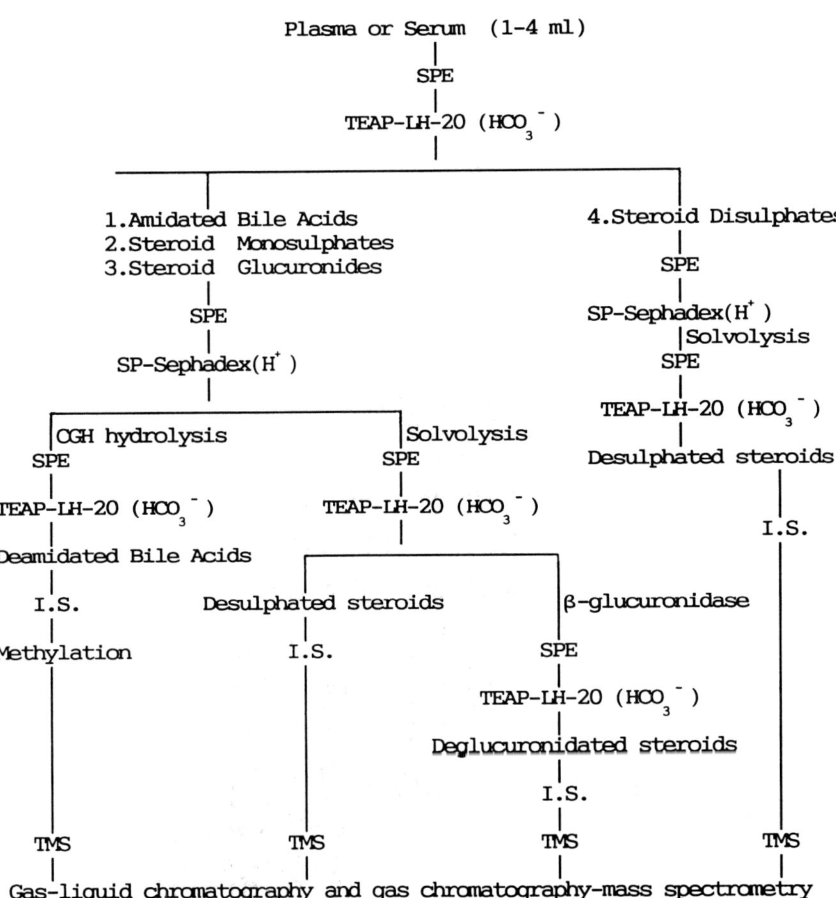

Fig. 1 Flow scheme of the analytical method. SPE, solid-phase extraction; TEAP-LH-20, triethylaminohydroxypropyl Sephadex LH-20; CGH, cholylglycine hydrolase; I.S., internal standard for GLC, n-$C_{36}H_{74}$ and n-$C_{32}H_{66}$ for bile acid and steroid derivatives, respectively

were little or not at all affected by either ICP or UDCA, neither with regard to composition nor to concentration.

In the patient who received two periods of treatment with UDCA, the levels of bile acids and steroids in serum increased 3.1 and 3.8 times, respectively, when drug administration had been discontinued for 14 days. They then decreased again (bile acids 15%, steroids 28%) when UDCA was readministered for 2 weeks.

DISCUSSION

This study shows for the first time that treatment with UDCA can effectively reduce the levels of both bile acids and sulphated steroids in the serum of patients with ICP. Not only is the total concentration of steroid sulphates

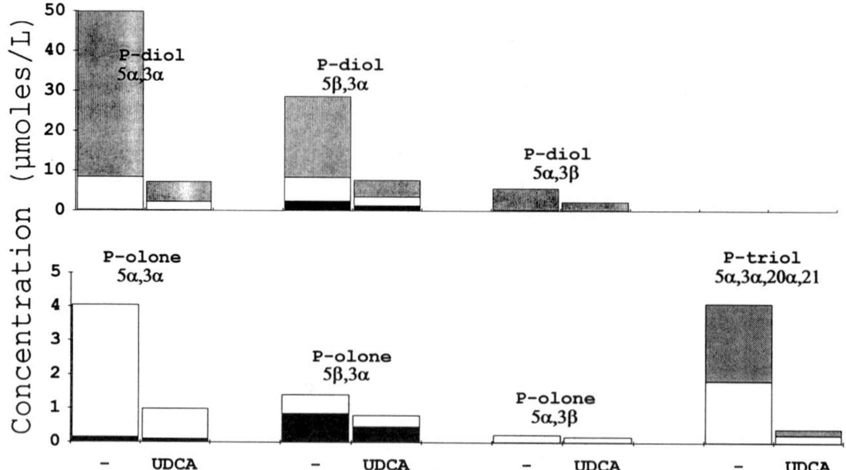

Fig. 2 Effect of UDCA on the levels of monosulphated (unfilled areas), disulphated (stippled areas) and glucuronidated (filled areas) progesterone metabolites in serum of a patient with ICP. The level of endogenous bile acids was 36.9 μmol/l before UDCA and 2.23 μmol/l after 20 days of UDCA

reduced, the relative composition of different isomers and their mono- and disulphates (the metabolic profile) also changes towards normal during UDCA administration. These results are in good agreement with the clinical improvement of pruritus and conventional liver function tests[6], and support the conclusion that oral UDCA can decrease cholestasis and improve liver function in patients with ICP. In the patient who received UDCA during two periods with a 14-day interval, the levels of bile acids and steroids increased after 2 weeks of drug withdrawal and decreased again when UDCA was readministered. Thus, the effect of UDCA was transient at least in this case.

Steroid mono- and disulphates are excreted in bile during pregnancy[7]. This is likely to be at least one reason for their increased levels in serum in ICP[5,8,9]. By stimulating bile flow, UDCA could increase the capacity for biliary elimination of steroid sulphates. Pregnanolone and pregnanediol glucuronides are excreted mainly by the kidney, and this could explain the small or absent effect of UDCA on steroid glucuronide levels in serum.

It cannot be excluded that UDCA also has an effect on the metabolism of progesterone in the liver cells. The increased proportions of 3α,5α and 3α,5β isomers and of pregnanediol disulphates with these configurations in serum of patients with ICP could indicate an abnormality in the reductive metabolism of progesterone and of the extent of sulphation[5]. UDCA might affect these reactions, since it changed the steroid sulphate pattern in serum towards normal. Alternatively, UDCA had a selective effect on the transport system(s) involved in the biliary excretion of steroid sulphate isomers.

Regardless of the mechanism behind the development of ICP, and whether the changes in steroid sulphate pattern reflect a primary metabolic defect or are secondary to some unknown liver affection, our results show that the pattern of progesterone metabolites in serum changes towards normal when the clinical condition is improved by the administration of UDCA.

Acknowledgements

This work was supported by the Swedish Medical Research Council (grant no. 13X-219) and Fondecyt (grant no. 91-1107).

References

1. Solomon S, Fuchs F. Progesterone and related neutral steroids. In: Fuchs F, Klopper A, editors. Endocrinology of pregnancy. New York: Harper & Row; 1971:66–100.
2. Sjövall K. Gas chromatographic determination of steroid sulphates in plasma during pregnancy. Ann Clin Res. 1970;2:393–408.
3. Baillie TA, Curstedt T, Sjövall K, Sjövall J. Production rates and metabolism of sulphates of 3β-hydroxy-5α-pregnane derivatives in pregnant women. J Steroid Biochem. 1980;13: 1473–88.
4. Anderson RA, Baillie TA, Axelson M, Cronholm T, Sjövall K, Sjövall J. Stable isotope studies on steroid metabolism and kinetics: sulfates of 3α-hydroxy-5α-pregnane derivatives in human pregnancy. Steroids. 1990;55:443–57.
5. Sjövall J, Sjövall K. Steroid sulphates in plasma from pregnant women with pruritus and elevated plasma bile acid levels. Ann Clin Res. 1970;2:321–38.
6. Palma J, Reyes H, Ribalta J et al. Effects of ursodeoxycholic acid in patients with intrahepatic cholestasis of pregnancy. Hepatology. 1992;15:1043–7.
7. Laatikainen T, Karjalainen O. Excretion of conjugates of neutral steroids in human bile during late pregnancy. Acta Endocrinol. 1972;69:775–88.
8. Eriksson H, Gustafsson J-Å, Sjövall J, Sjövall K. Excretion of neutral steroids in urine and faeces of women with intrahepatic cholestasis of pregnancy. Steroids Lipids Res. 1972;3: 30–48.
9. Laatikainen T, Karjalainen O, Jänne O. Excretion of progesterone metabolites in urine and bile of pregnant women with intrahepatic cholestasis. J Steroid Biochem. 1973;4:641–8.

Section II
Hepatocellular transport and mechanisms of cholestasis

6
Bilirubin metabolism in cholestasis

N. BLANCKAERT

Excretion of bilirubin requires esterification with sugar moieties. In humans, both mono-esterified and di-esterified bilirubins are formed. This esterification occurs virtually exclusively in the liver and is catalysed by microsomal UDP-glucuronosyltransferase. Conjugation with glucuronic acid predominates, while glucose and xylose conjugates are also formed in small amounts. Under normal conditions of hepatic excretion, esterified bilirubins are rapidly transferred from the hepatocytes into the bile canaliculus and disposed of in bile and the gastrointestinal tract, with little reflux in the plasma compartment. Because bidirectional transport of bilirubin and its ester conjugates occurs across the sinusoidal membrane, concentration changes for the various bilirubins in the hepatocytes are reflected in changes in concentration and composition of serum bilirubins. Hence, analysis of serum bilirubins provides information on pathophysiological changes in bilirubin conjugation and excretion in the liver.

Detailed analysis of serum bilirubins requires a highly specific and sensitive method for fractionation and determination. Using such methodology we found that normal human serum contains *unconjugated bilirubin* (UCB) and small concentrations ($\sim 4\%$ of total bilirubins) of *bilirubin glucuronides* (BGLUC). A second conjugated form of bilirubin, tentatively identified as *bilirubin–protein conjugates* (BPC), with pharmacokinetic properties that are clearly distinct from those of BGLUC, occurs in serum of patients in whom hepatic elimination of BGLUC is, or recently has been, impaired.

The major types of disorders of bilirubin metabolism producing hyperbilirubinaemia include: (1) bilirubin overproduction, (2) deficient hepatic clearance of UCB as a result of defective hepatic uptake or glucuronidation, and (3) impaired hepatobiliary excretion of BGLUC. Typical patterns of serum bilirubins appear to be associated with each of these broadly defined pathophysiological mechanisms and are defined by the extent to which UCB and/or BGLUC are increased in serum. A raised UCB/BGLUC ratio reflects impaired hepatic clearance of UCB. Bilirubin overproduction produces hyperbilirubinaemia with a proportional increase of both UCB and BGLUC. Impaired hepatobiliary excretion primarily affects the serum level of BGLUC and results in an increased BGLUC/UCB ratio.

Appearance of BPC in serum does not immediately and directly reflect hepatic function, since it appears to be the result of non-enzymatic conversion of BGLUC to BPC in serum, and occurs with some delay following a rise of serum BGLUC. Disappearance of BPC from plasma does not depend on hepatobiliary excretion, but on catabolism of the respective protein moiety, which has a relatively long half-life. Therefore, conjugated hyperbilirubin-aemia may persist for a limited time after hepatobiliary pigment excretion has returned to normal and the serum BGLUC concentrations have fallen. On the contrary, in the early phase of cholestasis, BGLUC may be selectively increased in serum without concomitant presence of significant concentrations of BPC, because conversion of BGLUC to BPC occurs slowly.

In addition to transformation to BPC, BLUC in cholestatic patients undergo positional isomerization, which is another non-enzymatic process and involves alkali-catalysed acyl shifting of the glucuronide moiety. Esterified bilirubins also undergo hydrolysis in the hepatocyte and the plasma compartment, leading to an increased level of UCB.

As a result of the various transformations in bilirubin conjugates during cholestasis, body fluids of patients with conjugated hyperbilirubinaemia may contain an extremely complex mixture of bilirubins.

Accurate determination of UCB, and particularly of BGLUC, requires highly specific and sensitive methodology, which is available but not yet suitable for routine application in the clinical laboratory. Results of fractionation of serum bilirubins by conventional diazo methods are highly procedure-dependent and are analytically unreliable, particularly when the level of total bilirubins is normal or only slightly raised. Interpretation of the results for serum bilirubins in cholestasis obtained with conventional methods used in clinical laboratories will be discussed.

7
Molecular mechanisms of bile acid transport in hepatocytes

P. J. MEIER

BASOLATERAL BILE ACID UPTAKE SYSTEMS

Basolateral uptake of bile acids into hepatocytes is mediated by both Na^+-dependent and Na^+-independent transport systems[1]. Both these uptake processes have been well characterized by means of conventional transport studies in a variety of experimental systems including the isolated perfused rat liver[2], isolated and cultured hepatocytes[3,4], and basolateral rat liver plasma membrane vesicles[5,6]. In addition, photoaffinity and chemical labelling, as well as immunological techniques, have been used in attempts to identify and isolate the bile acid-transporting polypeptides[7-12]. These studies suggested proteins in the molecular weight range of 48 000–54 000 as essential components of the basolateral bile acid uptake systems.

Na^+-dependent bile acid uptake

Na^+-coupled co-transport represents the most important hepatocellular uptake process for conjugated bile acids in mammalian liver[1]. It is driven by the physiological out to in Na^+-gradient and most probably is an electrogenic transport process with a Na^+ to bile acid stoichiometry[1] of greater than 1 to 1. Although a 49 kDa polypeptide has been identified[10], immunopurified and apparently reconstituted into proteoliposomes[11], this candidate bile acid transporter has never been convincingly shown to mediate true Na^+-dependent bile acid transport across the basolateral membrane of hepatocytes, since no clear-cut distinction between membrane binding and Na^+-dependent intravesicular accumulation of taurocholate could be obtained in the reconstitution experiments[11]. Furthermore, the same group of investigators demonstrated recently that their 49 kDa bile acid-binding protein is identical with microsomal epoxide hydrolase[13], which may serve a role in the intracellular sequestration of free cytoplasmic bile acids (e.g. under high bile salt load conditions) within the endoplasmic reticulum[14].

Uncertainty also exists with respect to an independently identified and isolated ontogenetically regulated 48 kDa protein, the immunoprecipitation of which has been suggested to be associated with loss of Na^+-dependent taurocholate transport in reconstituted basolateral proteoliposomes[12]. However, also in this latter study it was impossible to reconstitute Na^+-dependent bile acid co-transport by direct incorporation of the immunoprecipitated 48 kDa protein into liposomes. Hence, whether, how and to what extent these identified 48/49 kDa bile acid-binding polypeptides can indeed mediate Na^+-dependent bile acid uptake into rat hepatocytes remains controversial.

Because of the limitations of the classical biochemical techniques in the identification and isolation of the Na^+-dependent hepatocellular bile acid uptake system we adopted the strategy of expression cloning in *Xenopus laevis* oocytes to more definitely identify, isolate and clone the Na^+-coupled taurocholate co-transporting polypeptide of rat liver. This procedure first involved the functional expression of Na^+-dependent taurocholate uptake in mRNA-injected oocytes[15]. Second, a cDNA library was constructed from the active mRNA size-class and the library subdivided into pools from which recombinant plasmids were isolated. Third, plasmid DNA was *in vitro* transcribed into cRNA, which was injected into oocytes and tested for expression of Na^+-dependent taurocholate uptake function. Fourth, positive pools were further subdivided and tested until a single clone encoding the rat liver Na^+/taurocholate co-transporting polypeptide (Ntcp) could be isolated[16]. When injected into oocytes the cloned Ntcp–cRNA expressed selective Na^+-dependent taurocholate and cholate uptake. Ntcp is present only in mammalian liver, and does not occur in the liver of lower vertebrates[17]. During ontogenesis of rat liver it is expressed at days 18–21 of gestation[17]. In addition, Ntcp is present only in differentiated hepatocytes and absent in hepatoma cell lines such as HTC and Hep G2[17]. In primary cultures of rat hepatocytes the Ntcp–mRNA is lost to virtually undetectable levels[18] within 72 h. Structurally the cloned Ntcp is composed of 362 amino acids with five possible N-linked glycosylation sites. However, recent experiments using site-directed mutagenesis indicate that only positions 5 and 11 are glycosylated (Fig. 1)[19]. Consequently the amino-terminal end of the transporter has to be located on the extracellular side of the hepatocyte. Furthermore, studies with a polyclonal antibody against the C-terminal end of the transporter indicate that the COOH-terminal end of Ntcp is probably located intracellularly[19]. These studies confirm our originally proposed model of a protein with seven transmembrane domains[16] (Fig. 1). Although initial *in-vitro* translation experiments[16] indicated an apparent molecular mass of glycosylated Ntcp of 39 kDa, more recent immunoprecipitation experiments favour an M_r of ~ 50 kDa for the native Ntcp in the basolateral membrane of rat hepatocytes. Finally, the human NTCP analogue has recently also been cloned and shown to exhibit a 77% amino acid homology with the rat Ntcp[20]. Although these studies do not exclude the presence of additional Na^+-dependent bile acid uptake systems in the basolateral hepatocytic membrane, the cloned rat and human Na^+-taurocholate co-transporting polypeptides most probably represent different gene products than the 48/49 kDa bile acid-binding proteins previously identified[7–12].

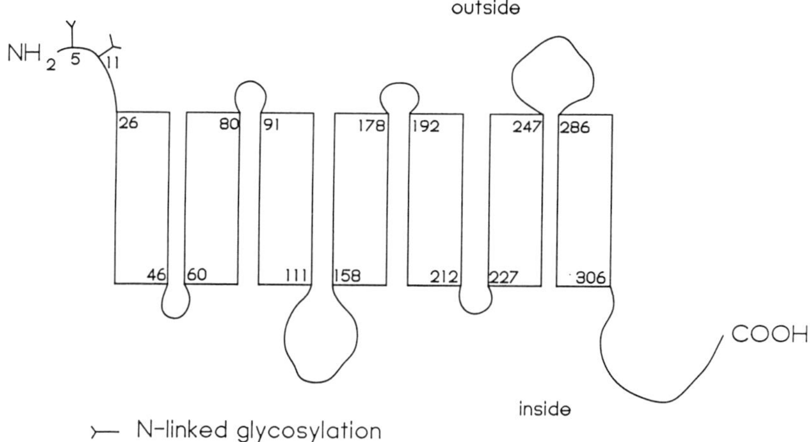

Fig. 1   Model of the Na$^+$/taurocholate co-transporting polypeptide (Ntcp) of rat liver

Na$^+$-independent bile acid uptake

Previous studies in the isolated perfused liver and in isolated rat hepatocytes have repeatedly suggested that a portion of hepatocellular bile acid uptake occurs via Na$^+$-independent pathways[1]. Although the exact mechanisms involved remain uncertain, both anion exchange and non-ionic diffusion have been implicated to contribute to overall bile acid influx[1]. Furthermore, a 54 kDa protein has been identified by photoaffinity labelling studies as a candidate Na$^+$-independent bile acid carrier[21]. Using expression cloning in *Xenopus laevis* oocytes we have recently also cloned a 74 kDa rat liver protein that mediates Na$^+$-independent bile acid as well as bromosulpho-phthalein (BSP) uptake when expressed in frog oocytes[22]. This organic anion-transporting polypeptide (oatp) consists of 670 amino acids with four potential N-linked glycosylation sites. The hypothetical model of oatp as based on hydropathy plotting is illustrated in Fig. 2. Oatp-mediated BSP and taurocholate transport can be inhibited by a variety of bile acid derivatives and bilirubin, but not by more hydrophilic organic anions such as oxalate, α-ketoglutarate and *p*-aminohippurate[23]. Furthermore, Northern plot analyses indicate that both liver and kidney of rat, mouse and rabbit may contain additional oatp-related membrane transport systems[22]. It remains to be seen to what extent these presumptive oatp-related carriers relate to the various organic anion-binding proteins previously identified and characterized by more classical biochemical techniques[24].

INTRACELLULAR BILE ACID TRANSPORT

Once taken up into hepatocytes a portion of bile acids is bound to cytoplasmic binding proteins; for example 3α-hydroxysteroid dehydrogenase in rat liver[25]. However, under high bile acid load conditions an increasing amount of free

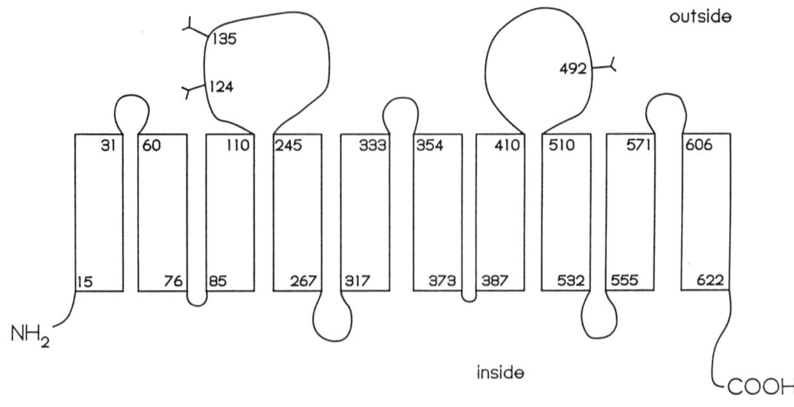

Fig. 2 Model of a cloned Na⁺-independent 'organic anion transporting polypeptide' (oatp) of rat liver

intracellular bile acids appears to associate with intracellular membrane-bound compartments, including the endoplasmic reticulum and the Golgi complex[26]. It is now well established that the endoplasmic reticulum (ER) contains a conductive organic anion pathway through which bile acids could segregate into the ER[14,27]. Furthermore, a presumptive 'precanalicular' vesicle fraction has recently been isolated that could play a role in the colchicine-sensitive vesicle-associated portion of canalicular bile acid secretion[27]. However, the exact mechanism of microtubule-dependent and vesicle-mediated canalicular bile acid secretion under various physiological and pathophysiological conditions remains to be determined.

CANALICULAR BILE ACID SECRETION

This topic has recently been reviewed in some detail[28,29]. Most importantly, two ATP-dependent transport systems have been described for the canalicular secretion of amidated monoanionic and glucuronidated or sulphated divalent bile acid conjugates, respectively[28,29]. The first system represents a high-affinity primary active transporter with an apparent K_m for taurocholate[1,28,29] between 2 and 50 μmol/l. It functions independently of the membrane potential and also appears to be localized in a precanalicular vesicle subfraction that is essentially free of canalicular ecto-ATPase[27]. Hence, these latter studies argue against the possibility of the canalicular ecto-ATPase being identical with the ATP-dependent bile acid efflux pump[30]. The second system represents the so-called 'multiple organic anion transporter' (MOAT) that transports a variety of divalent organic anion conjugates including glutathione–drug conjugates, bilirubin diglucuronide and divalent bile acid conjugates[28,29]. The function of MOAT is defective in three independently characterized rat strains[28,29], and most probably also in the human Dubin–Johnson syndrome.

In addition to these ATP-dependent bile acid transport systems, canalicular bile acid secretion has also repeatedly been suggested to be driven by the intracellular negative potential of approximately −40 mV in all the isolated perfused rat liver[31], isolated hepatocyte couplets[32] and isolated canalicular mmbrane vesicles[33,34]. Furthermore, a 100 kDa canalicular membrane protein with biochemical properties similar to the ecto-ATPase has been indicated to be involved in the mediation of electrogenic canalicular bile acid secretion[35]. This concept has recently been challenged by the findings that further subfractionation of isolated canalicular membrane vesicles by free-flow electrophoresis resulted in a complete loss of electrogenic taurocholate transport from the further purified canalicular membrane subfraction and in a parallel enrichment in the contaminating ER membranes[27]. From these studies it has been concluded that electrogenic bile acid transport is an intrinsic function of the endoplasmic reticulum rather than of the canalicular membrane. If these observations can be further validated in future experiments, the observed effects of the membrane potential on the biliary excretion of taurocholate in intact hepatocytes[31,32] must be explained by more complex interactions between intracellular homeostatic and canalicular excretory mechanisms. For example, it may well be that hyperpolarization of the cell interior may stimulate canalicular vesicle exocytosis and thereby increase the number of functional bile acid carriers at the canalicular membrane[36]. This hypothesis, however, requires further experimental validation including identification, isolation and quantitation of the so far mostly phenomenologically characterized canalicular bile acid carrier(s).

CONCLUSIONS

Our current view of the hepatocytic bile acid transport polarity is summarized in Fig. 3. Undoubtedly, the past decade has witnessed significant advances in our understanding of the mechanisms responsible for transcellular bile acid transport in mammalian liver. On the other hand we are faced with the fact that cloning of the first two basolateral bile acid uptake systems (Figs 1 and 2) yielded transporting polypeptides of unexpected size and molecular structure when compared with the previously labelled bile acid-binding proteins. In addition, the molecular mechanisms of intracellular bile acid transport, as well as the number and exact types of transport mechanisms involved in the canalicular secretion of bile acids, remain to be elucidated by molecular cloning techniques. Only if these challenges can be solved in the near future will it become possible to investigate definitely the pathophysiological mechanisms underlying various inherited and acquired forms of cholestatic liver disease.

References

1. Suchy FJ. Hepatocellular transport of bile acids. Semin Liver Dis. 1993;13:235–47.
2. Reichen J, Paumgartner G. Uptake of bile acids by perfused rat liver. Am J Physiol. 1976;231:734–42.

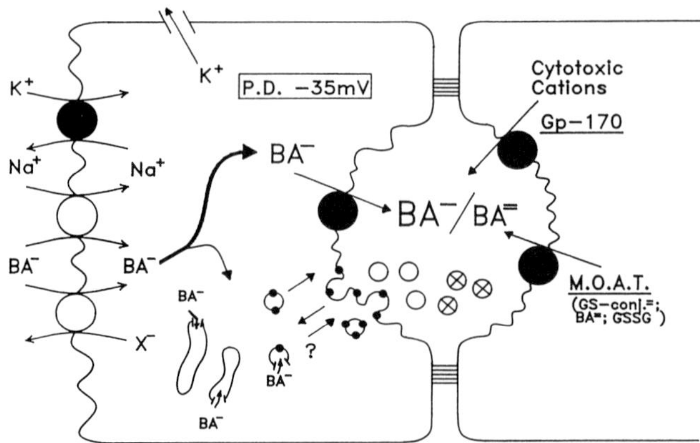

Fig. 3 Scheme of the hepatocellular bile salt transport polarity of rat liver. For explanation see text and ref. 28. *Abbreviations*: BA$^-$, monovalent bile salts; BA$^=$, sulphated and glucuronidated bile salts; Gp-170, *p*-glycoprotein of which mdr 2 and mdr 3 have been shown to be present at the canalicular membrane

3. Schwarz LR, Burr R, Schwenk M, Pfaff E, Greim H. Uptake of taurocholic acid into isolated rat liver cells. Eur J Biochem. 1975;55:617–23.
4. Van Dyke RW, Stephens JE, Scharschmidt BF. Bile acid transport in cultured rat hepatocytes. Am J Physiol. 1982;243:G484–92.
5. Inoue M, Kinne R, Tran T, Arias M. Taurocholate transport by rat liver sinusoidal membrane vesicles: evidence for sodium cotransport. Hepatology. 1982;2:572–9.
6. Zimmerli B, Valantinas J, Meier PJ. Multispecificity of Na$^+$-dependent taurocholate uptake in basolateral (sinusoidal) rat liver plasma membrane vesicles. J Pharmacol Exp Ther. 1989;250:301–8.
7. Kramer W, Bickel U, Buscher H-P, Gerok W, Kurz G. Bile-salt-binding polypeptides in plasma membranes of hepatocytes revealed by photoaffinity labelling. Eur J Biochem. 1982;129:13–24.
8. Wieland T, Nassal M, Kramer W, Fricker G, Bickel U, Kurz G. Identity of hepatic membrane transport systems for bile salts, phalloidin, and antamanide by photoaffinity labeling. Proc Natl Acad Sci USA. 1984;81:5232–6.
9. von Dippe P, Levy D. Characterization of the bile acid transport system in normal and transformed hepatocytes. J Biol Chem. 1983;258:8896–901.
10. Ananthanarayanan M, von Dippe P, Levy D. Identification of the hepatocyte Na$^+$-dependent bile acid transport protein using monoclonal antibodies. J Biol Chem. 1988;263:8338–43.
11. von Dippe P, Levy D. Reconstitution of the immunopurified 49-kDa sodium-dependent bile acid transport protein derived from hepatocytes sinusoidal plasma membrane. J Biol Chem. 1990;265:14812–16.
12. Ananthanarayanan M, Bucuvalas JC, Shneider BL, Sippel CJ, Suchy FJ. An ontogenically regulated 48-kDa protein is a component of the Na$^+$-bile acid cotransporter of rat liver. Am J Physiol. 1991;261:G810–17.
13. von Dippe P, Arnoni M, Alves Ch, Levy D. Na$^+$-dependent bile acid transport by hepatocytes is mediated by a protein similar to microsomal epoxide hydrolase. Am J Physiol. 1993;264:G528–34.
14. Alves CH, von Dippe P, Arnoni M, Levy D. Bile acid transport into hepatocyte smooth endoplasmic reticulum vesicles is mediated by microsomal epoxide hydrolase, a membrane protein exhibiting two distinct topological orientations. J Biol Chem. 1993;268:20148–55.
15. Hagenbuch B, Luebbert H, Stieger B, Meier PJ. Expression of the hepatocyte Na$^+$/bile acid cotransporter in Xenopus laevis oocytes. J Biol Chem. 1990;265:5357–60.
16. Hagenbuch B, Stieger B, Foguet M, Luebbert H, Meier PJ. Functional expression cloning

and characterization of the hepatocyte Na^+/bile acid cotransport system. Proc Natl Acad Sci USA. 1991;88:10629–33.

17. Boyer JL, Hagenbuch B, Ananthanarayanan M, Suchy F, Stieger B, Meier PJ. Phylogenic and ontogenic expression of hepatocellular bile acid transport. Proc Natl Acad Sci USA. 1993;90:435–8.

18. Liang D, Hagenbuch B, Stieger B, Meier PJ. Parallel decrease of Na^+/taurocholate cotransport and its encoding mRNA in primary cultures of rat hepatocytes. Hepatology. 1993 (In press).

19. Stieger B, Hagenbuch B, Cornacchia L, Schroeder A, Landmann L, Meier PJ. Molecular properties of the Na^+-dependent taurocholate cotransporting polypeptide (Ntcp) of rat liver. Hepatology. 1993;18:143A.

20. Hagenbuch B, Meier PJ. Molecular cloning, chromosomal localization and functional characterization of a human liver Na^+/bile acid cotransporter. J Clin Invest. 1994 (In press).

21. Fricker G, Hugentobler G, Meier PJ, Kurz G, Boyer JL. Identifiation of a single sinusoidal bile salt uptake system in skate liver. Am J Physiol. 1987;253:G816–22.

22. Jacquemin E, Hagenbuch B, Stieger B, Wolkoff AW, Meier PJ. Expression cloning of a rat liver sodium-independent organic anion transporter. Proc Natl Acad Sci USA. 1993 (In press).

23. Kullak-Ublick GA, Hagenbuch B, Stieger B, Meier PJ. Functional characterization of the recently cloned basolateral rat liver organic anion transporting polypeptide (oatp). J Hepatol. 1993;18:S6.

24. Tiribelli C, Lunazzi GC, Sottocasa GL. Biochemical and molecular aspects of the hepatic uptake of organic anions. Biochim Biophys Acta. 1990;1031:261–75.

25. Stolz A, Takikawa H, Ookthens M, Kaplowitz N. The role of cytoplasmic proteins in hepatic bile acid transport. Annu Rev Physiol. 1989;51:161–76.

26. Crawford JM. Transcellular transport of organic anions in hepatocytes: still a long way to go. Hepatology. 1991;14:192–7.

27. Kast Ch, Stieger B, Winterhalter KH, Meier PJ. Hepatocellular transport of bile acids. Evidence for distinct subcellular localizations of electrogenic and ATP-dependent taurocholate transport in rat hepatocytes. J Biol Chem. 1994 (In press).

28. Meier PJ, Stieger B. Canalicular membrane adenosine triphosphate-dependent transport system. Progr Liver Dis. 1993;11:27–44.

29. Arias IM, Che M, Gatmaitan Z, Leveille C, Nishida T, St Pierre M. The biology of the bile canaliculus, 1993. Hepatology. 1993;17:318–29.

30. Sippel CJ, Suchy FJ, Ananthanarayanan M, Perlmutter DH. The rat liver ecto-ATPase is also a canalicular bile acid transport protein. J Biol Chem. 1993;268:2083–91.

31. Veith CM, Thalhammer T, Felberbauer FX, Graf J. Relationship of hepatic cholate transport to regulation of intracellular pH and potassium. Biochim Biophys Acta. 1992;1021:70–6.

32. Weinmann SA, Graf J, Boyer JL. Voltage-driven taurocholate-dependent secretion in isolated hepatocyte couplets. Am J Physiol. 1987;256:G826–32.

33. Inoue M, Kinne R, Tran T, Arias IM. Taurocholate transport by rat liver canalicular membrane vesicles. J Clin Invest. 1984;73:659–63.

34. Meier PJ, Meier-Abt AS, Boyer JL. Properties of the canalicular bile acid transport system in rat liver. Biochem J. 1987;242:465–9.

35. Ruetz S, Hugentobler G, Meier PJ. Functional reconstitution of the canalicular bile salt transport system of rat liver. Proc Natl Acad Sci USA. 1988;85:6147–52.

36. Bruck R, Haddad P, Graf J, Boyer JL. Regulatory volume decrease stimulates bile flow, bile acid excretion and exocytosis in isolated perfused rat liver. Am J Physiol. 1992;262:G806–12.

8
Pathways of bile acid conjugation

S. MATERN, H.-U. MARSCHALL, H. HEINEMANN, C. GARTUNG,
H. WIETHOLTZ, H. MATERN and J. SJÖVALL

INTRODUCTION

The metabolism of bile acids in humans includes various conjugation reactions. Besides aminoacyl amidation with glycine or taurine[1] and sulphation[2], three glycosidic conjugation pathways have been established during recent years: glucuronidation, glucosidation and N-acetylglucosaminidation. This chapter summarizes major data on glycosidic conjugation of bile acids in humans, and focuses on recent advances in this field.

GLUCURONIDATION

Bile acids conjugated with glucuronic acid were first detected in the urine of man by Back *et al.*[3] and were then found in serum, urine and bile of patients with cholestatic liver diseases and intestinal malabsorption[4,5]. Bile acid glucuronides were also identified in the urine of healthy humans, where they constitute 12–36% of the total bile acids[6].

Three types of bile acid glucuronides are known at present: two ether glucuronides at position 3 and at position 6 of the steroid nucleus and an ester glucuronide in which the glucuronic acid is linked to the carboxyl group of the side-chain. Carboxyl-linked bile acid glucuronides were first detected for atypical short-chain bile acids in *in-vitro* studies with rat liver microsomes[7] and later with human liver microsomes[8]. Recently, conventional C_{24} bile acids were also shown to form carboxyl-linked glucuronides in *in-vitro* studies with microsomes from livers of experimental animals[9] or human liver[10]. However, the biological significance of this type of bile acid glucuronides is not known at present, since the *in-vivo* existence of carboxyl-linked bile acid glucuronides has not been demonstrated.

Hydroxyl-linked glucuronides are therefore the only types of bile acid glucuronides detected at present in humans under normal and pathological conditions. Within the urinary bile acid glucuronide fraction major primary and secondary bile acids could be identified as 3-*O*-glucuronides, whereas

6α-hydroxy bile acids were present as 6-*O*-glucuronides and constituted a major part of urinary bile acid glucuronides in humans[6]. In subsequent work it was shown that the 6α-hydroxy bile acids hyodeoxycholic and hyocholic acids (3α,6α-dihydroxy-5β-cholanoic and 3α,6α,7α-trihydroxy-5β-cholanoic) can be distinguished from major primary and secondary bile acids lacking 6α-hydroxy groups by their high rate of glucuronidation[11–13] and urinary excretion[14]. The *in-vitro* glucuronidation of 6α-hydroxy bile acids was shown to occur exclusively at the C-6 position with microsomes from human liver, kidney and intestine[12,13], thus confirming results from structural analysis of glucuronides of 6α-hydroxy bile acids *in vivo*[6].

In contrast to 3-*O*-glucuronidation of major primary and secondary bile acids[15,16], formation of bile acid 6-*O*-glucuronides appears to be a major detoxication pathway of potentially toxic bile acids, such as lithocholic and chenodeoxycholic acids (3α-hydroxy-5β-cholanoic and 3α,7α-dihydroxy-5β-cholanoic). Thus, lithocholic acid is either eliminated by sulphation[2] or by 6α-hydroxylation to hyodeoxycholic acid[17] followed by 6-*O*-glucuronidation[11–13] and excretion of the sulphates or corresponding 6-*O*-glucuronides. In contrast, lithocholic acid 3-*O*-glucuronide is poorly formed in the human[12,16] and has been shown to have more cholestatic potential than its parent compound[18]. The two-step pathway for detoxication of bile acids in which 6α-hydroxylation is followed by 6-*O*-glucuronidation could be triggered under conditions where 6α-hydroxylation of bile acids has been shown to be stimulated, e.g. in cholestasis[19] or after treatment of patients with certain drugs. This is supported by a recent study in healthy humans where an increased urinary excretion of glucuronides of the 6α-hydroxy bile acids hyodeoxycholic and hyocholic acids, as well as a diminished excretion of lithocholic acid sulphate, was observed after oral administration of the antibiotic rifampicin[20].

Extensive studies on the enzymology of bile acid glucuronidation from human tissues have shown that there is not a single bile acid UDP-glucuronosyltransferase, but that multiple isoforms exist with distinct substrate specificities. The enzymes responsible for formation of 3-*O*-glucuronides of conventional bile acids or carboxyl-linked bile acid glucuronides in human tissues have not been isolated to date, or cloned and expressed in cultured cells. In contrast, three human liver cDNA clones were identified encoding UDP-glucuronosyltransferases which catalyse the formation of bile acid 6-*O*-glucuronides. Two of these isoforms, UGT2B7[21] and UGT2B7 variant[22], have been shown to glucuronidate the bile acid hyodeoxycholic acid, as well as various other substrates such as certain oestrogens. With regard to the substrate specificity of the third isoform, UGT2B4, a controversy exists in the literature. This enzyme was described to have a restricted specificity towards hyodeoxycholic acid after expression of the UGT2B4 cDNA in mammalian cells[23,24] or from immunological studies[25]. In contrast to these results, other authors described a broad substrate specificity for UGT2B4 which conjugated hyodeoxycholic acid and certain oestrogens after expression of the cloned cDNA in mammalian cells[21]. On the basis of purification of the protein a human liver UDP-glucuronosyltransferase has been characterized which catalysed the glucuronidation of hyodeoxycholic acid and exhibited minor activity towards hyocholic acid and oestriol[26]. Therefore, further studies are needed to clarify the substrate specificity of the enzymes responsible for the formation of bile acid 6-*O*-glucuronides, a pathway which appears to be a major detoxication mechanism of potentially toxic bile acids.

GLUCOSIDATION

Bile acid glucosidation was first described *in vitro* by the isolation and characterization of a bile acid glucosyltransferase from human liver microsomes[27]. In contrast to other glycosidic conjugation reactions this bile acid glucosyltransferase is sugar nucleotide-independent and catalyses the sugar transfer from the lipid intermediate dolichyl phosphoglucose as natural cosubstrate or long-chain akyl-*β*-D-glucopyranosides as artificial cosubstrates to major primary and secondary bile acids[27,28]. The natural sugar donor dolichyl phosphoglucose is formed from UDP-glucose and dolichylphosphate via UDP-glucose dolichylphosphate glucosyltransferase, which is known from its role in glycoprotein biosynthesis[29] and has been recently purified to apparent homogeneity from human liver[30]. Both UDP-glucose dolichyl-phosphate glucosyltransferase and the sugar nucleotide-independent bile acid glucosyltransferase were shown to be localized in microsomal fractions from human liver, kidney cortex and intestinal mucosa[28] and were detectable in human liver and kidney tumours[31]. After subfractionation of human liver microsomal preparations both enzymes were found to be exclusively confined to the endoplasmic reticulum[32]. Bile acid glucosides formed *in vitro* by sugar nucleotide-independent glucosidation were exclusively conjugated at the C-3 position[33].

The physiological significance of bile acid glucosidation is suggested by the identification of glucosides of unconjugated, as well as glycine- and taurine-conjugated, bile acids in urine from healthy humans[34] and patients with extrahepatic cholestasis[35]. Bile acid glucosides were excreted into urine of healthy subjects in similar amounts as bile acid glucuronides[34]. In extrahepatic cholestasis total urinary bile acid glucoside excretion showed only a small increment compared to healthy subjects, and was significantly lower than bile acid glucuronide excretion[35]. This finding questions the role of bile acid glucosidation as a detoxication mechanism.

Recently, a human liver *β*-glucosidase activity has been identified which hydrolyses 3-*O*-glucosides of bile acids[36]. The enzyme occurs predominantly in the microsomal fraction of human liver[36]. Studies on the submicrosomal localization of the *β*-glucosidase in human liver showed that the enzyme is associated with the smooth endoplasmic reticulum[37], and is therefore localized in the same submicrosomal compartment as bile acid glucosyl-transferase (Fig. 1). From these results a pathway of bile acid glucosidation and deglucosidation exists in human liver microsomes, as shown in Fig. 2. Whether such a bile acid cycle plays a biological role *in vivo* needs clarification by further studies.

In addition to formation of bile acid 3-*O*-glucosides the enzymatic synthesis of bile acid 6-*O*-glucosides has been recently reported from *in-vitro* incubations

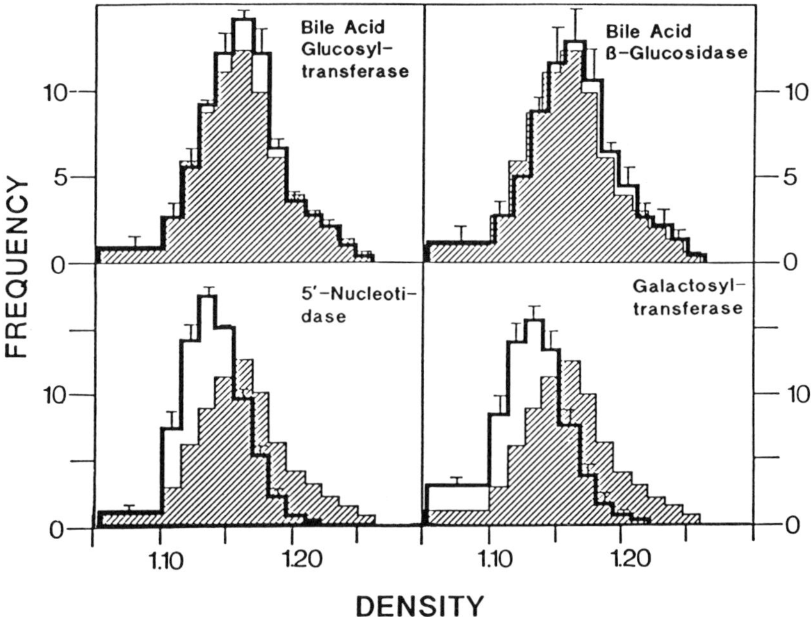

Fig. 1 Submicrosomal localization of bile acid β-glucosidase and bile acid glucosyltransferase in human liver. Frequency–density histograms of microsomal constituents were obtained after isopycnic centrifugation of microsomes on a continuous sucrose density gradient as described in ref. 32. Galactosyltransferase and 5'-nucleotidase were determined as marker enzymes of Golgi-complex and plasma membranes, respectively. The distribution of NADPH-cytochrome-c reductase (marker enzyme of smooth endoplasmic reticulum) is superimposed on each plot by shading. Density is given in g/cm^3. For the definition of frequency, see ref. 32

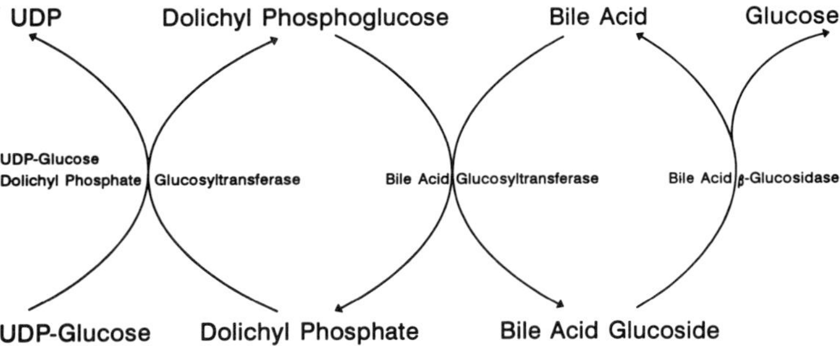

Fig. 2 Pathway of bile acid glucosidation and deglucosidation in human liver microsomes

with human liver microsomes[38]. This pathway was shown to be dependent on UDP-glucose as cosubstrate and was highly specific for the 6α-hydroxy bile acid hyodeoxycholic acid[38]. Thus, the C-6 position of hyodeoxycholic acid can be conjugated with glucuronic acid[12,13] or glucose as demonstrated *in vitro*[38]. The glucose-conjugating transferase was shown to be different from the UDP-glucuronosyltransferase isoform 2B4 catalysing formation of hyodeoxycholic acid 6-*O*-glucuronide[38].

N-ACETYLGLUCOSAMINIDATION

Bile acid *N*-acetylglucosaminides were first described to be constituents of normal human urine by Marschall *et al.*[39]. Subsequently, these novel glycosidic bile acid conjugates could be identified as derivatives of 7β-hydroxylated bile acids such as ursodeoxycholic (3α,7β-dihydroxy-5β-cholanoic), isoursodeoxycholic (3β,7β-dihydroxy-5β-cholanoic) or alloisoursodeoxycholic acids (3β,7β-dihydroxy-5α-cholanoic) in normal urine, as well as in the urine of patients with cholestatic liver diseases[40,41]. Conjugation of 7β-hydroxy bile acids with *N*-acetylglucosamine was shown to result in efficient urinary excretion of these bile acid conjugates, since after oral administration of [24-^{13}C]ursodeoxycholic acid[42] to a patient with extrahepatic cholestasis, 32% of the total ursodeoxycholic acid excreted in urine was conjugated with *N*-acetylglucosamine[41]. Urinary *N*-acetylglucosaminides of ursodeoxycholic acid were otherwise unconjugated or detectable as double-conjugates with glycine or taurine[43]. In healthy humans the urinary excretion rate for bile acid *N*-acetylglucosaminides was comparable to the excretion rates for bile acid glucosides and glucuronides[40].

The selective conjugation of 7β-hydroxy bile acids with *N*-acetylglucosamine observed *in vivo* could be confirmed *in vitro* by characterization of human liver and kidney microsomal UDP-*N*-acetylglucosaminyltransferases[44]. These enzymes showed significant *N*-acetylglucosamine-conjugating activity only with 7β-hydroxy bile acids in the presence of UDP-*N*-acetylglucosamine as cosubstrate[44]. The highest enzyme activity was observed with isoursodeoxycholic acid[41]. *N*-Acetylglucosamine was shown to be exclusively hydroxyl-linked at the 7β-position of bile acids after *in-vitro* synthesis[33], as well as *in vivo* after extraction from normal human urine[43].

In conclusion, *in-vivo* and *in-vitro* studies have shown that *N*-acetylglucosaminidation is a highly selective conjugation reaction for ursodeoxycholic acid and its isomers in humans, which leads to efficient urinary excretion of these bile acid derivatives. Ursodeoxycholic acid has been shown to improve the clinical and biochemical indices in patients with primary biliary cirrhosis and other cholestatic liver diseases. The possibility that *N*-acetylglucosaminidation is related to the physiological and therapeutic effects of ursodeoxycholic acid in patients with liver diseases remains to be explored.

Acknowledgement

This work was supported by the Deutsche Forschungsgemeinschaft (grant No. He 906/18-1).

References

1. Killenberg PG, Jordan JT. Purification and characterization bile acid-CoA: amino acid N-acyltransferase from rat liver. J Biol Chem. 1978;253:1005–10.
2. Palmer RH. The formation of bile acid sulfates: a new pathway of bile acid metabolism in humans. Proc Natl Acad Sci USA. 1967;58:1047–50.
3. Back P, Spaczynski K, Gerok W. Bile-salt glucuronides in urine. Hoppe-Seyler's Z Physiol Chem. 1974;355:749–52.
4. Fröhling W, Stiehl A. Bile acid glucuronides: identification and quantitative analysis in the urine of patients with cholestasis. Eur J Clin Invest. 1976;6:67–74.
5. Almé B, Nordén Å, Sjövall J. Glucuronides of unconjugated 6-hydroxylated bile acids in urine of a patient with malabsorption. Clin Chim Acta. 1978;86:251–9.
6. Almé B, Sjövall J. Analysis of bile acid glucuronides in urine. Identification of 3α,6α,12α-trihydroxy-5β-cholanoic acid. J Steroid Biochem. 1980;13:907–16.
7. Radominska-Pyrek A, Zimniak P, Chari M, Golunski E, Lester R, Pyrek J St. Glucuronides of monohydroxylated bile acids: specificity of microsomal glucuronyltransferase for the glucuronidation site, C-3 configuration, and side chain length. J Lipid Res. 1986;27:89–101.
8. Irshaid YM, Radominska A, Zimniak P, Zimniak A, Lester R, Tephly TR. Glucuronidation of monohydroxylated short chain bile acids by human liver microsomes and purified human liver UDP-glucuronosyltransferases. Drug Met Dis. 1991;19:173–7.
9. Zimniak PA, Radominska A, Zimniak M, Lester R. Formation of three types of glucuronides of 6-hydroxy bile acids by rat liver microsomes. J Lipid Res. 1988;29:183–90.
10. Zimniak P, Radominska A, Lester R. Phase I and II biotransformations of bile acids. In: Bock KW, Gerok W, Matern S, Schmid R, editors. Hepatic metabolism and disposition of endo- and xenobiotics. Dordrecht: Kluwer; 1991:183–92.
11. Parquet M, Pessah M, Saquet E, Salvat C, Raizman A, Infante R. Glucuronidation of bile acids in human liver, intestine and kidney. An *in vitro* study on hyodeoxycholic acid. FEBS Lett. 1985;189:183–7.
12. Marschall H.-U, Matern H, Egestad B, Matern S, Sjövall J. 6α-Glucuronidation of hyodeoxycholic acid by human liver, kidney and small bowel microsomes. Biochim Biophys Acta. 1987;921:392–7.
13. Radominska-Pyrek A, Zimniak P, Irshaid YM, Lester R, Tephly TR, Pyrek J St. Glucuronidation of 6α-hydroxy bile acids by human liver microsomes. J Clin Invest. 1987;80:234–41.
14. Sacquet E, Parquet M, Riottot M, Raizman A, Jarrige P, Huguet C, Infante R. Intestinal absorption, excretion and biotransformation of hyodeoxycholic acid in man. J Lipid Res. 1983;24:604–13.
15. Matern H, Matern S, Schelzig Ch, Gerok W. Bile acid UDP-glucuronyltransferase from human liver. Properties and studies on aglycone substrate specificity. FEBS Lett. 1980;118:251–4.
16. Matern S, Matern H, Farthmann EH, Gerok W. Hepatic and extrahepatic glucuronidation of bile acids in man. Characterization of bile acid uridine 5'-diphosphate-glucuronosyltransferase in hepatic, renal and intestinal microsomes. J Clin Invest. 1984;74:402–10.
17. Trülzsch D, Roboz J, Greim H, *et al.* Hydroxylation of taurolithocholate by isolated human liver microsomes. I. Identification of metabolic product. Biochem Med. 1974;9:158–66.
18. Oelberg DG, Chari MV, Little JM, Adcock EW, Lester R. Lithocholate glucuronide is a cholestatic agent. J Clin Invest. 1984;73:1507–14.
19. Summerfield JA, Billing BH, Shackleton CHL. Identification of bile acids in the serum and urine in cholestasis. Evidence for 6α-hydroxylation of bile acids in man. Biochem J. 1986;154:507–16.
20. Wietholtz H, Marschall H-U, Kern S, Matern H, Sjövall J, Matern S. Rifampin lowers urinary excretion of lithocholic acid by stimulation of 6α-hydroxylation and glucuronidation. Hepatology. 1992;16:120A.
21. Ritter JR, Chen F, Sheen YY, Lubet RA, Owens IS. Two human liver cDNAs encode UDP-glucuronosyltransferases with 2 log differences in activity toward parallel substrates including hyodeoxycholic acid and certain estrogen derivatives. Biochemistry. 1992;31:3409–14.
22. Jin C, Miners GO, Lillywhite KJ, Mackenzie PL. Complementary deoxyribonucleic

acid cloning and expression of human liver uridine diphosphate–glucuronosyltransferase glucuronidating carboxylic acid-containing drugs. J Pharm Exp Ther. 1993;264:475–9.

23. Fournel-Gigleux S, Jackson MR, Wooster R, Burchell B. Expression of a human liver cDNA encoding a UDP-glucuronosyltransferase catalysing the glucuronidation of hyodeoxycholic acid in cell culture. FEBS Lett. 1989;243:119–22.

24. Fournel-Gigleux S, Sutherland L, Sabolovic N, Burchell B, Siest G. Stable expression of two human UDP-glucuronosyltransferase cDNAs in V79 cell cultures. Mol Pharmacol. 1991;39:177–83.

25. Pillot T, Ouzzine M, Fournel-Gigleux S et al. Glucuronidation of hyodeoxycholic acid in human liver. Evidence for a selective role of UDP-glucuronosyltransferase 2B4. J Biol Chem. 1993;268:25636–42.

26. Matern H, Lappas N, Matern S. Isolation and characterization of hyodeoxycholic acid: UDP-glucuronosyltransferase from human liver. Eur J Biochem. 1991;200:393–400.

27. Matern H, Matern S, Gerok W. Formation of bile acid glucosides by a sugar nucleotide-independent glucosyltransferase isolated from human liver microsomes. Proc Natl Acad Sci USA. 1984;81:7036–40.

28. Matern H, Matern S. Formation of bile acid glucosides and dolichyl phosphoglucose by microsomal glucosyltransferases in liver, kidney and intestine of man. Biochim Biophys Acta. 1987;921:1–6.

29. Behrens NH, Leloir LF. Dolichol monophosphate glucose: an intermediate in glucose transfer in liver. Proc Natl Acad Sci USA. 1970;66:153–9.

30. Matern H, Bolz R, Matern S. Isolation and characterization of UDP-glucose dolichyl-phosphate glucosyltransferase from human liver. Eur J Biochem. 1990;190:99–105.

31. Matern H, Fiebig H-H, Matern S. Glycoside conjugation in microsomes from hepatic and renal carcinoma of man. Hepatology. 1987;7:931–6.

32. Gartung C, Matern S, Matern H. The submicrosomal localization of UDP-glucose dolichyl-phosphate glucosyltransferase and bile acid glucosyltransferase in the human liver. J Hepatol. 1994;20:32–40.

33. Marschall H-U, Griffiths WJ, Zhang J et al. The positions of conjugation of bile acids with glucose and N-acetylglucosamine in vitro. J Lipid Res. 1994 (In press).

34. Marschall H-U, Egestad B, Matern H, Matern S, Sjövall J. Evidence for bile acid glucosides as normal constituents in human urine. FEBS Lett. 1987;213:411–14.

35. Wietholtz H, Marschall H-U, Reuschenbach R, Matern H, Matern S. Urinary excretion of bile acid glucosides and glucuronides in extrahepatic cholestasis. Hepatology. 1991;13:656–62.

36. Matern H, Gartzen R, Matern S. β-Glucosidase activity towards a bile acid glucoside in human liver. FEBS Lett. 1992;314:183–6.

37. Gartung C, Matern S, Matern H. Synthesis and hydrolysis of bile acid glucosides both occur in the smooth endoplasmic reticulum of human liver. Gastroenterology. 1993;104:A905.

38. Radominska A, Little J, Pyrek JS et al. A novel UDP-glc-specific glucosyltransferase catalyzing the biosynthesis of 6-O-glucosides of bile acids in human liver microsomes. J Biol Chem. 1993;268:15127–35.

39. Marschall H-U, Green G, Egestad B, Sjövall J. Isolation of bile acid glucosides and N-acetylglucosaminides from human urine by ion-exchange chromatography and reversed-phase high-performance liquid chromatography. J Chromatogr. 1988;452:459–68.

40. Marschall H-U, Egestad B, Matern H, Matern S, Sjövall J. N-Acetylglucosaminides: a new type of bile acid conjugate in man. J Biol Chem. 1989;264:12989–93.

41. Marschall H-U, Matern H, Wietholtz H, Egestad B, Matern S, Sjövall J. Bile acid N-acetylglucosaminidation. In vivo and in vitro evidence for a selective conjugation reaction of 7β-hydroxylated bile acids in man. J Clin Invest. 1992;89:1981–7.

42. Matern S, Marschall H-U, Schill A et al. Synthesis of ¹³C-labeled chenodeoxycholic, hyodeoxycholic, and ursodeoxycholic acids for the study of bile acid metabolism in liver disease. Clin Chim Acta. 1991;203:77–90.

43. Marschall H-U, Griffiths WJ, Zhang J et al. Ursodeoxycholic acid is in vivo conjugated with N-acetylglucosamine at the 7β-position. Hepatology. 1993;18:307A.

44. Matern H, Bolz R, Marschall H-U, Sjövall J, Matern S. Bile acid N-acetylglucosaminides. Formation by microsomal N-acetylglucosaminyltransferases in human liver and kidney. FEBS Lett. 1990;270:11–14.

9
Characterization of the mechanism of glucuronidation using photoaffinity labelling

A. RADOMINSKA, R. R. DRAKE, S. TREAT and R. LESTER

The UDP-glucuronosyltransferases (UGT) are a superfamily of enzymes which utilize the glucuronic acid donor, uridine diphosphoglucuronic acid (UDPGlcA), to catalyse the glucuronidation of a group of structurally diverse substrates (aglycones). UGT are found in liver (and other tissues) bound to the membranes of the endoplasmic reticulum (ER). Certain of the enzymes have been cloned and expressed, but a number of problems relative to their characterization remain to be solved. Enzyme characterization is hampered by the tendency for denaturation during isolation procedures. The elucidation of enzyme physicochemical properties, catalytic properties and substrate specificity needs further study. Orientation of the active catalytic site in the membrane has been the subject of debate, and definition of the site needs to be performed. If, as previous work suggests, the catalytic site is oriented luminally, the mechanism for the transport of enzyme substrates from the cytoplasmic to the luminal membrane surface needs to be examined.

Consideration of these questions has been advanced by the development in our laboratory of sugar-nucleotide photoaffinity probes which can be used in the characterization of sugar-nucleotide-binding proteins. $[\beta\text{-}^{32}\text{P}]5$-azido-UDPGlcA and -UDPGlc (azido-UDPGA and -UDPGlc) along with other azido-sugar-nucleotide derivatives were prepared[1] and utilized in the studies briefly described below.

First, the probes were used to label UDPGlcA and UDPGlc-binding proteins in microsomal membranes. Human and rat liver microsomes were mixed with probe, exposed to UV light, proteins were extracted, the extracts were processed by SDS-PAGE, and autoradiographs were developed. Photolabelled bands were seen in two principal areas. The first corresponded to the 37 kDa protein, UDP-Glc:dolichylphosphate glucosyltransferase (Glc-P-Dol synthase), and the second to the 50–56 kDa region, the region of the UGT. In the presence of detergent (microsomal disruption) both azido-UDPGlcA and UDPGlc labelled both bands. Unlabelled UDPGlcA and

UDPGlc inhibited photolabelling of both bands by both probes, thus establishing the specificity of labelling. In rats, labelling of the band corresponding to the UGT (but not Glc-P-Dol synthase) was increased by pretreatment with phenobarbital.

The labelling of Glc-P-Dol synthase with the UDPGlcA probe and its inhibition with unlabelled UDPGlcA and UDPGlc was surprising, since UDPGlcA is not a known substrate of the enzyme. Equally surprising, both probes also labelled 50–56 kDa proteins. Labelling of the proteins in the UGT region was explored further[2]. It was shown that, although photolabelling with the two probes appeared in approximately the same (50–56 kDa) regions, the patterns of photolabelling, that is the specific bands within the region labelled, were distinct. These data suggested the existence of distinctive UDPGlc-binding protein(s) with mass(es) similar to those of UGT. This impression was supported when it was shown that activity of an hitherto unrecognized UDPGlc-dependent transferase was demonstrable in human (but not rat) microsomes. Substrate specificity for the enzyme was sharply delimited. The 6α-hydroxylated bile acid, hyodeoxycholic acid (HDCA), was glucosidated by human liver microsomes in the presence of UDPGlc, but its 6β-isomer was not. The 6-O-glucoside derivative was rigorously identified by FAB-MS and NMR. The apparent specific activity of the enzyme in microsomes was similar to that of 6α-glucuronidation. Enzyme kinetics were determined. Enzyme activity was strongly inhibited by UDPGlcA (apparent $K_i = 7\,\mu mol/l$). Studies performed with HDCA-specific UGT (clone UGT2B4) expressed in V79 cells showed that this enzyme is not photolabelled with azido-UDPGlc (but *is* with azido-UGPGlcA). Thus the presence of a novel UDPGlc-specific glucosyltransferase catalysing the biosynthesis of 6α-O-glucosides of bile acids was demonstrated in human liver microsomes. The role of this enzyme(s) in health and disease remains to be determined.

Photoaffinity techniques were utilized to determine the active site orientation of UGT. Photolabelling of human and rat liver microsomes was performed in the absence and presence of detergents; that is, in intact and disrupted microsomes. It was shown that photolabelling of Glc-P-Dol synthase was largely unaffected by the presence of detergents, as would be expected because of the cytosolic orientation of the enzymatic active site. Photolabelling of UGT was increased only slightly by microsome disruption. This would be compatible with either a cytosolic orientation of the active enzymatic site, or with a luminal orientation in association with a UDPGlcA transport mechanism. The latter view was confirmed by demonstrating that trypsin did not alter the mass of photolabelled UGT in intact microsomes, but *did* in disrupted microsomes. The view was further confirmed by the following: photolabelling in intact microsomes was found to be time- and temperature-dependent. It was diminished by the inclusion of the non-penetrating transport inhibitor, DIDS, in the incubation medium. In contrast to these results, photolabelling with azido-UDPGlc was minimal in intact microsomes, but was 14-fold increased by detergent disruption of microsomes. Taken together, these results suggest that the orientation of the enzymatic site of UGT is luminal rather than cytoplasmic (albeit the suggested intramembrane orientation[3] cannot be absolutely ruled out). They further suggest that UDPGlcA is transported across the microsomal membrane by a specific transport mechanism. Finally, they suggest that the mechanisms of transport for UDPGlcA and UDPGlc are distinct.

The mechanism of microsomal transport of sugar-nucleotides was further pursued by Berg, Gollan and co-workers[4,5]. Studies of the uptake of radiolabelled UDPGlcA were performed using rapid filtration techniques. Uptake was time-dependent and saturable, was osmotically sensitive, and was inhibited by DIDS and SITS. Unlike the postulated Golgi transporter, transport was not inhibited by UMP or UDP, but was *trans*-stimulated and *cis*-inhibited by UDPGlcNAc. Thus, the presence of a hepatic microsomal UDPGLcA transporter, suggested by the results of photoaffinity labelling studies, is confirmed by direct studies of microsomal transport.

Photoaffinity labelling was used in studies of the action of inhibitors. The examination of inhibitors through the measurement of their effect on enzymatic activity is cumbersome and time-consuming. A preliminary evaluation of inhibitor activity is facilitated through the study of the effect of inhibitors on photoaffinity labelling of suitable substrates. A series of potential UGT inhibitors with *N*-acyl phenylaminoalcohol derivatives linked to uridine or isopropylideneuridine were prepared[6]. Their effects on photolabelling with azido-UDPGlcA and -UDPGlc, and on the enzymatic formation of the hydroxyl and carboxyl derivatives of lithocholic acid, were examined[7]. The degree of inhibition of the two processes by the set of inhibitors was characterized. Overall, inhibition of both processes showed similarities, but quantitative distinctions were also evident. It should be kept in mind that photoaffinity labelling does not give stoichiometric results, and labels only a small percentage of active enzymatic sites. The results confirm that photolabelling with the probes can be used as a qualitative tool with which to screen inhibitors of UGT without performing the tedious examination of inhibition of enzymatic activity.

Studies of the effect of several members of the same set of inhibitors were extended to examine their effects on the enzymatic activity of UGT1*6, cloned and expressed in V79 cells[8]. The most effective inhibitor was found to be competitively inhibitory to both UDPGlcA and an aglycone. The results suggested that the compound and other members of the set may be transition state analogue inhibitors of the recombinant enzyme.

Finally, UGT2B4 was produced as a catalytically active protein A fusion protein in *E. coli* by Siest's group[9]. The protein was shown to photolabel by azido-UDPGlcA and enzyme kinetics were characterized. Using this protein and suitable fragments, and making use of photolabelling techniques, it was possible to characterize a specific UDP-binding site between amino acids 299 and 446. Further, an interaction between the amino-terminal part of the protein and glucuronic acid (but not glucose) was demonstrated. Certain of the properties of this latter site were determined. These results were confirmed using studies of antibody specific for the UGT2B4 isoform, and are in agreement with the studies described above demonstrating the utilization of UDPGlcA, but not UDPGlc, as a substrate by this UGT.

The work described above demonstrates the broad uses of photoaffinity labelling with azido-sugar-nucleotide probes in the study of UGT and other sugar-nucleotide-binding proteins. Together, these studies form the basis for future work in which the mechanism of glucuronidation will be characterized in normals and individuals with cholestatic liver disease.

References

1. Drake RR, Zimniak P, Haley BE, Lester R, Elbein AD, Radominska A. Synthesis and characterization of 5-azido-UDP-glucuronidic acid. A new photoaffinity probe for UDP-glucuronic acid-utilizing proteins. J Biol Chem. 1991;266:23257–60.
2. Drake R, Igari I, Lester R, Elbein A, Radominska A. Application of 5-azido-UDP-glucose and 5-azido-UDP-glucuronic acid photoaffinity probes for the determination of the active site orientation of microsomal UDP-glucosyltransferases and UDP-glucuronosyltransferases. J Biol Chem. 1992;267:11360–5.
3. Zakim D, Dannenberg AJ. How does the microsomal membrane regulate UDP-glucuronosyl-transferases? Biochem Pharmacol. 1992;43:1385–93.
4. Hauser SC, Ziurys JC, Gollan JL. A membrane transporter mediates access of uridine 5'-diphosphoglucuronic acid from the cytosol into the endoplasmic reticulum of rat hepatocytes: implications for glucuronidation reaction. Biochim Biophys Acta. 1988;967:149–57.
5. Berg C, Radominska A, Lester R, Gollan J. Membrane translocation of uridine diphospho-glucuronic acid in rat liver microsomal vesicles: regulation and implications for glucuronid-ation. 1994 (Submitted).
6. Paul P, Lutz T, Osborn C et al. Synthesis and characterization of a new class of inhibitors of membrane-associated UDP-glycosyltransferases. J Biol Chem. 1993;268:12933–8.
7. Radominska A, Paul P, Treat S et al. Photoaffinity labelling for evaluation of uridinyl analogs as specific inhibitors of rat liver microsomal UDP-glucuronosyltransferases. Biochim Biophys Acta. 1994 (In press).
8. Battaglia E, Elass A, Drake RR et al. Characterization of a new class of inhibitors of a recombinant human liver UDP-glucuronosyltransferase, UGT1*6. Biochim Biophys Acta. 1993 (Submitted).
9. Pillot T, Ouzzine M, Fournel-Gigleux S et al. Purification and characterization of a catalytically active human liver UDP-glucuronosyltransferase expressed as a fusion protein in E. coli. Biochem Biophys Res Commun. 1993;196:473–9.

10
Drugs, chemicals and cellular mechanisms of cholestasis

I. M. ARIAS, Z. GATMAITAN, J. F. DUFOUR, M. ST PIERRE,
L. EPSTEIN, M. CHE, Y. MATSUDA and C. LEVEILLE-WEBSTER

INTRODUCTION

'Cholestasis' (i.e. bile secretory failure) has a multifactorial pathogenesis involving impairment in cellular mechanisms utilized in normal bile formation and secretion. New information regarding hepatobiliary motility, secretion and transport provides novel potential cholestatic mechanisms.

THE BILE CANALICULUS IS A CONTRACTILE MECHANISM AND CONTAINS AT LEAST FOUR ATP-DRIVEN TRANSPORT SYSTEMS

The bile canaliculus contains about 10% of the plasma membrane of the mammalian hepatocyte and $5\,\mu l$ per gram of liver. Despite many attempts its contents have never been sampled *in vivo* or in cultured hepatocytes. Recent studies of bile canalicular biology provide new information regarding membrane transport and cytoskeletal function in relation to bile secretion and cholestasis[1].

Bile canalicular contraction occurs *in vivo* and in cultured cells. What is its function? Is it related to cholestasis?

Phillips and his group were the first to demonstrate bile canalicular contraction in response to increased intracellular calcium concentration[2]. ATP, vasopressin and other agonists prompt a signal cascade which results in myosin light-chain phosphorylation and canalicular contraction[3]. Nitric oxide prevents this response by inhibiting inositol triphosphate-mediated release of calcium from intracellular stores[4]. Theoretically, canalicular paralysis may reduce the activity of ATP-dependent transporters, much as cholera toxin affects the intestinal tract. An experimental model of cholestasis related to such a phenomenon results from the effect of cytochalasin, which blocks cytoskeletal polymerization and produces canalicular atony but does not inhibit ATP-mediated transport of bile acids or non-bile acid organic anions into the bile canaliculus in hepatocyte doublets in culture[5]. Phillips and co-workers have postulated that cholestasis in rats treated with cytochalasin or phalloidin may result from the effect of these drugs on canalicular contraction[6,7].

Bile canalicular ectoenzymes are functionally linked to conservation transporters. Are they related to cholestasis?

Ca^{2+},Mg^{2+}-ATPase, the most abundant ATPase activity in the bile canaliculus, was identified as an ectoenzyme because its ability to hydrolyse ATP disappears when cells containing the enzyme are treated with proteases which act only outside the cell. Cloning and sequencing of the cDNA and protein indicate that it is a single polypeptide with one transmembrane domain[8]. ATP hydrolysis is a property of the extracellular domain. More than 10 ectoenzymes have been identified in the canalicular plasma membrane. Although ecto-ATPase properties and primary structure have been studied, the physiological role of the enzyme is less certain. One function is to hydrolyse extracellular ATP, which is a ligand for P_2-purinergic receptors. The second function protects cells from deleterious effects of extracellular ATP and, in concert with 5'-nucleotidase (AMPase), another canalicular ectoenzyme, forms adenosine, which is recaptured by a canalicular nucleoside transporter[9]. Because the ecto-ATPase has sequence homology with Cell CAM 105, a role in cell adhesion has also been proposed[10]. Recently these two proteins have been separated and shown to have different functions (unpublished).

Other investigators have proposed that Ca^{2+},Mg^{2+}-ATPase may be an ATP-dependent bile acid transporter[11-13]. Transfection of COS cells with the cDNA resulted in energy-dependent taurocholate transport, which was not observed when a truncated form of the cDNA was used for transfection. These provocative studies have raised many questions which require additional research to resolve.

Whether ATP is present in the bile canaliculus is also unknown; however, the hepatocyte is the likely source for canalicular ATP. Hypoxia produces rapid decline in hepatocellular ATP content, increased ATP release, extracellular ATP accumulation in the bile canaliculus and cholestasis.

Recently, a Na^+ gradient-energized, concentrative nucleoside transport system was localized to canalicular membranes[9]. Transport is primarily driven by the high sodium gradient between bile (140 mmol/l) and hepatocyte (14 mmol/l) and is specific for purines. The co-localization of ecto-ATPase, 5'-nucleotidase and a sodium-dependent nucleoside transport system in canalicular membranes suggests a functional link between extracellular nucleotide degradation and nucleoside conservation in hepatocytes.

The bile canalicular plasma membrane is enriched in other ectoenzymes which can degrade glutathione (i.e. GGTP) and other peptides (i.e. dipeptidyl peptidase, COOH terminal peptidase, LAP and aminopeptidase M)[13]. Ecto-GGTPase and dipeptidyl peptidase degrade extracellular glutathione into cysteine, glutamic acid and glycine, which are conserved by sodium gradient-driven amino acid transporters in the bile canalicular membrane. It is likely that the entire repertoire of ectoenzymes in the canaliculus is linked with unidirectional transporters which conserve amino acids, purines and pyrimidines. Thus, the cell may secrete hydrophobic peptides, some of which are potentially damaging and – following digestion by ectoenzymes in the bile canaliculus – amino acids, purines and pyrimidines are conserved.

THE BILE CANALICULUS CONTAINS AT LEAST FOUR SPECIFIC ATP-DEPENDENT TRANSPORT MECHANISMS WHICH PROBABLY PROVIDE CHOLESTATIC MECHANISMS

Bile is a major route for the excretion of endogenous compounds, such as bile acids, bile pigments, metabolites and xenobiotics which are predominantly hydrophobic compounds with molecular weight exceeding 400. Oxidative metabolism of these compounds is followed by conjugation with amino acids, glucuronic acid, sulphate or glutathione prior to biliary secretion.

The discovery of ATP-dependent transporters for bile acids, non-bile acid organic anions and organic cations opens opportunities for understanding biliary physiology and the pathobiology of cholestasis and other disorders[1,14].

Multidrug resistance gene products as canalicular ATP-dependent transporters

Multidrug resistance (MDR) in cultured cells results from overexpression of a small group of 170 kDa membrane phosphoglycoproteins, termed Pgp, which bind ATP and drug analogues and have intrinsic ATPase activity suggesting that they function as energy-dependent efflux pumps in drug-resistant cells. Normal human and murine tissues revealed Pgp expression in liver, small intestine, colon, adrenal and kidney with lesser amounts in other tissues. In liver, small intestine and kidney the gene product is restricted to the secretory domain of the cell. In hepatocytes it is present only in the bile canalicular membrane.

Pgp was the first ATP-dependent transporter identified in the bile canalicular plasma membrane[15]. Temperature-dependent saturable, ATP-dependent transport of daunomycin and other cationic hydrophobic anticancer drugs and other compounds with molecular weight of 400–1200 was demonstrated. The K_m of ATP-dependent transport of daunomycin is in the micromolar range. The process requires hydrolysable ATP, is restricted to inside-out CMV and absent from SMV. Hydrophobic bile acids and progesterone inhibit the transport process non-competitively and are not substrates. Non-bile acid organic anions, such as glutathione conjugates, glucuronides and various dyes, do not inhibit ATP-dependent daunomycin transport by CMV.

Pgp are encoded by a small multigene family consisting of three genes in rodents and man. Pgp have high intra-species sequence homology with 75–85% identity among the three mouse genes. Mouse mdr1 and mdr3 and human MDR1 confer drug resistance to drug-sensitive cells but mouse mdr2 and the human MDR2 homologue (termed MDR3) do not[7,16].

Mdr2 is responsible for most Pgp in the bile canaliculus; Mdr3 is present in small amount and there is no mdr1 expressed in normal liver[18]. Mdr2 does not not confer the multidrug resistance phenotype but has considerable sequence homology with other MDR proteins and corrected the defect in mutant yeast which lacks a transporter for the *a* mating factor. Based upon the structure of substrates for Mdr1 and 3, hydrophobic cations with molecular weight of 400–1500 were sought as substrates for Mdr2. Various hydrophobic peptides were shown not to be substrates.

The search for an endogenous substrate(s) for the hepatic Mdr2 was unproductive until recent observations were made in mice in which mdr1, mdr2 and mdr3 were selectively 'knocked out' by homologous recombination[19]. Mdr1 and mdr3 'knock-out' mice did not reveal an abnormal phenotype. Mdr2 'knock-out' mice revealed progressive damage to small bile ducts with resulting obstructive-type jaundice and eventual destruction of the bile ducts and fibrosis. The morphological picture resembles that seen in various vanishing bile duct syndromes. Analysis of bile in normal and Mdr2 'knock-out' mice revealed virtual absence of phospholipids from the bile of the latter. These remarkable studies suggest that phospholipids may be transported into bile by a process which involves a 'flippase' (which transports phosphatidyl choline from the inner to the outer layer of the plasma membrane) and/or a potential ATP-dependent transporter. The precise mechanism is uncertain, but offers exciting opportunities to understand phospholipid and cholesterol transport from hepatocyte into bile. In addition, an attractive hypothesis for the hepatic phenotype is that bile acids are not converted into micelles due to the absence of phospholipids and consequently damage the small bile duct epithelial cells. The relationship of these observations to vanishing bile duct and cholestatic syndromes in man remains to be explored.

The precise mechanism whereby Pgp act as transporters is not known. Hydrolysable ATP is required. A recent report describes volume-regulated, ATP-dependent chloride channel activity associated with Pgp in MDR1-transfected fibroblasts. CFTR and MDR appear to be novel proteins which have substrate transport and chloride channel activities. An MDR-like transport function for CFTR has been proposed but not demonstrated.

ATP-dependent transport of bile acids

In the 1980s the driving force for bile secretion was presumed to be the electrochemical membrane potential ($-35\,mV$); however, approximately $-100\,mV$ would be required to sustain the taurocholate concentration gradient between bile and hepatocyte (approximately 100:1) *in vivo*. The missing component was described in 1991 when ATP-dependent, vanadate-sensitive and unidirectional (i.e. present in inside-out but not right-side-out vesicles) was demonstrated in rat CMV but not in SMV[20-23]. The system is specific for bile acids and requires hydrolysable ATP. Inhibition of ATP-dependent taurocholate transport was not observed with Pgp substrates, such as daunomycin, verapamil or doxorubicin, or various non-bile acid organic anions, such as bilirubin glucuronide, glutathione adducts, GSH, GSSG or leukotriene metabolites. A putative 110 kDa carrier for ATP-dependent bile acid transport was identified following immunoprecipitation by monoclonal antibodies against canalicular transformation-sensitive glyco-proteins. The relationship between this protein and a 100 kDa canalicular protein previously characterized as a membrane potential-driven taurochol-ate transporter is unknown. The large number of canalicular proteins of approximately 100 kDa, including the abundant Ca^{2+},Mg^{2+} ecto-ATPase, may account for the difficulty in purifying these candidate transporters for structural, functional and molecular studies. As mentioned previously, one study suggests that the ecto-ATPase may be a bile acid transporter, but this has been challenged.

ATP-dependent transport of non-bile acid organic anions defects result in the Dubin–Johnson syndrome but not in cholestasis

Ten years ago, electrogenic carrier-mediated transport of several non-bile acid organic anions was demonstrated in CMV with an apparent K_m in the millimolar range, whereas concentrations encountered physiologically are micromolar. An exception is reduced glutathione, which may attain millimolar concentrations in bile. Recently, ATP-dependent transport of BSP-GSH, DNP-SG and cysteinyl leukotriene C4 was demonstrated in CMV but not SMV[24-28]. ATP-dependent transport of bilirubin monoglucuronides and diglucuronides in CMV was subsequently demonstrated[28]. Some bile acids and non-bile acid organic anions may interact with more than one ATP-dependent transport system; however, purification of individual transporters is required before differential substrate specificity can be demonstrated. The ATP-dependent transporter for non-bile acid organic anions has also been called the multispecific organic anion transporter (MOAT), as well as the leukotriene transporter, because leukotriene C4 is a natural substrate having very high affinity for the system. The ATP-dependent non-bile acid organic anion transporter has not been purified; however, progress has been reported based upon description of ATP-dependent transport of GSH adducts in other tissues.

Study of ATP-dependent transport of non-bile acid organic anions was enhanced by the serendipitous discovery of a strain of jaundiced mutant Wistar rats. The mutant rats (termed TR⁻) manifest predominantly conju-gated hyperbilirubinaemia, and are defective in the biliary secretion of many non-bile acid organic anions including bilirubin conjugates; sulphated and glucuronidated bile acids; anionic epinephrine metabolites and GSH conjugates of BSP, DNP and leukotriene C4, but not taurocholate or Pgp substrates[24,25,28,29]. The functional defect is transmitted with the characteristics of an autosomal recessively inherited abnormality. CMV from TR⁻ rats retain membrane potential-dependent transport of non-bile acid organic anions at the same activity level observed in CMV from normal rats[28]. This observation suggests that different transporters may be responsible for ATP-dependent and membrane potential-dependent transport of non-bile acid organic anions in CMV. The transport defect in the Dubin–Johnson syndrome and the comparable disorder in TR⁻ and EHBR rats[30], mutant Corriedale sheep and mutant Golden Lion Tamarin monkeys[31] is phenotypically manifested by mild conjugated hyperbilirubinaemia and impaired biliary secretion of several non-bile acid organic anions, but not bile acids or organic cations. The mild degree of conjugated hyperbilirubinaemia and presence of bilirubin glucuronides in the bile of these mutants may result from the transport of bilirubin glucuronides by a membrane potential-driven canalicular transport system.

Relation of ATP-dependent transporters to drug-associated cholestasis

Although the relation of these transporters to specific diseases has not been fully explored, defects in ATP-dependent bile acid transport may underlie various inheritable and acquired forms of cholestasis. Several examples are provided by recent studies on the effect of cholestatic drugs and chemicals on these transporters[30]. Cyclosporin A is a mdr1,3 substrate, inhibited daunomycin and taurocholate transport competitively (K_i 5 μmol/l and 7 μmol/l respectively) and DNP-GSH transport non-competitively. Similar results were obtained with FK 506; however, K_i was substantially greater. These results are in agreement with studies reported by Keppler *et al.* using membrane preparations from human liver[33,34]. The results are consistent with doses of cyclosporin which produce cholestasis in patients and the relative rarity of cholestasis after FK 506 treatment. In canalicular membrane vesicles, 20–200 μmol/l taurolithocholate inhibited all systems non-competitively. Pretreatment of rats with ethinyl oestradiol selectively and competitively inhibited ATP-dependent but not potential-dependent taurocholate transport in canalicular membrane vesicles. Similar treatment of TR⁻ rats did not affect serum bilirubin concentrations or potential-driven taurocholate transport. Thus, cholestatic compounds may affect some or all ATP-dependent canalicular transporters. Ethinyl oestradiol *in vivo* selectively affects ATP-dependent but not potential-dependent bile acid transport[31].

HOW ARE TRANSPORTERS AND ECTOENZYMES RECRUITED TO THE BILE CANALICULUS? DO THEY RECYCLE BETWEEN GOLGI AND CANALICULAR MEMBRANE? IS SUCH A PROCESS INVOLVED IN CHOLESTASIS?

Several investigators have demonstrated that apical domain ectoenzymes are synthesized in the endoplasmic reticulum, processed in the Golgi and targeted to the basolateral plasma membrane domain, from which they are transcytosed to the apical domain[35,36]. These processes involve vesicular trafficking, and are associated with the cytoskeleton, possibly involving ATP-activated motors, such as dynein. This complex process involves the participation of many small GTPases which are conserved in yeast and mammalian cells. Temperature-sensitive yeast mutants have been identified which are defective in each of several specific steps in membrane fusion from Golgi release to the plasma membrane. To date, the trafficking of ATP-dependent canalicular transporter proteins has not been established. In temperature-sensitive mutant *S. cerevisae* transfected with mdr1, mdr2 or mdr3 cDNA, the gene product appears in cytoplasmic membrane vacuoles which fail to fuse with the plasma membrane. A similar situation exists in mammalian polarized cells. Specific GTPases are probably required for the fusion of Golgi-derived vesicles with the apical domain, and may account for direct targeting of apical transporters from the Golgi. Support for this view was obtained from studies in which fluorescent derivatives of bile acids or non-bile acid organic anions localized to Golgi-derived vesicles prior to delivery to the plasama membrane[5,37]. Furthermore, this process was affected by colchicine and vinblastin, which inhibit cytoskeletal organization and traffic patterns[5]. Other studies reveal that canalicular membrane components are internalized into the hepatocyte following biliary obstruction. The prescient studies of Coleman originally demonstrated that biliary lipids are derived from the plasma membrane (i.e. canalicular domain), and may be replaced by movement of additional lipids from the Golgi to the plasma membrane[38]. These observations suggest that a regulated system may exist between lipid loss into the canalicular lumen and replacement. Canalicular transport proteins may participate in a similar regulated internal cycle between Golgi and plasma membrane. If so, it is reasonable to speculate that disruption of the cytoskeleton and targeting molecules could impair the steady-state level of specific canalicular transporters resulting in cholestasis.

Rapid developments in cell biology with regard to intracellular and membrane transport have expanded the scope of potential 'primary' defects in cholestasis.

References

1. Arias IM, Che M, Gatmaitan Z, Leveille C, Nishida T, St-Pierre MV. The biology of the bile canaliculus, 1993. Hepatology. 1993;17:318–29.
2. Watanabe N, Tsukada N, Smith CR, Phillips MJ. Motility of bile canaliculi in the living animal: implications for bile flow. J Cell Biol. 1991;113:1069–80.
3. Kitamura T, Brauneis U, Gatmaitan Z, Arias IM. Extracellular ATP, intracellular calcium and canalicular contraction in rat hepatocyte doublets. Hepatology. 1991;14:640–7.
4. Dufour J-F, Arias IM. The mechanism whereby nitric oxide inhibits bile canalicular contraction. (In press).
5. St-Pierre MV, Arias IM. Disruption of actin organization by cytochalasin D does not impair biliary secretion of organic anions. Hepatology. 1992;17:145A (abstr.).
6. Phillips MJ. Biology and pathobiology of actin in the liver. In: Arias IM, Boyer JC, Fausto N, Jakoby WB, Schacter D, Shafritz D, editors. The liver: biology and pathobiology, 3rd edn. New York: Raven Press; 1994:19–33.
7. Phillips MJ. Cytoskeleton: actin. In: Arias IM, Boyer JL, Fausto N, Jakoby WB, Schachter

DA, Shafritz DA, editors. The liver: biology and pathobiology, 3rd edn. New York: Raven Press; 1994 (In press).

8. Lin SH, Guidotti G. Cloning and expression of a cDNA coding for a rat liver plasma membrane ecto-ATPase. J Biol Chem. 1989;264:14408–14.

9. Che M, Nishida T, Gatmaitan Z, Arias IM. A nucleoside transporter is functionally linked to ectonucleotidases in rat liver canalicular membrane. J Biol Chem. 1992;267:9684–8.

10. Lin SH, Bulic O, Flanagan D, Hixson D. Immunochemical characterization of two isoforms of rat liver ecto-ATPase which show an immunological and structural identity to cell CAM105. Biochem J. 1991;278:155–61.

11. Sippel CJ, Ananthanarayanan M, Suchy FJ. Isolation and characterization of the canalicular membrane bile acid transport protein of rat liver. Am J Physiol. 1990;258:G728–37.

12. Sippel CJ, Suchy FJ, Ananthanarayanan M, Perlmutter DH. The rat liver ecto-ATPase is also a canalicular bile acid transport protein. J Biol Chem. 1993;268:2083–91.

13. Sippel CJ, McCollum MJ, Perlmutter DH. Bile acid transport by the rat liver canalicular bile acid transport/eco-ATPase protein is dependent on ATP but not on its own ecto-ATPase activity. J Biol Chem. 1994;269:2800–26.

14. Arias IM. Multidrug resistance genes, P-glycoprotein and the liver. Hepatology. 1990;12:159–65.

15. Kamimoto Y, Gatmaitan Z, Hsu J, Arias IM. The function of Gp 170, the multidrug resistance gene product, in rat liver canalicular membrane vesicles. J Biol Chem. 1989;264:11693–8.

16. DeVault A, Gros P. Two members of the mouse mdr gene family confer multidrug resistance with overlapping but distinct specificities. Mol Cell Biol. 1990;10:1652–63.

17. Buschman E, Gros P. Functional analysis of chimeric genes obtained by exchanging homologous domains of the mouse *mdr*1 and *mdr*2 genes. Mol Cell Biol. 1991;11:595–603.

18. Buschman E, Areci R, Croop J *et al.* Mouse mdr 2 encodes P-glycoprotein expression in the bile canalicular membrane as determined by isoform specific antibodies. J Biol Chem. 1992;267:18093–9.

19. Smit JJM, Schinkel AH, Oude Elferink RPJ *et al.* Homozygous disruption of the murine mdr2 P-glycoprotein gene leads to a complete absence of phospholipid from bile to liver disease. *Cell.* 1994 (In press).

20. Nishida T, Gatmaitan Z, Che M, Arias IM. Rat liver canalicular membrane vesicles contain an ATP-dependent bile acid transport system. Proc Natl Acad Sci USA. 1991;88:6590–4.

21. Muller M, Ishikawa R, Berger U *et al.* ATP-dependent transport of taurocholate across the hepatocyte canalicular membrane mediated by a 110-kDa glycoprotein binding ATP and bile salt. J Biol Chem. 1991;266:18920–6.

22. Adachi Y, Kobayashi H, Kurumi Y, Shouji M, Kitano M, Yamamoto T. ATP-dependent taurocholate transport by rat liver canalicular membrane vesicles. Hepatology. 1991;14:655–9.

23. Stieger B, O'Neill B, Meier PJ. ATP-dependent bile-salt transport in canalicular rat liver plasma-membrane vesicles. Biochem J. 1992;284:67–74.

24. Kitamura T, Jansen P, Hardenbrook C, Kamimoto UC, Gatmaitan Z, Arias IM. Defective ATP-dependent bile canalicular transport of organic anions in mutant (TR⁻) rats with conjugated hyperbilirubinemia. Proc Natl Acad Sci USA. 1990;87:3557–61.

25. Nishida T, Hardenbrook C, Gatmaitan Z, Arias IM. ATP-dependent organic anion transport system in normal and TR⁻ rat liver canalicular membranes. Am J Physiol. 1992;262:G629–35.

26. Kobayashi J, Sogame Y, Hara H, Hayashi K. Mechanism of glutathione S-conjugate transport in canalicular and basolateral rat liver plasma membranes. J Biol Chem. 1990;265:7737–41.

27. Ishikawa T, Muller M, Klunemann C, Schaub T, Keppler D. ATP-dependent primary active transport of cysteinyl leukotrienes across liver canalicular membranes. J Biol Chem. 1990;265:19279–86.

28. Nishida T, Gatmaitan Z, Roy-Chowdhury J, Arias I. Two distinct mechanisms for bilirubin glucuronide transport by rat bile canalicular membrane vesicles: demonstration of defective ATP-dependent transport in rats (TR⁻) with inherited conjugated hyperbilirubinemia. J Clin Invest. 1992;90:227–32.

29. Oude Elferink RPJ, Ottenhoff R, Liefting W, DeHaan J, Jansen PLM. Hepatobiliary transport of glutathione and glutathione conjugate in rats with hereditary hyperbilirubinemia. J Clin Invest. 1989;84:476–83.

30. Kitamura T, Gatmaitan Z, Alroy J *et al.* The pathogenesis of hepatic pigmentation in mutant rats with the Dubin–Johnson syndrome. Hepatology. 1990;12:871.
31. Schulman FY, Montali RJ, Bush M *et al.* Dubin–Johnson-like syndrome in Golden Lion Tamarins (*Leonthopitheous rosalia rosalia*). Vet Pathol. 1993;30:491–8.
32. Romanelli R, Che M, Leveille C, Gatmaitan Z, Arias IM. Effect of cholestatic compounds on bile canalicular ATP-dependent transport systems. AASLD. 1993 (abstr.).
33. Kadmon M, Klunemann C, Bohme T *et al.* Inhibition by cyclosporin A of adenosine triphosphate-dependent transport from the hepatocyte into bile. Gastroenterology. 1993;104:1507–14.
34. Arias IM. Cyclosporin, the biology of the bile canaliculus, and cholestasis. Gastroenterology. 1993;104:1558–9.
35. Bartles JR, Feracci HM, Steiger B, Hubbard AL. Biogenesis of the rat hepatocyte plasma membrane *in vivo*: comparison of the pathways taken by apical and basolateral proteins using subcellular fractionation. J Cell Biol. 1987;105:1241–51.
36. Hubbard AL, Barr V, Scott LM. Hepatocyte surface polarity. In: Arias IM, Boyer JL, Fausto N, Jakoby WB, Schaechter DA, Shafritz DA, editors. The liver: biology and pathobiology, 3rd edn. New York: Raven Press; 1994 (In press).
37. Oude Elferink RPJ, Bakker CTM, Roelofsen H *et al.* Accumulation of organic anion in intracellular vesicles of cultured rat hepatocytes is mediated by the canalicular multispecific organic anion transporter. Hepatology. 1993;17:434–44.
38. Coleman R. Lipid transport into bile. Biochem J. 1987;244:249–61.

11
Transport of taurine conjugates of 7α-hydroxy-3-oxo-4-cholenoic acid and 3β,7α-dihydroxy-5-cholenoic acid in rat liver plasma membrane vesicles

B. STIEGER, J. ZHANG, B. O'NEILL, J. SJÖVALL and P. J. MEIER

INTRODUCTION

Patients with genetic or acquired defects in bile acid biosynthesis frequently suffer from intrahepatic cholestasis. In patients with a deficiency of 3β-hydroxy-Δ^5-C_{27}-steroid dehydrogenase/isomerase, $3\beta,7\alpha$-dihydroxy- and $3\beta,7\alpha,12\alpha$-trihydroxy-5-cholenoic acids are formed, and are found in urine and in bile as sulphated and partially glycine-conjugated forms[1,2]. Patients deficient in 5β-reductase excrete 3-oxo-Δ^4 bile acids in urine and also have cholestasis. This association between formation of abnormal bile acids and cholestatic liver disease in childhood has led to the suggestion that abnormal bile acids might be cholestatic agents[1-4].

This hypothesis is difficult to test *in vivo* since the abnormal bile acids might be metabolized by those enzymes lacking in patients. The development of methods to isolate plasma membrane vesicles from liver has opened the possibility to test the hypothesis that abnormal bile acids interfere with transport and secretion of normal bile acids *in vitro* under well-defined conditions, and in the absence of interfering metabolic activities. Since there is evidence that bile acid transport in human and rat liver is similar[5-7], such experiments can be performed with readily available plasma membrane vesicles from rat liver.

In the present study we have addressed the question whether taurine conjugates of $3\beta,7\alpha$-dihydroxy-5-cholenoic acid (5CA-tau) and 7α-hydroxy-3-oxo-4-cholenoic acid (4CA-tau) inhibit transport of cholyltaurine in rat liver basolateral and/or canalicular plasma membrane vesicles, and whether they are transported by the previously characterized bile acid transport systems[8-13].

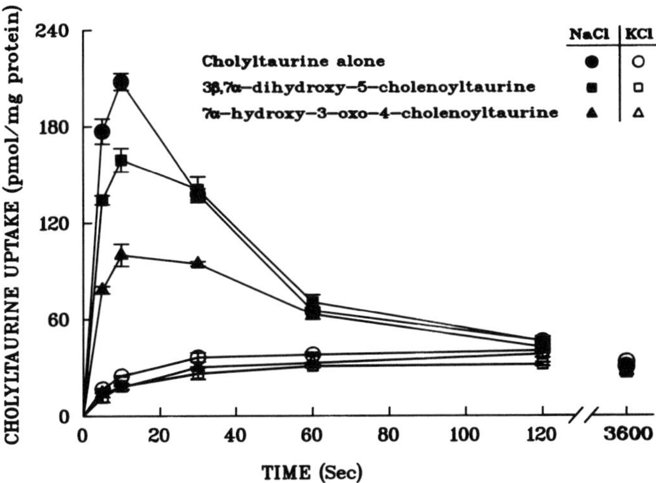

Fig. 1 Effects of synthetic bile acids on sodium-driven cholyltaurine transport in basolateral plasma membrane vesicles. Basolateral rat liver plasma membrane vesicles were resuspended in 250 mmol/l sucrose, 0.2 mmol/l CaCl$_2$, 20 mmol/l HEPES/KOH, pH 7.4. The incubation medium consisted of 50 mmol/l sucrose, 100 mmol/l NaCl or KCl, 5 mmol/l MgCl$_2$, 0.2 mmol/l CaCl$_2$, 20 mmol/l HEPES/KOH, pH 7.4. The uptake of 2.5 μmol/l cholyltaurine was determined at 37°C. The concentration of the inhibitors was 10 μmol/l. Data represent means $\pm$ SD of triplicate determinations

EFFECT OF 7α-HYDROXY-3-OXO-4-CHOLENOYLTAURINE AND OF 3β,7α-DIHYDROXY-5-CHOLENOYLTAURINE ON SODIUM-DEPENDENT CHOLYLTAURINE TRANSPORT IN BASOLATERAL PLASMA MEMBRANE VESICLES

Rat liver plasma membrane vesicles isolated as described in ref. 14 were used to perform transport experiments with radiolabelled cholyltaurine by a rapid filtration technique[15]. First we assayed for the possible interference of 4CA-tau and 5CA-tau, which were synthesized as detailed in refs 16 and 17 with the sodium-dependent bile acid uptake system in basolateral plasma membrane vesicles. As shown in Fig. 1, 10 μmol/l 4CA-tau inhibited sodium-dependent cholyltaurine uptake by 60% at 5 s, whereas the corresponding value for 5CA-tau was only 23%. This indicated that 4CA-tau may indeed be an inhibitor of the basolateral sodium-dependent cholyltaurine transport system. Dixon plot experiments with 4CA-tau gave an apparent K_i value of 16 μmol/l. On the contrary, 5CA-tau yielded no conclusive Dixon plots confirming its weak inhibitory potency apparent from Fig. 1. In order to rule out inhibitory effects related to byproducts of the synthesis of 4CA-tau and 5CA-tau on cholyltaurine transport, a blank synthesis without product was performed. This material did not inhibit sodium-dependent bile acid transport (data not shown). To also rule out an unspecific cholyltaurine transport inhibition by the two bile acids, their influence on sodium-dependent L-alanine transport was tested and found to be negative (data not shown). Thus, the data indicate a specific inhibition of the sodium-dependent

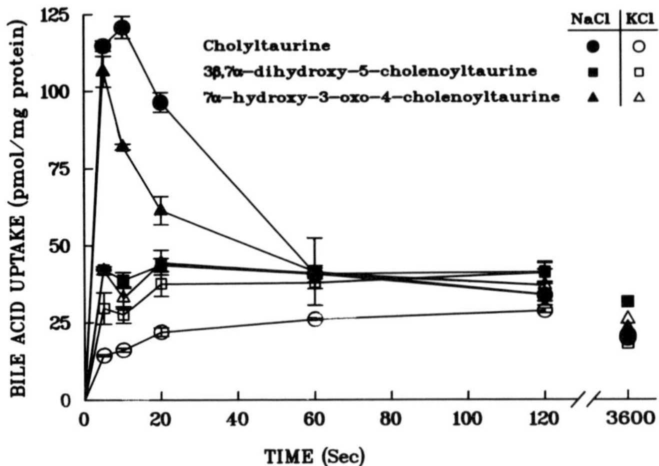

Fig. 2 Sodium-driven transport of synthetic bile acids in basolateral plasma membrane vesicles. Basolateral rat liver plasma membrane vesicles were resuspended and incubated as given in Fig. 1. The concentration of cholyltaurine and of the synthetic bile acids was 2.5 μmol/l. Data represent means $\pm$ SD of triplicate determinations

bile acid transport system in basolateral plasma membrane vesicles.

Since inhibitory substances are not necessarily transported by the same carrier we also performed transport experiments with radiolabelled 4CA-tau and 5CA-tau in basolateral plasma membrane vesicles and compared the results to the transport of the physiological substrate cholyltaurine. This result is given in Fig. 2. Sodium-dependent transport of 4CA-tau was comparable to that of cholyltaurine, whereas no sodium-dependent transport was observed for 5CA-tau. This result is in keeping with the data from the inhibition experiments which showed only a marked interaction of 4CA-tau with the sodium-dependent transport system for cholyltaurine in basolateral plasma membrane vesicles.

EFFECT OF 7α-HYDROXY-3-OXO-4-CHOLENOYLTAURINE AND OF 3β,7α-DIHYDROXY-5-CHOLENOYLTAURINE ON ATP-DEPENDENT CHOLYLTAURINE TRANSPORT IN CANALICULAR PLASMA MEMBRANE VESICLES

After having established the inhibitory pattern for 4CA-tau and 5CA-tau in basolateral plasma membrane vesicles we next determined whether these compounds would also be inhibitors of the ATP-dependent transport system for bile acids in the canalicular plasma membrane of hepatocytes. The results in Fig. 3 show that both 10 μmol/l 4CA-tau (36% inhibition at 30 s) and 10 μmol/l 5CA-tau (47% inhibition at 30 s) inhibited the ATP-dependent transport of cholyltaurine in canalicular plasma membrane vesicles. Dixon plot experiments of two independent experiments yielded K_i values of 16 and 15 μmol/l for 4CA-tau and 5CA-tau, respectively. Finally, we used

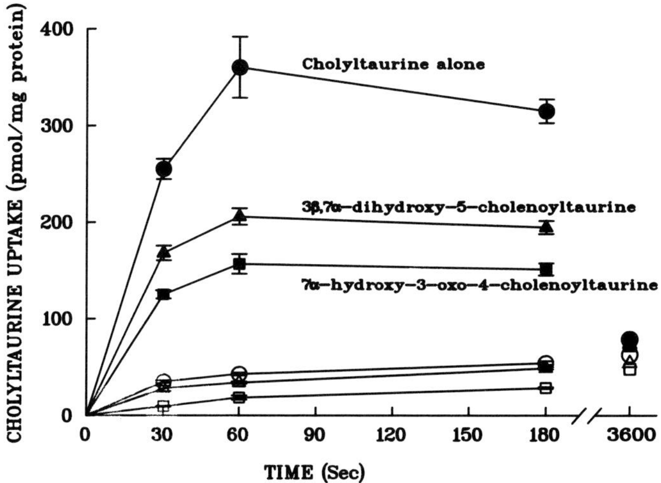

Fig. 3 Effects of synthetic bile acids on ATP-driven cholyltaurine transport in canalicular plasma membrane vesicles. Rat liver canalicular plasma membrane vesicles were resuspended in 50 mmol/l sucrose, 100 mmol/l KNO_3, 10 mmol/l HEPES/Tris, pH 7.4. The incubation medium consisted of 50 mmol/l sucrose, 100 mmol/l KNO_3, 10 mmol/l $Mg(NO_3)_2$, 10 mmol/l HEPES/Tris, pH 7.4. The uptake of 2 μmol/l cholyltaurine was determined at 37°C in the presence (closed symbols) or absence (open symbols) of 5 mmol/l ATP. The concentration of the synthetic bile acids was 10 μmol/l. Data represent means ± SD of triplicate determinations

radiolabelled 4CA-tau and 5CA-tau to test whether they exhibit ATP-dependent transport in canalicular plasma membrane vesicles. Figure 4 shows that, in comparison to cholyltaurine, neither 4CA-tau nor 5CA-tau is taken up in an ATP-dependent manner by canalicular plasma membrane vesicles. Thus, both synthetic bile acids are inhibitors without being transported by the canalicular bile acid transporter, indicating that they could exert a cholestatic action in intact hepatocytes.

DISCUSSION

In the present study we investigated the interaction of the two synthetic bile acids 4CA-tau and 5CA-tau with the bile acid transport systems involved in bile acid uptake into and secretion from hepatocytes. The most important finding is that both synthetic bile acids inhibit the ATP-dependent bile acid transport system located in the canalicular plasma membrane. However, neither of the two bile acids was transported in an ATP-dependent way into canalicular plasma membrane vesicles. Although these studies were performed *in vitro* with rat liver plasma membrane vesicles it is nevertheless possible to extend the results to the situation *in vivo* in humans, since the transport systems for bile acids are similar in human and rat liver[5-7]. The analysis of bile in patients with defects in the biosynthesis of bile acids revealed that neither of the two bile acids used in this study is excreted into bile, although 5CA-tau is excreted in sulphated form[1-4]. This agrees well with the finding

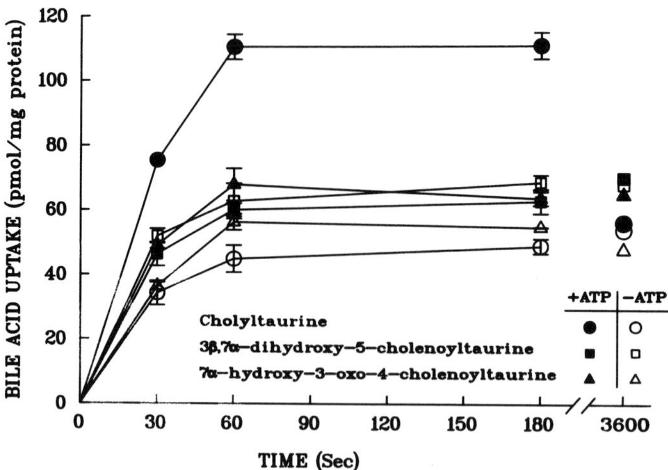

Fig. 4 ATP-driven transport of synthetic bile acids in canalicular plasma membrane vesicles. Canalicular rat liver plasma membrane vesicles were resuspended and incubated as given in Fig. 3. The concentration of cholyltaurine and of the synthetic bile acids was $2\,\mu\text{mol/l}$. Data represent means $\pm$ SD of triplicate determinations

that they are not transported by the canalicular transport system, and is further evidence for the similarity of rat and human bile acid transport systems. In addition, the inhibition of the ATP-dependent bile acid transport system in the canalicular plasma membrane of hepatocytes by 4CA-tau and 5CA-tau may explain their cholestatic effects, because the transport of bile acids across the canalicular plasma membrane is the rate-limiting step in hepatic bile formation[18].

A second interesting finding from this study was the result that the two synthetic bile acids interact differently with the transport systems for cholyltaurine in the basolateral and in the canalicular plasma membrane. In contrast to the canalicular transport system, the sodium-dependent transport system in the basolateral plasma membrane was inhibited only by 4CA-tau. Furthermore, 4CA-tau was transported in a sodium-dependent way in basolateral plasma membrane vesicles. This may indicate that the basolateral and canalicular transport systems for bile acids exhibit a slightly different substrate specificity.

Acknowledgements

This study was supported by Swiss National Science Foundation Grants 31-33520.92 (to B.S.) and 32-29878.90 (to P.J.M.). It was also supported by grants from the Swedish Medical Research Council (No. 03X-219) and from the Karolinska Institutet (to J.S.).

References

1. Clayton PT, Leonard JV, Lawson AM *et al*. Familial giant cell hepatitis associated with synthesis of $3\beta,7\alpha$-dihydroxy- and $3\beta,7\alpha,12\alpha$-trihydroxy-5-cholenoic acids. J Clin Invest. 1987;79:1031–8.
2. Ichimiya H, Egestad B, Nazer H, Baginski ES, Clayton PT, Sjövall J. Bile acids and bile alcohols in a child with hepatic 3β-hydroxy-Δ^5-C_{27}-steroid dehydrogenase deficiency: effects of chenodeoxycholic acid treatment. J Lipid Res. 1991;32:829–41.
3. Setchell KDR, Suchy FJ, Welsh MB, Zimmer-Nechemias L, Heubi J, Balistreri WF. Δ^4-3-oxosteroid 5β-reductase deficiency described in identical twins with neonatal hepatitis. J Clin Invest. 1988;82:2148–57.
4. Clayton PT, Patel E, Lawson AM *et al*. 3-oxo-Δ^4 bile acids in liver disease. Lancet. 1988;2:1283–4.
5. Novak DA, Ryckman FC, Suchy FJ. Taurocholate transport by basolateral plasma membrane vesicles isolated from human liver. Hepatology. 1988;10:447–53.
6. Wolters H, Kuipers F, Sloof MJH, Vonk RJ. Adenosine triphosphate-dependent taurocholate transport in human liver plasma membranes. J Clin Invest. 1992;90:2321–6.
7. Suchy FJ. Hepatocellular transport of bile acids. Semin Liver Dis. 1993;13:235–47.
8. Hagenbuch B, Stieger B, Foguet M, Lübbert H, Meier PJ. Functional expression cloning and characterization of the hepatocyte Na^+/bile acid cotransport system. Proc Natl Acad Sci USA. 1991;88:10629–33.
9. Nishida T, Gatmaitan Z, Che M, Arias IW. Rat liver canalicular membrane vesicles contain an ATP-dependent bile acid transport system. Proc Natl Acad Sci USA. 1991;88:6590–4.
10. Müller M, Ishikawa T, Berger U *et al*. ATP-dependent transport of taurocholate across the hepatocyte canalicular membrane mediated by a 110-kDa glycoprotein binding ATP and bile salt. J Biol Chem. 1991;266:18920–6.
11. Adachi Y, Kobayashi H, Kurumi Y, Shouji M, Kitano M, Yamamoto T. ATP-dependent taurocholate transport by rat liver canalicular membrane vesicles. Hepatology. 1991;14:655–9.
12. Stieger B, O'Neill B, Meier PJ. ATP-dependent bile-salt transport in canalicular rat liver plasma-membrane vesicles. Biochem J. 1992;284:67–74.
13. Meier PJ, Stieger B. Canalicular membrane adenosine triphosphate-dependent transport systems. Progr Liver Dis. 1993;11:27–44.
14. Meier PJ, Sztul ES, Reuben A, Boyer JL. Structural and functional polarity of canalicular and basolateral plasma membrane vesicles isolated in high yield from rat liver. J Cell Biol. 1984;98:991–1000.
15. Meier PJ, Meier-Abt AS, Barrett C, Boyer JL. Mechanisms of taurocholate transport in canalicular and basolateral rat liver plasma membrane vesicles. Evidence for an electrogenic canalicular organic anion carrier. J Biol Chem. 1984;259:10614–22.
16. Shoda J, Axelson M, Sjövall J. Synthesis of C_{27}-intermediates in bile acid biosynthesis and their deuterium labeled analogues. Steroids. 1993;58:119–25.
17. Zhang J, Griffiths WJ, Bergman T, Sjövall J. Derivatization of bile acids with taurine for analysis by fast atom bombardment mass spectrometry with collision-induced fragmentation. J Lipid Res. 1993;34:1895–1900.
18. Reichen J, Paumgartner G. Kinetics of taurocholate uptake by the perfused rat liver. Gastroenterology. 1975;68:132–6.

Section III
Mechanisms of gallstone formation and cholestasis

12
Biliary lipid secretion and cholesterol transport: new insights

M. C. CAREY

INTRODUCTION

The *raison d'être* of biliary lipid secretion is to provide the principal excretory route for steroidal lipids, thereby maintaining homeostatic control over cholesterol metabolism and disposition in the organism[1]. Three lipids are involved; (a) a mixture of bile salt congeners, that are synthesized from cholesterol and modified by anaerobic bacterial enzymes in the large intestine; (b) a mixture of phospholipids that are mostly phosphatidylcholines (PC, lecithins); and (c) cholesterol itself. Bile is also the sole excretory route for bilirubin conjugates and for trace amounts of other sterols, including cholesterol precursors and dietary phytosterols[1]. Although a remarkable amount of information is available about bile salt secretion[2] and osmotically entrailed bile water and electrolyte flow[3], relatively little is known concerning the origins and movement of biliary PC and cholesterol and their secretion into bile[1,2]. This review will focus principally on what is known about biliary secretion of these two lipid classes and their transport throughout the biliary tree. There are many lacunae in our knowledge[1] and my ulterior motive for this review is to highlight fruitful directions for further investigation. This article will be structured as follows: (1) origins of biliary lipids and lipid movement to the canalicular membrane, the highly specialized bile secretory domain of the hepatocyte[4]; these will be grouped as *pre-canalicular events*; (2) lipid secretion across the canalicular membrane and the physical–chemical events in the canalicular space that are putatively involved in biliary lipid secretion[5]; these will be grouped as *canalicular events*; and (3) the physical–chemical state of lipids and phase transitions that occur in and distal to the canalicular space[6]; these will be grouped as *post-canalicular events*.

PRE-CANALICULAR EVENTS

Bile salts

Bile salts are remarkably well conserved in the organism by means of an enterohepatic circulation[1]. This circulation conserves most bile salt molecules secreted into bile and the alimentary canal by virtue of active and passive absorption mechanisms from both small and large intestines[1]. Approximately 98% of the bile salt flux across the hepatocyte and secretion into bile returns again to the liver in the portal vein. At the level of sinusoidal (basolateral) membranes of hepatocytes, bile salts are efficiently cleared by means of several protein carrier mechanisms[7]. To balance the obligatory faecal bile salt loss from the enterohepatic circulation, only 2% of *de-novo* synthesis is required each day for maintenance of bile salt secretion, and this is derived solely from cholesterol in the liver[1]. As far as is known, bile salts are extensively bound to a number of soluble proteins within hepatocytes, and move to the canalicular pole by cytosolic diffusion[8]. From there they are efficiently secreted into the canalicular space by ATP-driven active export carriers[9]. While in the liver cell, bile salts effect many regulatory functions by molecular mechanisms that are not well understood[1]. These include feedback inhibition of the rate-limiting enzymes in cholesterol and bile salt synthesis[10,11], as well as recruitment of PC and cholesterol molecules destined for secretion into bile[1]. The endoplasmic reticulum appears to be the principal target organelle where lipid recruitment takes place[12].

Biliary phosphatidylcholines

More than 95% of all biliary phospholipids are PC[13], trivially known as lecithins. Most (>80%) biliary PC has palmitic acid in the sn-1 position with linoleic, oleic, arachidonic acids in the sn-2 position in that rank order[14]. During bile salt flux through the liver cell, global synthesis of microsomal phospholipids takes place and apparently flux and synthesis are causally related[15]. Recent evidence from studies in the isolated perfused rat liver indicate that most PC destined for bile are synthesized by extensive reutilization of endogenous acylglyceride sources[16]. After acyl group remodelling of pre-existing PC and other acylglycerides[16], *de-novo* PC synthesis by the classic (Kennedy) pathway[17], *N*-methylation of phosphatidylethanolamine[18], base exchange[19], or transesterification of lysolecithin[20] make, in that rank order, smaller contributions to biliary PC synthesis[16].

How then, are the correct biliary-specific PC selected out of the highly heterogeneous mixture of PC molecular species, as well as other microsomal membrane lipids? New insights have come from an unexpected source[21]. An important observation showed that the binding affinity of the specific PC-transfer protein (PC-TP) of hepatocytes for PC with saturated sn-1 chains and long polyunsaturated sn-2 chains, i.e. biliary-specific PC, was higher than for other, especially more saturated, PC[22]. However, the relevance of this was not appreciated until recently[23], when it was demonstrated that the transfer function of PC-TP to ferry palmitoyl-pararinoyl PC, a biliary-type fluorescent species, in an equimolar complex to model canalicular membranes was stimulated strongly by micromolar concentrations of common bile salts in proportion to their hydrophobicity and concentration[23]. Moreover, the PC-TP transfer rates of PC as functions of bile salt hydrophobicity were shown to bear a strong positive correlation with biliary PC secretion rates *in vivo* using bile fistula laboratory animals infused with a wide hydrophobicity range of bile salt species[23]. These observations suggest, but do not prove, that the specific PC transfer protein of liver may have a physiological role in biliary PC selection and movement to the canalicular membrane[23,24].

Biliary cholesterol

All biliary cholesterol molecules are non-esterified, i.e. free cholesterol[13], derived principally from the free cholesterol on the surface coat of lipoprotein particles and from the cholesterol esters in their cores following endocytosis and lysosomal hydrolysis[24,25]. Whereas cholesterol of dietary origin which reaches the liver as part of chylomicron remnants, as well as newly synthesized cholesterol molecules in the liver, appear to play minor roles in contributing to biliary cholesterol secretion in health[26], there is emerging evidence to indicate that both of these sources are drawn upon appreciably in cholesterol gallstone subjects[27] who hypersecrete biliary cholesterol continuously throughout their adult lives[28]. Inbred mice acquiring cholesterol gallstones when fed a cholesterol/cholic acid diet appear to have a similar defect[29].

It has been estimated that more than 80% of cholesterol in hepatocytes (and at least 90% in other cells) resides in the plasma membrane[30,31], with the canalicular domain of liver cells being most enriched[4]. This appears to be maintained by movement of cholesterol molecules to the plasma membrane from both inside and outside the cell. There is rapid aqueous diffusion of free cholesterol molecules to the cell surface from the surface coats of lipoprotein particles as they reach the space of Disse in the transhepatic circulation[32,33]. Further, the sinusoidal membranes have receptors for essentially all lipoprotein particles[34], that are responsible for clearance of most plasma cholesterol[35]. It has been suggested that free cholesterol molecules released in lysosomes following lipoprotein endocytosis also move to the adjacent plasma membrane[36]. Cholesterol, newly synthesized in the endoplasmic reticulum, also escapes rapidly from these intracellular organelles, by mechanisms not fully understood[37], but may reach the plasma membrane in a sterol-rich organelle[38] and/or with sphingomyelin in recycling endosomes[39] derived from the plasma membrane itself (discussed below).

What is now the subject of considerable interest is whether the non-specific lipid transfer protein of liver[21], better known as sterol-carrier protein 2 (SCP-2)[40], which apparently has multiple intracellular functions[41], could play a role in cholesterol selection and delivery to the canalicular domain of the plasma membrane for secretion into bile. In most cells SCP-2 is principally a peroxisomal protein[42], but in enterocytes and hepatocytes, two cell systems where there is a great deal of transcytolic bile salt traffic[1], the cytosolic levels of SCP-2 as well as PC-TP are considerably higher than in other cells[43-45].

Whether SCP-2 has a physiological function in delivering cholesterol to the canalicular membrane is unknown, but in human livers from gallstone patients it has been shown that cytosolic SCP-2 levels are considerably higher than controls[46], and parallel increased cytosolic concentrations of free cholesterol[28,46]. This implies that in gallstone subjects there is enhanced intracellular transport of cholesterol to the canalicular membrane[24,28].

CANALICULAR EVENTS

Crossing the membrane

Of relevance to the present account is the well-established fact that an ATP-driven bile salt transporter which is present on canalicular membranes is capable of transporting uphill, into the canalicular space, monomeric bile salts with a single anionic charge[9]. Another transporter, of relevance to understanding the mechanism of biliary lipid secretion, is the multiorganic anion transporter (MOAT). This is also an ATP-driven transporter ferrying a wide variety of dianionic endo- and xenobiotic monomers into the canalicular space[9]. It is obvious that, while undergoing transmembrane transport, bile salt molecules are shielded by the canalicular membrane transporter and thereby their detergency is unexpressed[1]. This implies that while being ferried across the lipid membrane they cannot entrail cholesterol and phospholipid molecules physicochemically for secretion into bile[1]. Rather, the logic of an older hypothesis[47], resurrected recently[48], suggests that bile salts express their detergent action only in the canalicular space, and induce vesiculation of patches of the outer (exoplasmic) monomolecular layer of the canalicular membrane bilayer[47,49,50] where the appropriate PC and cholesterol molecules reside. This is an agreement with ultrafast morphological[51], as well as laser light scattering[52], observations of vesicle secretion into canalicular spaces of intact rat liver and rat hepatocyte couplets, respectively. The vesicle paradigm stems from the well-established observation that high secretion levels of organic dianions (including dianionic bile salts) that utilize the MOAT transporter, uncouple and down-regulate PC and cholesterol secretion rates from bile salt secretion rates in experimental animals (reviewed in ref. 5). The MOAT deficient $(-/-)$ rat does not exhibit this phenomenon, suggesting that bile salt-organic dianion binding within the canalicular lumen of normal rats prevents bile salt vesiculation of the outer monolayer leaflet of the canalicular membrane[5]. In addition to organic dianions, vesicle production rates, and hence biliary lipid secretion rates, fall off with decreasing bile salt concentrations and hydrophobicity, and with increases in the magnitude of bile salt-independent bile flow[47,50], all suggesting bile salt-induced biliary lipid secretion is an 'extracellular' event involving time and efficient detergency. Since there is no cell biological or morphological evidence for transcanalicular transcytosis of biliary lipids as vesicles[53,54], this hypothesis would be in keeping with the separate movements of biliary-specific PC and cholesterol molecules via lipid transport proteins[23] to the canalicular domain of the hepatocyte's plasma membrane.

The one missing element in this story is how biliary-specific PC and cholesterol molecules translocate to the exoplasmic leaflet of the relatively rigid canalicular membrane after their insertion into the cytoplasmic leaflet. In principle this should be simple, for cholesterol molecules, since transbilayer translocation (trivially known as 'flip-flop') is fast following insertion of cholesterol molecules into one hemileaflet of a membrane, provided a concentration gradient exists[31]. Insertion from outside the cell, i.e. from the surface coat of lipoproteins[34], would place cholesterol molecules on the correct hemileaflet for the molecules to reach the canalicular domain by lateral diffusion. This process is known to be very rapid, notwithstanding the presence of tight junctions that normally act as barriers to molecular diffusion in the exoplasmic monolayer[4,33]. However, it is likely that cholesterol molecules during lateral diffusion could do a double 'flip-flop' around them! The only problem with this construct is that cholesterol has a higher affinity for membrane sphingomyelin molecules compared with PC molecules because of an energetically more favourable steric fit (reviewed in ref. 39). In many cell types the content of exoplasmic leaflet cholesterol is very sensitive to the content of exoplasmic sphingomyelin[39], and this should also be typical of the canalicular membrane. Further, it has been suggested that another way in which cholesterol molecules could gain access to the outside monolayer of the plasma membrane is that the sterol could diffuse from intracellular organelles into recycling endosomal membranes during synthesis of sphingomyelin[39]. Since sphingomyelin synthesis occurs on the inner hemileaflet of recycling endosomes, cholesterol would thereby reside on the inner monolayer and, together with the sphingolipid, would arrive simultaneously and be in the correct topology to reside on the outer monolayer of the canalicular membrane following endosome–membrane fusion[39].

The problem with translocating lecithin molecules is very different, since the rate of spontaneous PC 'flip-flop', i.e. from inner to outer monolayer of membranes, is extraordinarily slow with corresponding $t_{\frac{1}{2}}$ values of days[55]. Functional evidence for a PC-specific 'flippase' has been established decisively on microsomal membranes, although no protein has been isolated[56]. Recently, on the basis of kinetic experiments with a short-chain PC, a similar ATP-independent 'flippase' has been proposed to exist on canalicular membranes of rat liver[57]. It is tempting to accept this proposal at face value, because it fits so many of the known facts, particularly the recent demonstration of the complete absence of lecithin from bile in the mdr2 knockout mouse[58]. However, a true 'flippase' may not be necessary, especially if bile salts themselves in the canalicular lumina are continually denuding the exoplasmic membrane of lipid patches via vesiculation[51,52]. Obviously, much more precise physical–chemical work on this important subject is needed, including verification of a protein translocator as well as the definition, purification and characterization of the proposed 'flippases' involved[59].

Getting lipids off the membrane

Several lines of indirect evidence suggest that the physical–chemical state of canalicular bile should be vesicular[60-63]. Nevertheless, only in very recent years have vesicles been visualized directly in canalicular spaces following rapid hepatocyte vitrification and electron spectroscopic imaging of intact rat liver[51], as well as microscope quasielastic laser light scattering spectroscopy of rat hepatocyte couplets[52]. How might intracanalicular vesicles form? It is well known that submicellar bile salts are capable of vesiculating artificial and native membranes[64,65]. Hydrated bile salt anions preferentially partition into membranes in a ratio of approximately 4:1 compared with water[61]. Recent evidence suggests that bile salt molecules should reside exclusively in the exoplasmic membrane lipids of the canalicular membrane, i.e. lumen facing monolayer[66], since 'flip-flop' of ionized bile salt conjugates to the inner monolayer is completely forbidden[67,68]. The asymmetric lateral pressure gradient of one hemimembrane on the other results in membrane blebbing and, like soap-bubbles[66], vesicles in various stages of vesiculation have been visualized on the luminal sides of 'living' canalicular membranes[51]. The vesiculation theory also helps to explain how an infused bile salt pulse as a secreted bile salt peak reaches the hepatic ducts a few minutes ahead of a crest of PC plus cholesterol molecules, which are invariably synchronous with each other[69]. Unfortunately (or fortunately for the investigator!) this is where our knowledge ends. We have no information on (a) how bile salts vesiculate the correct patches of biliary specific PC and not a mixture of PC or PC plus other membrane lipids; (b) how cholesterol, with its special binding affinity for sphingomeylin[39], elutes with bile-specific PC; (c) why cholesterol enters bile at all, if its affinity for sphingomyelin is so much higher than for PC; (d) how cholesterol molecules can enter bile if, having saturated sphingomyelin patches, they might stiffen putative PC patches on the exoplasmic hemimembrane[70]; (e) whether PC is vesiculated independently of cholesterol and whether cholesterol could, by diffusion, enter PC vesicles fast enough[69]; and (f) how the coupling ratios of cholesterol to PC in humans are generated differently and maintained at 0.34–0.38 in health and 0.45–0.48 in cholesterol gallstone disease[28].

POST-CANALICULAR EVENTS

Canaliculus as stopped-flow retort

The canalicular membrane is one of the stiffest membranes in the body, and encloses a sealed system with only one outlet[4]. The membrane rigidity is imparted by a high cholesterol to total phospholipid ratio (of about 0.6) and a high sphingomyelin to PC ratio (of about 0.3)[4]. Therefore, since it can be inferred from microscope laser light scattering spectroscopy of hepatocyte couplets[52] that micellar levels of bile salts are attained in canalicular spaces, no detergent damage occurs, since PC molecules are replaced rapidly following vesiculation and the membrane annealed, presumably by specific PC flipping activity and spontaneous transmembrane translocation of both lipids.

Bile, having remained sufficiently long in the canalicular space to induce vesiculation, flows rapidly caudad, during which many changes occur in the physical–chemical state[6]. It is well known that, in the healthy liver, canalicular contractions occur at frequent intervals[71,72]. Whether these contractions accelerate the processes of outer-membrane vesiculation and/or lipid 'flip-flop' is not known, but canalicular contractions certainly add to the hydrostatic forces involved in bile flow, since microfilament dysfunction is a possible cause of intrahepatic cholestasis[73]. The physical–chemical changes have their beginnings when the bile salt concentration in the canalicular space attains its critical micellar concentration (CMC)[74,75]. When vesicles are first formed, their sizes are approximately 800 Å in radius and the size distribution is remarkably small[52]. This monodispersity has been shown to occur *in vitro* by rapid phospholipid exchange between vesicles[76] induced by submicellar concentrations of bile salts[61,76]. Exactly at the CMC of the bile salt a phase transition is induced, so that the vesicle system produces, in part, rod-shaped particles forming a three-phase system with vesicles and bile salt monomers; at slightly higher bile salt concentration rod-shaped lipid particles coexist with micelles[74,75]. The rod-like particles are a fragment of a hexagonal liquid crystalline phase denoted by a roman numeral I to indicate that the PC head groups are all on the outside of the particle facing the water continuum[74,75]. During post-canalicular bile formation the occurrence of this rod-like phase is an obligate intermediate between vesicles and formation of micelles[6]. Although not yet visualized *in vivo* the rod-like phase has been detected in appropriately designed *in vitro* systems modelling the lipid concentration stages that correspond to the physical–chemical states of bile formation[77].

With the establishment of micelle formation, rod-like particles disappear, but the micelles that are formed initially are highly flexible and elongated 'worm-like' objects[78]. With progressive lipid concentration the long 'worm-like' objects break up into progressively smaller mixed micelles, and eventually these reach a limiting size of approximately 30–40 Å in radius. With physiological lipid compositions the mixed micelles are globular or spherical, and coexist with a population of smaller simple micelles without lecithin[79,80]. The structures of all of these micelles are still disputed, but it appears that in the elongated 'worm-like' micelles the lecithin molecules are radially oriented (diameters approximately 40 Å) with bile salt molecules capping the ends and 'plastered' infrequently between the PC head groups on the surfaces like 'marble fillers on a brick wall'[78]. The structure of physiologically relevant mixed micelles as in gallbladder bile is unknown. However, their PC molecules are loosely packed[81] and, because they can grow as 'worm-like' objects[78], this suggests a possible asymmetric arrangement of PC, cholesterol and bile salt molecules in the particles. Interestingly, bilayered disc structures as models for small mixed micelles[79] cannot be ruled out on the basis of a 'worm-like' growth pattern, since there is no *a-priori* hindrance to the way in which PC molecules can pack in small as opposed to rod-like mixed micelles[78].

Lipid compositional changes

During all of these phase transitions the PC and cholesterol compositions of the micelles and vesicles change[6,61]. It is likely that, at the time of vesicle formation, the lipid composition represents the cholesterol to PC ratio of the outer hemileaflet of the canalicular membranes. Whether this is a low value, possibly 0.25–0.35 in health[4], as in the normal canalicular membrane, or appreciably higher in cholesterol gallstone disease, as the cholesterol to PC coupling in bile would suggest[28], is not known. As the obligatory phase transitions occur, PC is transferred to the micelles in a 4:1 excess compared with cholesterol, simply because the phase diagram allows a solubility differential of exactly this magnitude with micelles solubilizing much more PC than cholesterol molecules[82]. Therefore cholesterol 'enrichment' of vesicles occurs only in the presence of micelles, and the coexisting vesicles can achieve a cholesterol to PC ratio of as high as 2:1[83,84]. For thermodynamic reasons, simple and mixed micelles that coexist with vesicles are cholesterol-supersaturated[84]. This sequence of events is time-dependent and, even in animals with cholesterol-unsaturated biles, traces of vesicles are detected in fresh hepatic biles, but disappear over several hours by micellar dissolution[60,63]. The situation is very different in humans, where the amount of cholesterol secreted into bile is in great excess of what biliary bile salts and PC can dissolve at equilibrium[24,28]. Therefore, the mature physical–chemical state of many human biles is a metastable system of cholesterol-rich vesicles coexisting with simple and mixed micelles that may be saturated or, more usually, supersaturated with cholesterol[84]. This sets the stage for nucleation, principally but not exclusively from vesicles, that can lead to precipitation and crystallization of cholesterol in the gallbladder, processes that can lead eventually to cholesterol gallstone formation[24,28].

CONCLUSIONS

I have attempted in this chapter to trace, in a non-technical way, the physical–chemical aspects of the selection and movement of the three principal biliary lipids through the liver cell, their 'secretion' across the canalicular membrane into bile and the phase transitions that occur during their flow through the biliary tree and in the gallbladder. I hope that I have made clear, in this account, that this field of enquiry is evolving rapidly, and that most of the new information I have presented represents information derived from many laboratories all in the space of the past few years. I trust that in this exercise I have conveyed to the reader much of the excitement of the new, and the anticipation of what is still to come concerning hepatocellular and canalicular events in bile formation. Since the principles underlying the physical chemistry of all these important events will reveal their secrets over the next few years, the basic knowledge acquired will undoubledly lead to new and better strategies for prevention and treatment of hepatobiliary and cholestatic diseases.

Acknowledgements

The author's work is supported in part by research grant number DK36588 and centre grant number DK34854 from the National Institutes of Health,

US Public Health Service. In the preparation of the manuscript, Ms Monika Leonard and Elaine O'Rourke provided expert technical and secretarial assistance, and Drs David E. Cohen and James M. Crawford graciously rendered insightful criticisms of the text.

References

1. Carey MC, Duane WC. Enterohepatic circulation. In: Arias IM, Boyer JL, Fausto N, Jakoby WB, Schachter D, Shafritz DA, editors. The liver, biology and pathobiology, 3rd edn. New York: Raven Press, 1994:719–67.
2. Roda E, Aldini R, Mazzella G, Festi D, Bazzoli F, Roda A. Hepatic secretion of bile acids. In: Tavoloni N, Berk PD, editors. Hepatic transport and bile secretion: physiology and pathophysiology. New York: Raven Press, 1993:553–69.
3. Lenzen R, Tarsetti F, Salvi R, Schuler E, Dembitzer R, Tavaloni N. Physiology of canalicular bile formation. In: Tavoloni N, Berk PD, editors. Hepatic transport and bile secretion: physiology and pathophysiology. New York: Raven Press, 1993:539–51.
4. Schacter D. The hepatocyte plasma membrane: organization and differentiation. In: Arias IM, Jakoby WB, Popper H, Schacter D, Shafritz DA, editors. The liver: biology and pathobiology, 2nd edn. New York: Raven Press, 1988:131–40.
5. Verkade HJ, Vonk RJ, Kuipers F. Mechanisms of bile acid-induced biliary lipid secretion. Hepatology. 1994 (In press).
6. Cohen DE, Kaler EW, Carey MC. Cholesterol carriers in human bile: Are 'lamellae' involved? Hepatology. 1993;18:1522–32.
7. Stremmel W, Tiribelli C, Vyske K. The multiplicity of sinusoidal membrane carrier system of organic anions. In: Tavoloni N, Berk PD, editors. Hepatic transport and bile secretion: physiology and pathophysiology. New York: Raven Press, 1993:225–33.
8. Erlinger S. Intracellular events in bile acid transport by the liver. In: Tavoloni N, Berk PD, editors. Hepatic transport and bile secretion: physiology and pathophysiology. New York: Raven Press, 1993:467–76.
9. Meier PJ, Stieger B. Canalicular membrane adenosine triphosphate-dependent transport systems. Prog Liver Dis. 1993;11:27–44.
10. Duckworth PF, Vlahcevic ZR, Studer EJ et al. Effect of hydrophobic bile acids on 3-hydroxy-3-methylglutaryl coenzyme A reductase activity and mRNA levels in the rat. J Biol Chem. 1994;266:9413–18.
11. Vlahcevic ZR, Pandak WM, Heuman DM, Hylemon PB. Function and regulation of hydroxylases involved in the bile acid biosynthesis pathways. Sem Liver Dis. 1992;12:403–19.
12. Carey MC, Robins SJ. Bile production and secretion. In: Stein JH, editor. Internal medicine, 3rd edn. Boston: Little-Brown, 1990:429–34.
13. Hay DW, Carey MC. Chemical species of lipids in bile. Hepatology. 1990;12:6S–14S.
14. Hay DW, Cahalane MJ, Timofeyeva N, Carey MC. Molecular species of lecithins in human gallbladder biles. J Lipid Res. 1993;34:759–68.
15. Cronholm T, Curstedt T, Sjövall J. Origin of biliary phosphatidylcholine studied by coenzyme labelling with $[1,1\text{-}^2H_2]$ ethanol. Biochim Biophys Acta. 1983;753:276–9.
16. Patton GM, Fasulo JM, Robins SJ. Hepatic phosphatidylcholines: evidence for synthesis in the rat by extensive reutilization of endogenous acylglycerides. J Lipid Res. 1994;35:1211–21.
17. Kennedy EP, Weiss SB. The function of cytidine coenzymes in the biosynthesis of phospholipids. J Biol Chem. 1956;222:193–214.
18. Bremer J, Greenberg DM. Methyl transferring enzyme system of microsomes in the biosynthesis of lecithin. Biochim Biophys Acta. 1961;46:205–16.
19. Bjerve KS. The Ca^{++}-dependent biosynthesis of lecithin, phosphatidylethanolamine and phosphatidylserine in rat liver subcellular particles. Biochim Biophys Acta. 1973;296:549–62.
20. Erbland J, Marinetti GV. The enzymatic acylation and hydrolysis of lyso-lecithin. Biochim Biophys Acta. 1965;106:128–38.

21. Wirtz KWA. Phospholipid transfer proteins. Annu Rev Biochem. 1991;60:73–99.
22. Kasurinen J, Van Paridon PA, Wirtz KWA, Somerharju P. Affinity of phosphatidylcholine molecular species for the bovine phosphatidylcholine and phosphatidylinositol transfer proteins. Properties of the sn-1 and sn-2 acyl binding sites. Biochemistry. 1990;29:8548–54.
23. Cohen DE, Leonard MR, Carey MC. In vitro evidence that phospholipid secretion into bile may be coordinated intracellularly by the combined actions of bile salts and the specific phosphatidylcholine transfer protein of liver. Biochemistry. 1994 (In press).
24. Carey MC, LaMont JT. Cholesterol gallstone formation. 1. Physical-chemistry of bile and biliary lipid secretion. Prog Liver Dis. 1992;10:139–63.
25. Robins SJ, Fasulo JM, Collins MA, Gatton GM. Evidence of separate pathways of newly synthesized and preformed cholesterol into bile. J Biol Chem. 1985;260:6511–13.
26. Duane WC. Effects of lovastatin and dietary cholesterol on bile acid kinetics and bile lipid composition in healthy male subjects. J Lipid Res. 1994;35:501–9.
27. Kern F Jr. Effects of dietary cholesterol on cholesterol and bile acid homeostasis in patients with cholesterol gallstones. J Clin Invest. 1994;93:1186–94.
28. LaMont JT, Carey MC. Cholesterol gallstone formation. 2. Pathobiology and pathomechanics. Prog Liver Dis. 1992;10:165–91.
29. Khanuja B, Cheah Y-C, Hunt M *et al. Lith 1*, a major gene affecting cholesterol gallstone formation among inbred strains of mice. Proc Natl Acad Sci USA. 1994 (Submitted).
30. Lange Y, Ramos BV. Analysis of the distribution of cholesterol in the intact cell. J Biol Chem. 1983;258:15130–4.
31. Lange Y. Tracking cell cholesterol with cholesterol oxidase. J Lipid Res. 1992;33:315–21.
32. Schwartz CC, Halloran LG, Vlahcevic ZR, Gregory DH, Swell L. High and low density lipoprotein metabolism in man: preferential utilization of HDL free cholesterol by the liver for biliary cholesterol secretion. Science 1978;200:62–4.
33. Schwartz CC, Berman M, Vlahcevic ZR, Halloran LG, Gregory DH, Swell L. Multicompartment analysis of cholesterol metabolism in man: characterization of the hepatic bile acid and biliary cholesterol precursor sites. J Clin Invest. 1978;61:408–23.
34. Cooper AD. Hepatic lipoprotein and cholesterol metabolism. In: Zakim D, Boyer TD, editors. Hepatology: a textbook of liver disease. Philadelphia: W.B. Saunders, 1990:96–123.
35. Brown MS, Goldstein JL. Lipoprotein receptor in the liver control signals for plasma cholesterol traffic. J Clin Invest. 1983;72:743–7.
36. Sleight RG. Intracellular lipid transport in eukaryotes. Annu Rev Physiol. 1987;49:193–208.
37. Lange Y, Matthies HJG. Transfer of cholesterol from its site of synthesis to the plasma membrane. J Biol Chem. 1984;259:14624–30.
38. Lange Y, Steck TL. Cholesterol-rich intracellular membranes: a precursor to the plasma membrane. J Biol Chem 1985;260:15592–7.
39. Allan D, Kallen K-J. Transport of lipids to the plasma membrane in animal cells. Prog Lipid Res. 1993;32:195–219.
40. van Amerongen A, Teerlink T, van Heusden GPH, Wirtz KWA. The non-specific lipid transfer protein (sterol carrier protein-2) from rat and bovine liver. Chem Phys Lipids. 1985;38:195–204.
41. Scallen TJ, Vahouny GV. Participation of sterol carrier protein in cholesterol biosynthesis, utilization and intracellular transfer. In: Danielsson H, Sjövall J, editors. Sterols and bile acids. Amsterdam: Elsevier, 1985:73–93.
42. Lazarow PB. Peroxisomes. In: Arias IM, Boyer JL, Fausto N, Jakoby WB, Schachter D, Shafritz DA, editors. The liver: biology and pathobiology, 3rd edn. New York: Raven Press, 1994:293–307.
43. Teerlink T, van der Krift TP, van Heusden GPH, Wirtz KWA. Determination of non-specific lipid transfer protein in rat tissues and morris hepatoma by enzyme immunoassay. Biochim Biophys Acta. 1984;793:251–9.
44. van Amerongen A, van Noort M, van Beckhoven JRCM, Rommerts FFG, Orly J, Wirtz KWA. The subcellular distribution of the nonspecific lipid transfer protein (sterol carrier protein 2) in rat liver and adrenal gland. Biochim Biophys Acta. 1989;1001:243–8.
45. Teerlink T, van der Krift TP, Post M, Wirtz KWA. Tissue distribution and subcellular localization of phosphatidylcholine transfer protein in rats as determined by radioimmunoassay. Biochim Biophys Acta. 1982;713:61–7.

46. Kawata S, Imai Y, Inada M *et al.* Modulation of cholesterol 7-α-hydroxylase activity by non-specific lipid transfer protein in human liver – possibly altered regulation of its cytosolic level in patients with gallstones. Clin Chim Acta. 1991;197:201–8.

47. Small DM. The formation of gallstones. Adv Intern Med. 1970;16:243–64.

48. Verkade HJ, Wolbers MJ, Havinga R, Uges DR, Vonk RJ, Kuipers F. The uncoupling of biliary lipid from bile acid secretion by organic anions in the rat. Gastroenterology. 1990;99:1485–92.

49. Verkade HJ, Wolters H, Gerding A *et al.* Mechanism of biliary lipid secretion in the rat: a role for bile acid-independent bile flow? Hepatology. 1993;17:1074–80.

50. Verkade HJ, Havinga R, Gerding A, Vonk RJ, Kuipers F. Mechanism of bile acid-induced biliary lipid secretion in the rat: effect of conjugated bilirubin. Am J Physiol. 1993;264:G462–9.

51. Crawford JM, Möckel GM, Godleski JJ, Hagen SJ, Carey MC. Imaging of biliary lipid secretion as vesicles in canalicular spaces. J Cell Biol. 1994 (In preparation).

52. Möckel GM, Gorti S, Tandon RK, Tanaka T, Carey MC. Microscope laser light scattering spectroscopy of vesicles within canaliculi of rat hepatocyte couplets. Am J Physiol. 1994 (In press).

53. Marks DL, LaRusso NF. Vesicle-dependent transport pathways in liver cells. In: Tavoloni N, Berk PD, editors. Hepatic transport and bile secretion: physiology and pathophysiology. New York: Raven Press, 1993;513–30.

54. Meier PJ. Transport polarity of hepatocytes. Sem Liver Dis. 1988;8:293–307.

55. de Kruijft B, Wirtz KWA. Induction of a relatively fast transbilayer movement of phosphatidylcholine in vesicles: a ^{13}C NMR study. Biochim Biophys Acta. 1977;468:318–26.

56. Bishop WR, Bell RM. Assembly of the endoplasmic reticulum phospholipid bilayer: The phosphatidylcholine transporter. Cell. 1985;42:51–6.

57. Berr F, Meier PJ, Stieger B. Evidence for the presence of a phosphatidylcholine translocator in isolated rat liver canalicular plasma membrane vesicles. J Biol Chem. 1993;268:3976–9.

58. Smit JJM, Schinkel AH, Oude Elferink RPJ *et al.* Homozygous disruption of the murine mdr2 P-glycoprotein gene leads to a complete absence of phospholipid from bile and to liver disease. Cell. 1993;75:451–62.

59. Devaux PF. Protein involvement in transmembrane lipid asymmetry. Annu Rev Biophys Biomol Struc. 1992;21:417–39.

60. Cohen DE, Angelico M, Carey MC. Quasielastic light scattering evidence for vesicular secretion of biliary lipids. Am J Physiol. 1989;257:G1–8.

61. Cohen DE, Angelico M, Carey MC. Structural alterations in lecithin–cholesterol vesicles following interactions with monomeric and micellar bile salts. Physical chemical basis for subselection of biliary lecithin species and aggregative states of biliary lipids during bile formation. J Lipid Res. 1990;31:55–70.

62. Cohen DE, Carey MC. Physical chemistry of biliary lipids during bile formation. Hepatology 1990;12:143–8S.

63. Cohen DE, Leighton LS, Carey MC. Bile salt hydrophobicity controls vesicle secretion rates and transformations in native bile. Am J Physiol. 1992;263:G386–95.

64. Coleman R, Rahman K. Lipid flow in bile formation. Biochim Biophys Acta. 1992;1125:113–33.

65. Coleman R. Bile salts and biliary lipids. Biochem Soc Trans. 1987;15(Suppl.):68–80S.

66. Small DM. 1992 Aspen Bile Acid/Cholesterol/Lipoprotein Conference. Report of a Conference. J Lipid Res. 1993;34:680–9.

67. Kamp F, Westerhoff HV, Hamilton JA. Movement of fatty acids, fatty acid analogues, and bile acids across phospholipid bilayers – kinetics of fatty acid-mediated proton movement across small unilamellar vesicles. Biochemistry. 1993;32:11074–86.

68. Cabral DJ, Small DM, Lilly HS, Hamilton JA. Transbilayer movement of bile acids in model membranes. Biochemistry. 1987;26:1801–4.

69. Lowe PJ, Barnwell SG, Coleman R. Rapid kinetic analysis of the bile salt-dependent secretion of phospholipid, cholesterol and a plasma membrane enzyme into bile. Biochem J. 1984;222:631–7.

70. Salvioli G, Carey MC. A novel *in vitro* perfusion system to study membrane dissolution by bile salts: different effects of taurochenodeoxycholate (TCDC) and tauroursdeoxycholate (TUDC) on lipid secretion and membrane resistance. Gastroenterology. 1982;82:1168(abstr.).

71. Oshio C, Phillips MJ. Contractility of bile canaliculi: implications for liver function. Science. 1981;212:1041–2.
72. Phillips MJ, Oshio C, Miyairi M, Watanabe S, Smith CR. What is actin doing in the liver cell. Hepatology. 1983;3:433–6.
73. Phillips MJ, Oda M, Mak E, Fisher MM, Jeejeebhoy KN. Microfilament dysfunction as a possible cause of intrahepatic cholestasis. Gastroenterology. 1975;69:48–58.
74. Cabral DJ, Small DM. Physical chemistry of bile. In: Schultz SG, Forte JG, Rauner BB, editors. Handbook of physiology – the gastrointestinal system III, Section 6. Baltimore, MD.: American Physiology Society/Waverly Press, 1989:621–2.
75. Carey MC. Lipid solubilization in bile. In: Northfield T, Jazrawi R, Zentler-Munro P, editors. Bile acids in health and disease. Dordrecht: Kluwer, 1988:61–82.
76. Nichols JW. Low concentrations of bile salts increase the rate of spontaneous phospholipid transfer between vesicles. Biochemistry. 1986;25:4596–601.
77. Walter A, Vinson PK, Kaplun A, Talmon Y. Intermediate structures in the cholate–phosphatidylcholine vesicle–micelle transition. Biophys J. 1991;60:1315–25.
78. Cohen DE, Chamberlin RA, Thurston GM, Carey MC. Laser light scattering evidence for 'worm-like' mixed micelles in both cholanoyl (bile salt) and acyl (octylglucoside) detergent-long chain phosphatidylcholine aqueous systems: new insights on the structure of bile. Biochemistry. 1994(Submitted).
79. Mazer NA, Benedek GB, Carey MC. Quasielastic light scattering studies of aqueous biliary lipid systems: mixed micelle formation in bile salt-lecithin solutions. Biochemistry. 1980;19:601–15.
80. Mazer NA, Schurtenberger P, Carey MC, Preisig R, Weigand K, Känzig W. Quasielastic light scattering studies of native hepatic bile from the dog: Comparison with aggregative behavior of model biliary lipid systems. Biochemistry. 1984;23:1994–2005.
81. Cohen DE, Carey MC. Acyl chain unsaturation modulates distribution of lecithin molecular species between mixed micelles and vesicles in model bile. Implications for particle structure and metastable cholesterol solubilities. J Lipid Res. 1991;32:1291–302.
82. Carey MC, Small DM. Physical chemistry of cholesterol solubility in bile: Relationship to gallstone formation and dissolution in man. J Clin Invest. 1978;61:998–1026.
83. Mazer NA, Carey MC. Quasi-elastic light-scattering studies of aqueous biliary lipid systems: cholesterol solubilization and precipitation in model bile solutions. Biochemistry. 1983;22:426–42.
84. Donovan JM, Carey MC. Separation and quantitation of cholesterol 'carriers' in bile. Hepatology. 1990;12:94–105S.

13
Control of biliary lipid secretion: studies in the *mdr2* P-glycoprotein knock-out mouse

A. K. GROEN, R. OTTENHOFF, M. J. A. VAN WIJLAND,
J. J. M. SMIT, A. H. SCHINKEL and R. P. J. OUDE ELFERINK

The mechanism of biliary lipid secretion has been the subject of considerable speculation during the past two decades. In classical studies Wheeler and King were, in 1972, the first who discussed the regulation of lipid secretion in mechanistic terms[1]. In careful studies in the dog they studied the relationship between biliary lecithin secretion and bile salt output, and in accordance with earlier studies of Balint *et al.*[2] they demonstrated tight coupling of lecithin to bile salt output. Applying a relatively simple model of lipid solubilization they predicted a hyperbolic relationship between biliary lipid output and bile salt secretion (BS_{sec}). In 1984 Mazer and Carey[3] used their own data and that of others to describe the relationships between bile salt secretion and biliary lipid secretion in a more sophisticated mathematical model. Although they describe the relationship between phospholipid secretion (PL_{sec}) and BS_{sec} as curvilinear, in their model the relation between BS_{sec} and phospholipid secretion was modelled by a rectangular hyperbola:

$$PL_{sec} = (PL_{max} \cdot BS_{sec})/(\beta/k + BS_{sec}) \tag{1}$$

where PL_{max} is the maximal rate of phospholipid synthesis, β represents feedback inhibition of hepatic phospholipid content on its synthesis and k refers to a coupling constant between PL_{sec} and BS_{sec}.

The model of Mazer and Carey[3], although nicely describing the data, did not yield further insight in factors underlying the regulation of lipid secretion, since at the time so little was known about processes controlling the different steps that the model parameters were rather phenomenological and did not lead to testable hypotheses. Recently we have discovered that a protein is involved in the hepatobiliary transport of phospholipid (PL)[4]. Mice with a disrupted gene for the P-glycoprotein (Pgp) *mdr2* were not able to secrete PL, and almost no Ch. This defect induced liver disease, most probably mediated by the formation of toxic (lipid-free) bile. The most prominent abnormality in young mice was portal expansion caused by extensive bile duct proliferation. Mice heterozygous for the defect showed no abnormalities, had normal levels of cholesterol in bile, but showed a 40% decrease in PL secretion. This result led us to conclude that the protein is primarily involved in mediating PL output[4]. The molecular mechanism by which *mdr2* Pgp catalyses PC secretion is not yet clear. In accordance with the mechanism proposed by Gottesman and Pastan[5] for the *mdr1* Pgp it could function as a flippase translocating PL molecules from the inner to the outer leaflet. Alternatively, the protein could act as a direct acceptor of PL or be involved in fusion of incoming transport vesicles with the canalicular membrane. In principle it could even exert an indirect effect, for instance, via the transport of a regulating ion. In this chapter we report studies on the control of *mdr2* Pgp on biliary lipid secretion.

Figure 1 shows the result of an experiment in which the bile salt pool of anaesthetized mice was drained by cannulating the gallbladder after distal ligation of the common bile duct. Bile was collected for 2 h and the contents of BS, Ch and PL were determined. In Fig. 2A the rate of PL secretion is plotted against BS secretion. In accordance with data from many groups for other animals curvilinear relations were observed for both $(+/+)$ and $(+/-)$ mice. The $(-/-)$ mice did not secrete PL at all rates of BS secretion. We have fitted the data in Fig. 2A using the equation of Mazer and Carey[3]. A good fit was obtained for the data from the $(+/+)$ mice ($r^2 = 0.93$). The values for the two constants L_{max} and β/k were 65 nmol/min per 100 g and 221 nmol/min per 100 g respectively. A decrease in *mdr2* Pgp activity will not directly influence maximal PL synthesis, hence we have kept PL_{max} constant when fitting the data for the $(+/-)$ mice. A direct effect of the protein on the kinetics of product inhibition is also not obvious but, depending on the molecular mechanism of *mdr2* Pgp, the protein could have an effect on the coupling constant k. We have therefore allowed free variation in the value of β/k in the fitting procedure. A rather good fit was obtained, $r^2 = 0.90$ at a value for β/k of 481 nmol/min per 100 g, which is about two-fold higher than the value for the $(+/+)$ mice. Assuming that the coupling is fully determined by *mdr2* secretion of lecithin is of course zero in the $(-/-)$ animal. Thus the Mazer and Carey model appears to be rather successful. At constant PL_{max}, variation in β/k is sufficient to explain the experimental data. Unfortunately, so far β and k lack a mechanistic basis, and they are not amenable to experimental verification. However, the assumption that maximal $PL_{sec} = PL_{max}$ is unaltered in the $(+/-)$ mice can be verified. We have therefore infused mice with large amounts of taurocholate to increase BS load and drive PL_{sec} to its maximum. Maximal PL_{sec} was reached at a rate of 800 nmol/min per 100 g of taurocholate infused in both the $(+/+)$ and $(+/-)$ mice (Table 1). One could argue that it is the toxicity of the bile salt which primarily determines maximal PL output. We have

---

Fig. 1 (*opposite*) Time-dependent decrease in bile salt secretion (**A**), bile flow (**B**) and phospholipid (**C**) and cholesterol (**D**) secretion after interruption of the enterohepatic cycle in the mouse. The figure shows a representative experiment with a control mouse. Directly after cannulation of the gallbladder bile was collected for the indicated time periods

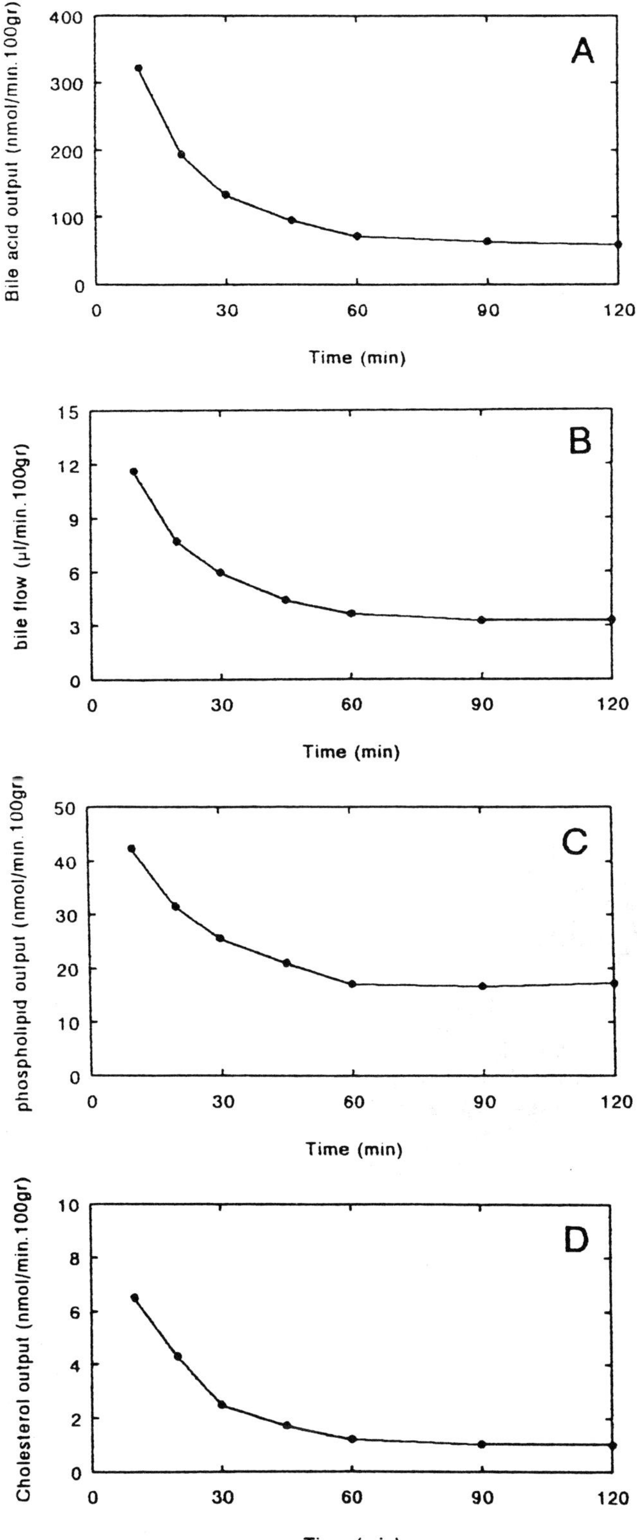

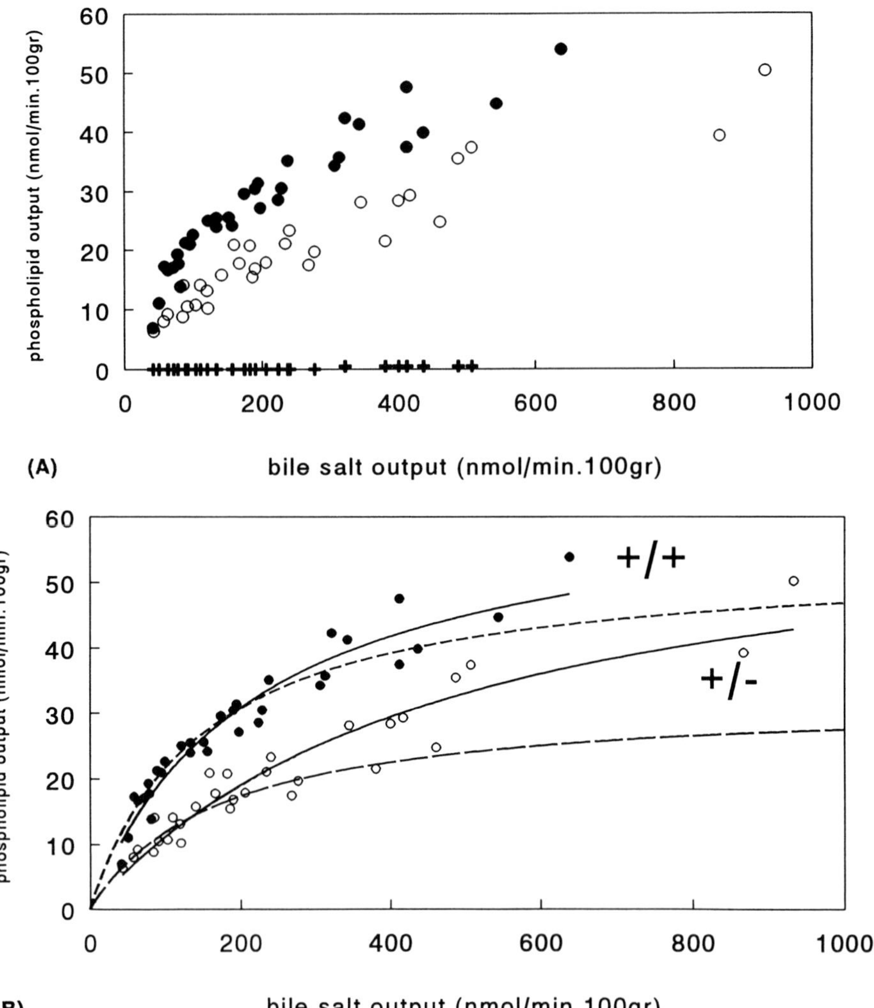

Fig. 2 **A**: Relation between bile salt and phospholipid secretion in the three mouse strains. The data represent all separate measurements from six animals of each strain in an experimental set-up as shown in Fig. 1. ●: $(+/+)$ mice; ○: $(+/-)$ mice; +: $(-/-)$ mice. **B**: Data of Fig. 2 fitted according to the equation of Mazer and Carey (solid lines) or after adjustment of the equation as described in the text (dashed lines)

therefore repeated the experiment with the hydrophilic BS tauroursodeoxycholate (TUDC) which does not cause cholestasis. As shown in Table 1, the values of PL_{max} were almost identical. Also with TUDC PL_{max} in the $(+/-)$ was about 40% lower than in the $(+/+)$. According to equation (1), maximal PL output is determined by maximal synthesis (PL_{max}). Since this assumption apparently does not hold, the model needs adjustment. An obvious adjustment to the model would be replacement of PL_{max} by V_{max} of *mdr2* Pgp.

Table 1 Maximal rate of phospholipid secretion (PL_{max}, nmol/min per 100 g) in $(+/+)$ and $(+/-)$ mice during infusion of taurocholate and tauroursodeoxycholate

Bile salt	n	$(+/+)$	$(+/-)$
Taurocholate	6	55 ± 2.1	28 ± 6.2
Tauroursodeoxycholate	4	54 ± 4.9	32 ± 2.2

Mice were cannulated in the gallbladder and directly after starting bile collection taurocholate or tauroursodeoxycholate was infused into the tail vein at a starting rate of 400 nmol/min per 100 g. In 30-min periods the rate was increased stepwise to 1200 nmol/min per 100 g in the case of taurocholate and 1600 nmol/min per 100 g in the case of TUDC. Maximal PL_{sec} was obtained at an infusion rate of 800 nmol/min per 100 g of TC and 1600 nmol/min per 100 g of TUDC. Data represent average $\pm$ SD from three mice of each strain

Thus

$$PL_{sec} = (V_{max} \cdot BS_{sec})/(Ks + BS_{sec}) \qquad (2)$$

where V_{max} is the maximal capacity of *mdr2* Pgp, and Ks refers to the value of BS_{sec} where PL_{sec} is half-maximal.

The results of this adjustment are given in Fig. 2B (dashed lines). Using the V_{max} values given in Table 1, fit is not satisfactory, particularly in the case of the heterozygotes. At high rates the theoretical curve deviates considerably from the experimental data. Closer inspection of the kinetic pattern revealed that the data can best be described by a curvilinear model, i.e. when a linear term is added to the equation. For instance

$$PL_{sec} = (V_{max} \cdot BS_{sec})/(Ks + BS_{sec}) + M \cdot BS_{sec} \qquad (3)$$

where M is a constant which could represent the aselective interaction of BS with the membrane.

The results for a straightforward curvilinear model are given in Fig. 2B. The model fits the data exceptionally well. In the case of the $(+/+)$ mice $r^2 = 0.94$; for the $(+/-)$ mice $r^2 = 0.93$. This model suggests that phospholipid secretion is only partly determined by *mdr2* Pgp. In addition there is a Pgp-independent linear component. The saturable component is then caused by the *mdr2* protein and the linear component could be the result of pure micellization of the membrane. In Fig. 3 these separate curves and lines have been drawn and the kinetic constants have been calculated. The hypothesis that the *mdr2* protein is responsible for the hyperbolic component of the curve bears out nicely, since in the $(+/-)$ mice the BS_{sec} at which half-maximal PL_{sec} is obtained remains unchanged while the maximal rate of PL_{sec} is half. The linear component of the curve is not affected in the heterozygote, suggesting that *mdr2* is not directly involved in the mechanism of this part of lipid extraction.

Although this model provides the best fit to the data for both the $(+/+)$ and $(+/-)$ mice it does not explain the absence of lecithin secretion in the $(-/-)$ mice. When the curvilinear model is correct and the *mdr2* Pgp is indeed a flippase the PL extracted in the linear part of the curve by definition arrives in the outer leaflet of the membrane by an *mdr2* Pgp-independent

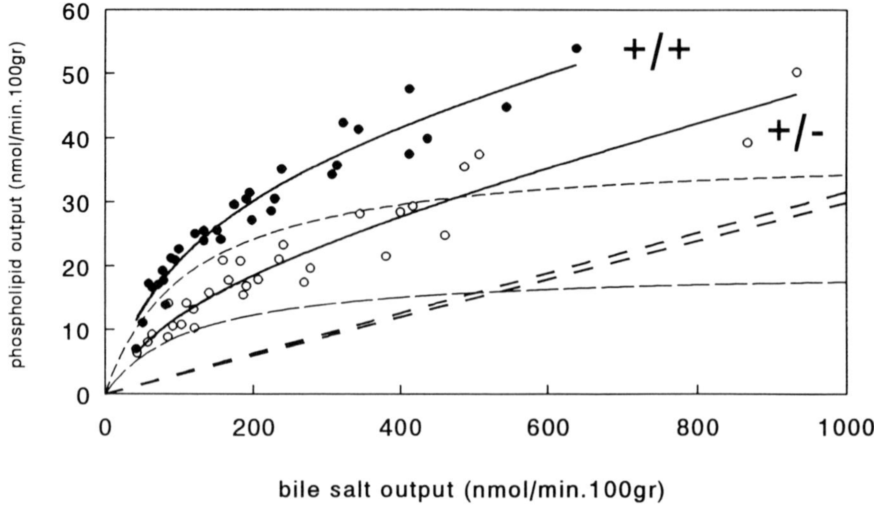

Fig. 3 Data of Fig. 2A were fitted using a curvilinear equation as described in the text.

mechanism. This is possible since there is (convincing) evidence for a microtubule-dependent vesicular pathway of PL transport to the canalicular membrane (see ref. 7 for review). This pathway could account for the PL extracted in the linear part of the curve, since up to half of this PL arrives directly in the outer leaflet of the membrane. When vesicular transport of PL is indeed operational the question arises why PL_{sec} is completely absent in the $(-/-)$ mice. There are at least two solutions to this problem. Firstly, the absence of *mdr2* Pgp leads to lack of extraction of PC from the inner leaflet of the membrane. The accumulation of PC in the inner leaflet of $(-/-)$ membrane may in turn lead to very efficient feedback inhibition of PC synthesis and vesicular transport to the canalicular membrane. Secondly, the 'linear term' in the curvilinear model is not correct, and the kinetics at high BS_{sec} may represent a second Pgp-dependent hyperbolic term, but with a much lower affinity towards BS extraction. The consequences of these different scenarios for the mechanism of biliary PL secretion are given in Fig. 4. PL arrives at the canalicular membrane either in the form of a vesicle or bound to PC-TP[6]. Depending on the relative contribution of the two pathways part of the PC arrives directly in the outer leaflet and is available for BS-mediated extraction. Activity of *mdr2* Pgp induces local excess of PL in the outer leaflet, which induces bulges that mediate very efficient extraction by BS. We hypothesize that only the outer leaflet of the membrane is directly involved in PL secretion. Selection of biliary PC species is either controlled by the affinity of BS to these PC species or is caused by a high specificity of *mdr2* Pgp.

The model does not explain the appearance of vesicles very early in bile formation. Current theories on the mechanism of biliary lipid secretion postulate vesiculation of microdomains in the canalicular membrane (see ref. 7 for review). In these microdomains specific PC species must be highly

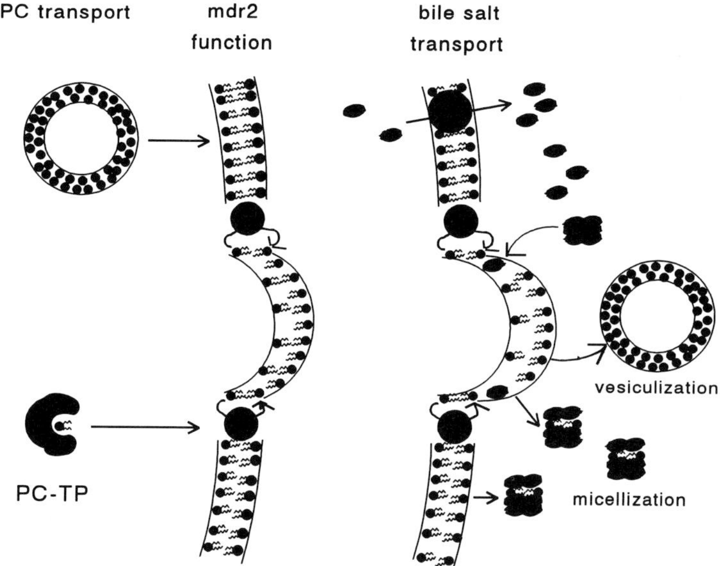

Fig. 4 Cartoon of hypothetical pathways involved in biliary lipid secretion

enriched in both inner and outer leaflet. In early studies with erythrocytes Billinton and Coleman[8] have shown that BS can induce vesicle formation from outer membrane phospholipids. In these interesting studies enrichment of biliary-type PC was found, suggesting that indeed BS play an important role in selecting PC species.

So far we have only discussed the mechanism of PL output. In the model of Mazer and Carey cholesterol secretion is fully coupled to PL. This coupling could be a consequence of vesicular co-transport from an intracellular compartment to the canalicular membrane. However, when intracellular cholesterol is transported independently from phospholipid, the coupling must be regulated at the site of secretion (e.g. the canalicular membrane). The rate of spontaneous flip-flop of cholesterol has been reported to be rather high, certainly compared to the flip-flop of PC. Since we do not know the flip-flop rate in a specialized membrane such as the canalicular membrane it cannot be concluded whether spontaneous flip-flop of Ch is fast enough to account for the rate of Ch secretion, or whether for cholesterol a specific flippase is also present. The rate of cholesterol secretion is described by Mazer and Carey as follows:

$$Ch_{sec} = (Ch_{max} \times PL_{sec})/((\beta_2 + \tau)k_2 + PL_{sec}) \tag{4}$$

where k_2 defines the coupling between PC and Ch secretion, β_2 refers to the feedback inhibition constant on Ch synthesis/input and τ is a rate constant defining the conversion of cholesterol to bile salts.

This equation predicts a hyperbolic relation between Ch_{sec} and PL_{sec}. In the experiment of Fig. 1 we also determined cholesterol output. In Fig. 5

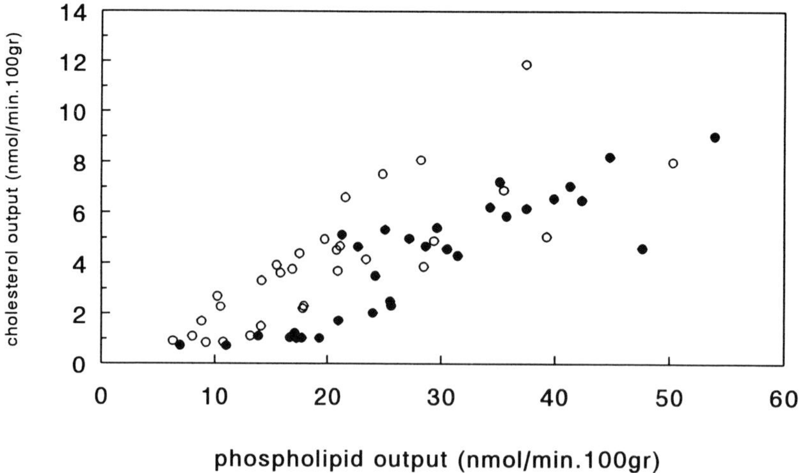

Fig. 5 Cholesterol secretion in the three mouse strains. Relation between cholesterol and phospholipid secretion. The data represent separate measurements from six animals of each strain in an experimental set-up as shown in Fig. 1. ●: $(+/+)$ mice; ○: $(+/-)$ mice

Ch_{sec} is plotted as a function of PL_{sec}. The coupling between PL_{sec} and Ch_{sec} seems unaltered in $(+/-)$ mice, although the relation is linear rather than curvilinear.

In conclusion, in this chapter we have shown that the *mdr2* Pgp transgenic mouse models provide an important tool in increasing our understanding of the mechanism of biliary lipid secretion. Analysis of the experimental data has enabled us to suggest refinements of current models of the regulation of biliary lipid secretion by bile salts.

Acknowledgement

We thank Professor P. Borst for stimulating discussions and for critically reading the manuscript. This study was partly supported by grants NKI 88-6 and NKI 92-41 to P. Borst.

References

1. Wheeler HO, King KK. Biliary excretion of lecithin and cholesterol in the dog. J Clin Invest. 1972;51:1337–50.
2. Balint JA, Beeler DA, Kyriakides EC, Treble DH. The effect of bile salts upon lecithin synthesis. J Lab Clin Med. 1971;77:122–33.
3. Mazer NA, Carey MC. Mathematical model of biliary lipid secretion: a quantiative analysis of physiological and biochemical data from man and other species. J Lipid Res. 1984;25: 932–53.
4. Smit JJM, Schinkel AH, Oude Elferink RPJ *et al*. Homozygous disruption of the murine *mdr2* P-glycoprotein gene leads to a complete absence of phospholipid from bile and to liver disease. Cell. 1993;75:451–62.

5. Gottesman MM, Pastan I. Biochemistry of multidrug resistance mediated by the multidrug transporter. Annu Rev Biochem. 1993;62:385–427.
6. Wirtz KWA. Phospholipid transfer proteins. Annu Rev Biochem. 1991;60:73–99.
7. Coleman R, Rahman K. Lipid flow in bile formation. Biochim Biophys Acta. 1992;1125: 113–33.
8. Billington B, Coleman R. Effects of bile salts on human erythrocytes. Plasma membrane vesiculation, phospholipid solubilization and their possible relationships to bile secretion. Biochim Biophys Acta. 1978;509:33–47.

14
Role of gallbladder motility in the pathogenesis of cholesterol gallstones

M. F. J. STOLK, P. PORTINCASA, K. J. VAN ERPECUM and
G. P. VAN BERGE HENEGOUWEN

BACKGROUND

Gallstone disease is a common disease throughout the world. In a large survey in Italy, gallstones were found in 6.7% of men and 14.6% of women[1]. Gallstones are found more often in females (male/female 1:2) and the incidence of gallstones increases with age[2]. In the Netherlands about 14 000 cholecystectomies are performed each year, and this heavily weighs upon health-care budgets[3].

Three different gallstone types can be distinguished: cholesterol gallstones (mainly composed of cholesterol monohydrate), pigment gallstones (composed of calcium bilirubinate) and mixed gallstones. In Western countries, approximately 70% of gallstones are cholesterol gallstones[4]. In contrast, approximately 70% of gallstones in Eastern Asia are pigment gallstones.

In this chapter we focus on the role of gallbladder motility (disorders) in the formation of cholesterol gallstones and review some of the newer insights in the regulation of postprandial and interdigestive gallbladder emptying.

SECRETION OF BILIARY LIPIDS AND CHOLESTEROL CRYSTAL NUCLEATION

Biliary secretion of cholesterol is the major mechanism for the body to excrete cholesterol. However, *hypersecretion* of hepatic cholesterol in bile is probably the major cause of supersaturated bile and gallstone formation in the Western world[5,6]. Cholesterol secretion is largely driven by bile salt secretion[5,7,8]. However, during the fasting state, when bile salt secretion is low, cholesterol secretion does not decrease proportionally and bile may become supersaturated with cholesterol[9,10]. Cholesterol is mainly secreted into the bile canaliculus as cholesterol/phospholipid vesicles.

Bile salts are amphiphatic molecules with detergent properties which are secreted in the bile canaliculus as monomers and simple micelles. Above the critical micellar concentration (CMC), mixed micelles can be formed with cholesterol and phospholipids derived from the vesicles. Mixed micelle formation requires the solubilization of 10–20 times more phospholipid than cholesterol. As a result the cholesterol concentration in the remaining vesicles will progressively increase and the cholesterol/phospholipid ratio will increase above one[8,11–13]. Cholesterol-rich vesicles are unstable and tend to aggregate into multilamellar vesicles of increasing size. In these multilamellar aggregates, domains with high cholesterol concentrations emerge (liquid crystals) and finally solid cholesterol monohydrate crystals may precipitate, as observed by video-enhanced time-lapse microscopy[14].

It is important to realize that native bile is not an equilibrium system and supersaturated vesicles and micelles can coexist for a long time before cholesterol crystals appear[15–17]. Therefore, it is not the fact that cholesterol-rich vesicles *exist* that is important, but it is the *rate* of cholesterol crystal formation which is an important discriminator between biles from healthy subjects and gallstone patients[18].

The process of mixed micelle formation starts in the biliary tree but is strongly promoted in the gallbladder[19]. The gallbladder absorbs electrolytes actively and water passively, thereby increasing the concentration of biliary lipids. High bile salt levels promote mixed micelle formation and hence the formation of cholesterol-rich vesicles. Increased retention time of bile, or an increased amount of bile in the gallbladder, due to impaired gallbladder emptying, might provide the time necessary for cholesterol crystal precipitation and subsequent gallstone formation. On the other hand, the gallbladder is also able to absorb cholesterol and phospholipids[20–22]. This might be a defence mechanism against biliary cholesterol supersaturation.

Many proteins with cholesterol nucleation *promoting* as well as *inhibiting* properties have been found. Lipoprotein Apo A-I inhibits nucleation[23]. Groen and co-workers isolated a concanavalin A binding protein of 130 kDa that promotes nucleation[24]. Recently, phospholipase C[25], immunoglobulins of the IgM and IgA classes[26], fibronectin[27], a biliary anionic polypeptide fraction (APF[28]), and a low-density lipoprotein[29] have been found to exert nucleation promoting effects *in vitro*. The liver probably secretes promoting and inhibiting factors at the same time. However, the contribution of these factors to cholesterol crystal nucleation and the relative effect of each of the factors *in vivo* is still a matter of debate.

Mucin, produced by the gallbladder wall, also promotes nucleation of cholesterol crystals[30,31]. In animals, cholesterol crystal precipitation might be prevented by the administration of aspirin[32], although this has recently been disputed[33]. In obese patients, who have an increased risk of gallstone formation during rapid weight loss, aspirin prevented the formation of gallstones during low-calorie dieting[34,35]. Interestingly, deoxycholate promotes the secretion of bile rich in arachidonate, which is a precursor of prostaglandin synthesis[36]. Mucin concentrations in gallstone patients are increased[37] or normal compared with healthy subjects[38].

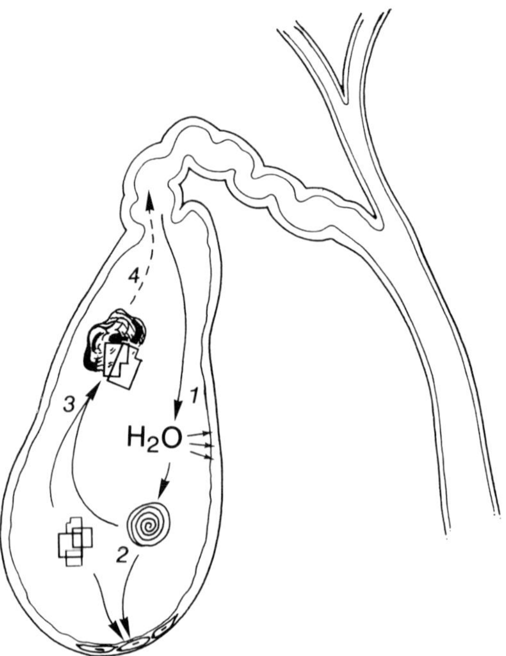

Fig. 1 Role of gallbladder hypomotility in cholesterol gallstone formation: (1) water absorption with increased formation of mixed micelles and increased vesicular cholesterol/phospholipid ratio; (2) precipitation of cholesterol monohydrate crystals; (3) crystal aggregation and stone formation, gallbladder wall inflammation, decreased smooth muscle contractility; (4) incomplete evacuation of bile

The generally accepted theories on cholesterol gallstone formation assume that the pathogenesis of cholesterol gallstones is a multifactorial process, in which hepatic cholesterol hypersecretion, unstable cholesterol-rich vesicles, nucleation promoting and inhibiting factors are involved (Fig. 1). Decreased gallbladder emptying may further contribute to vesicular instability and provide the time for the cholesterol nucleation process to evolve. Recent progress in the understanding of the regulation of postprandial and interdigestive gallbladder emptying may shed new light on the role of gallbladder motility in the pathogenesis of cholesterol gallstone disease.

ROLE OF GALLBLADDER HYPOMOTILITY IN CHOLESTEROL GALLSTONE FORMATION

Supersaturation of bile with cholesterol is a prerequisite for cholesterol crystal precipitation. In healthy man, gallbladder bile becomes frequently supersaturated, especially during the night when gallbladder emptying is small[9,10]. However, most people do not get gallstones. Prolonged stasis of bile in the gallbladder is probably one of the most important factors in the pathogenesis of gallstone formation. In stagnant bile, continuous concentration through water absorption by the gallbladder mucosa will take place. This will increase the cholesterol concentration in gallbladder bile and facilitate the precipitation of cholesterol monohydrate crystals from unstable cholesterol-rich vesicles. Moreover, stasis of bile may provide the time for cholesterol crystal growth and aggregation to gallstones. Finally, defective gallbladder function prevents the evacuation of cystals and stones from the gallbladder.

In some studies it has been shown that disturbed gallbladder motility occurs *before* cholesterol crystal formation. However, other studies suggested that the presence of gallstones (and sometimes cholecystitis) may *induce* disturbed gallbladder motility. In the following sections both possibilities will be discussed.

GALLBLADDER MOTILITY DISORDERS IN THE EARLY STAGE OF CHOLESTEROL GALLSTONE FORMATION

Most studies in this field have been performed in animals, mainly prairie dogs and guinea pigs. Feeding of prairie dogs with a lithogenic diet (0.4–1.2% cholesterol added), results in the formation of cholesterol gallstones within a few weeks[39].

DenBesten and co-workers convincingly showed that cholesterol feeding in prairie dogs reduced gallbladder emptying *before* cholesterol crystals and gallstone formation occurred[40–43]. Fridhandler made similar observations in ground squirrels and demonstrated that *in vitro* gallbladder muscle contractility to CCK-8 was reduced by 42% before gallstones developed and by 65% when gallstones had developed[44]. Poston *et al.* demonstrated that in the early stage the sensitivity of the isolated gallbladder to CCK was decreased[45]. However, stimulation of the gallbladder *in vivo* by frequent lipid–protein emulsion feeding or CCK infusion prevented the formation of gallstones[46,47].

Almost simultaneously, several other changes in biliary function were observed. Enhanced absorption of electrolytes and water by the gallbladder[48,49], increased cystic duct closing pressure, increased resistance to bile outflow through the cystic duct[50] and increased blood flow to the gallbladder mucosa[51] before gallstones were found.

It has also been demonstrated that impaired gallbladder muscle contraction precedes excessive mucin secretion. In its turn, mucin production precedes or coincides with cholesterol crystal formation[52–54]. In man, increased secretion of gallbladder mucin precedes cholesterol crystal precipitation, as observed in duodenal bile obtained from obese patients on a low-calorie diet who have an increased risk for gallstone formation[55]. It has been suggested that mucin promotes nucleation and that the presence of cholesterol crystals irritates the gallbladder mucosa and further enhances mucin production[30,31]. The concomitant concentration of bile and the changes in bile composition (relatively more deoxycholate and more arachidonate) may contribute to gallbladder wall inflammation. Chapman and co-workers demonstrated that prostaglandin synthesis increased in the early stage of gallstone formation[56].

Although prostaglandins have a strong stimulatory effect on gallbladder contractility[57] it is possible that their net effect is a diminished bile outflow due to enhanced cystic duct resistance. Finally, gallbladder wall inflammation and progressive fibrosis may further deteriorate gallbladder emptying.

Li and co-workers found no changes in total actin and myosin concentrations after 8 days of cholesterol feeding to prairie dogs[58]. However, further qualitative analysis revealed a shift from α to γ-actin filaments in prairie dog gallbladder smooth muscle[59]. This observation may point to a biochemical basis for decreased gallbladder contractility in the very early stage of cholesterol gallstone formation.

Although it is very difficult to study the events *before* gallstones become manifest in humans, some prospective studies have been performed. Van der Linden assessed gallbladder function with oral cholecystography in 21 subjects without gallstones and found weak contracting gallbladders in 12 subjects. He repeated this investigation after 14 years and found that 7/12 of subjects with weak contracting gallbladders developed gallstones, whereas only one of the subjects with a strong contracting gallbladder developed gallstones[60]. Brugge demonstrated that the postprandial gallbladder ejection fraction was 26% in subjects with cholesterol crystals in bile but without gallstones, and 60% in subjects without crystals or stones[61].

In conclusion, in the early stage of gallstone formation, changes take place in gallbladder muscle composition and function which precede the formation of cholesterol crystals. Cholesterol crystals may further deteriorate gallbladder function and enhance mucin production. In this sense the early events in gallstone formation might be regarded as parts of a self-reinforcing process.

CONDITIONS ASSOCIATED WITH AN INCREASED RISK OF CHOLESTEROL GALLSTONES AND WITH DECREASED GALLBLADDER EMPTYING

In some diseases or conditions an increased incidence of gallstones is observed, together with decreased gallbladder emptying (Table 1). These situations give the opportunity to study the early events that are involved in the formation of gallstones in a prospective way.

An increased incidence of gallstones has been observed in pregnancy[62]. After the first trimester of pregnancy, gallbladder fasting and residual volume increase and ejection fraction decreases[63]. This might be attributed to a direct inhibitory effect of progestagens on gallbladder contraction[64]. A recent study showed that, after giving birth, gallstones spontaneously disappeared in 30% of subjects[65]. This might be due to restoration of gallbladder emptying after normalization of the progestagen state.

In patients on total parenteral nutrition, maximal gallbladder filling and prolonged bile stasis with subsequent gallstone formation is found[66,67]. The prevention of sludge and gallstone formation by regular CCK infusions strongly suggests that abolished gallbladder emptying is crucial in the process of gallstone formation[68].

Table 1 Factors, conditions and treatments associated with cholesterol cholelithiasis

	References
Factors associated with cholesterol cholelithiasis	
Ethnic differences	115
Familiarity	116
Age	2
Sex	1,117
Legume intake	118,119
Diet?	39,46,119–121
Conditions associated with cholesterol cholelithiasis and decreased gallbladder emptying	
Pregnancy	63,65,122,123
Somatostatinoma	124
Spinal cord injury	125
Hypertriglyceridaemia	126–128
Obesity	129–132
Cystic fibrosis?	133,134
Inflammatory bowel disease?	135–137
Diabetes mellitus?	138–141
Treatments associated with cholesterol cholelithiasis and decreased gallbladder emptying	
Very low calorie dieting	55,130,142,143
Sex hormone	63,144,145
Total parenteral nutrition	66,67
Gastric surgery/(truncal) vagotomy	146,147
Fibric acid	148
Octreotide	69,149–151

Treatment of acromegaly patients with octreotide (a somatostatin analogue) results in the formation of cholesterol gallstones in 50% of patients after 1 year of treatment[69]. In this way octreotide treatment can serve as a model for (prospective) investigations into the pathogenesis of cholesterol gallstones. Octreotide injections result in suppression of postprandial gallbladder contraction and CCK release, and increase the lithogenic index of bile[70–73]. We recently showed that the timing of injections, in relation to meals, might be important for the preservation of postprandial gallbladder emptying[72].

Gallstone formation during rapid weight loss in obese subjects also allowed prospective studying of the events involved. Rapid weight loss increases cholesterol secretion and reduces bile salt and phospholipid secretion, resulting in increased CSI[34]. Biliary prostaglandin E_2, arachidonate and glycoprotein also increase[74]. These factors promote cholesterol gallstone formation as outlined above. Moreover, increased fasting and postprandial residual gallbladder volumes and reduced gallbladder emptying have been observed in obese patients[75–79], allowing progressive concentration of gallbladder bile and formation of cholesterol-rich unstable vesicles. Two recent studies convincingly showed that addition of no more than 10 g of fat to the diet completely restored gallbladder emptying and prevented the formation of gallstones during low-calorie dieting[80,81]. Taken together, these data indicate that intact gallbladder emptying is important in the prevention of cholesterol gallstone formation.

GALLBLADDER MOTILITY DISORDERS IN THE PRESENCE OF CHOLESTEROL GALLSTONES: EVOLVING HYPOTHESIS

Few studies assessed the effect of the presence or absence of (prosthetic) gallstones on gallbladder motility. In guinea pigs, implantation of glass beads in the gallbladder diminished *in-vitro* gallbladder contractility by 20% and left bile composition unchanged[82]. The impairment of gallbladder motility in gallstone patients persists after successful extracorporeal shock-wave lithotripsy and stone dissolution[83]. In addition, Berr and co-workers demonstrated that incomplete evacuation of the gallbladder upon CCK infusion was associated with an increased risk for gallbladder stone recurrence after initially successful clearance of stones with shock-wave lithotripsy[84].

The first studies on gallbladder motility were performed in gallstone patients at the moment when stones became clinically apparent. From these studies no definite conclusions can be drawn about the causal relationship between gallbladder motility disorders and gallstones, although many studies point to a role for diminished gallbladder motility in cholesterol gallstone formation. Several methods are used to assess gallbladder function. Initially, X-ray studies were performed[85], and Van der Linden was one of the first to discriminate between strong and weak postprandial gallbladder emptying in gallstone patients[60]. With the advent of radioisotope techniques and real-time ultrasonography, dynamic gallbladder studies improved[86,87]. The advantage of real-time ultrasonography is that it is non-invasive, that no radiation is involved and that measurements of gallbladder *volume*, and not only gallbladder function, can be made. Radionuclide studies confirmed that among gallstone patients a subgroup with severely impaired postprandial gallbladder emptying exists[88,89], while gallbladder emptying values of the other patients are in the normal range or even larger than in healthy controls[87,90]. *In-vitro* studies on the contractility of human gallbladder muscle strips showed that contractility was substantially reduced in the case of cholesterol gallstones as compared with pigment gallstones[91]. Moreover, we also demonstrated that *in-vitro* strong and weak contractor cholesterol gallstone patients can be distinguished[92].

From real-time ultrasonography studies it appeared that gallstone patients have high residual postprandial gallbladder volumes and increased fasting gallbladder volumes[90,93]. Interestingly, high postprandial CCK levels in patients with weak contracting gallbladders were also observed[90]. This may be explained by impaired negative feedback of intraduodenal bile salts on CCK release[94,95]. Although increased fasting and residual gallbladder volumes may be epiphenomena, they may contribute substantially to the pathogenesis of cholesterol gallstones by providing the residual bile mass and the time for progressive nucleation and stone growth. Furthermore, increased fasting gallbladder volume may point to disturbed interdigestive gallbladder emptying in gallstone patients.

Therefore, attention was focused on the regulation of fasting gallbladder volume. In fasting healthy volunteers it has been observed that gallbladder volume fluctuated in accordance with the migrating motor complex[96]. The MMC is a cyclic triphasic pattern of contractile activity in the interdigestive state, with a cycling frequency of 1–3 h. Three phases can be distinguished: in phase I no contractile activity is observed; in phase II irregular contractile activity is present; in phase III rhythmic contractions, with a maximum frequency of two or three contractions/min in antrum and 10–12 contractions/min in duodenum and jejunum are observed (Fig. 2). Phase III originates in 50% of cases in the lower oesophageal sphincter or stomach and migrates to the small intestines. In the other 50%, phase III originates in the small intestines and migrates aborally. We recently observed that only *antral* phase III was preceded by significant gallbladder emptying and motilin release, whereas phase III starting at the level of the *duodenum* was not preceded by gallbladder emptying and motilin peaks (Fig. 3[97]). We therefore hypothesized that cholesterol gallstone patients might have disturbed MMC patterns with reduced occurrence of antral phase III. Preliminary observations by our group revealed that antral phase III was still present in gallstone patients but that MMC cycle length was increased. Interdigestive gallbladder emptying was absent and motilin release patterns were disturbed in gallstone patients. In addition, in six acromegaly patients on 2 months of octreotide treatment, we observed that octreotide abolished interdigestive gallbladder emptying and suppressed motilin levels. Octreotide also abolished antral phase III, and fasting gallbladder volume increased from 40 to 60 ml (unpublished data).

These studies indicate that fasting gallbladder volume regulation is closely related to the MMC, and that MMC pattern disturbances are associated with decreased interdigestive gallbladder emptying and increased fasting gallbladder volume.

Interdigestive gallbladder emptying is linked to the MMC, and bile salt output may have an important regulatory effect on the MMC. As demonstrated by Qvist and co-workers, the MMC is largely responsible for the transport of intraluminal bile salts to the terminal ileum[98]. In this way the MMC and the enterohepatic circulation (EHC) are closely linked. Bile salt homeostasis is maintained by regulation of synthesis and uptake in the enterohepatic circulation. In the fasting state 50–90% of the bile salt pool is stored in the gallbladder[99,100]. In patients with severe Crohn's disease or ileal resection, decreased bile salt pool size has been associated with cholesterol supersaturation and subsequent gallstone formation[101,102]. In cholesterol gallstone patients a decreased bile salt pool size is also observed[103,104]. However, in the prairie-dog model, reduced pool size is found only *after* the formation of cholesterol gallstones[40,41], and may be considered as an epiphenomenon. It is conceivable that changes in bile salt pool size or composition, changes of the MMC and changes of interdigestive gallbladder emptying are interrelated. However, no conclusive data on this subject are yet available.

Taking all these data together, the scheme shown in Fig. 4, on the role of gallbladder motility in the formation of gallstones, can be proposed.

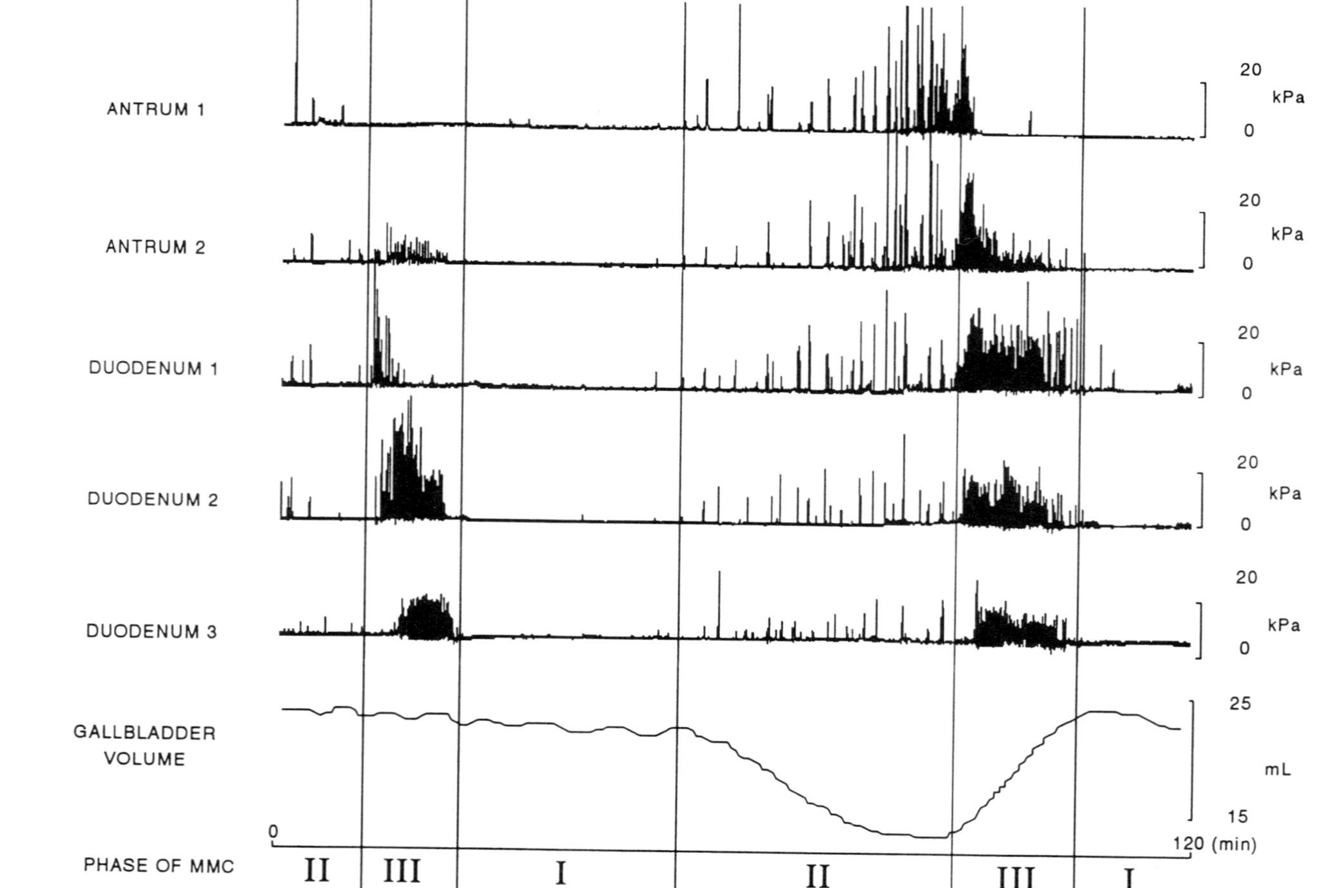

Fig. 2 Relationship between the phases of the migrating motor complex (MMC) and interdigestive gallbladder emptying. Note the presence of gallbladder emptying before antral phase III and its absence before duodenal phase III

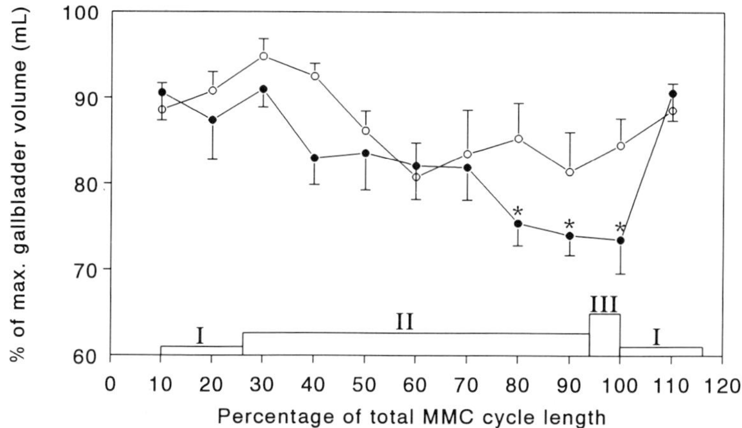

Fig. 3 Relationship between interdigestive gallbladder emptying and MMC in 10 healthy volunteers. Gallbladder emptying is expressed as percentage of maximal gallbladder volume during the cycle. Percentiles denote fraction of elapsed total cycle length. Closed dots show cycles with phase III starting in antrum. Open dots show cycles with phase III starting in duodenum. *Significantly different from p50, p60 and p70, from ref. 97

PROSPECTS FOR IMPROVEMENT OF DEFECTIVE GALLBLADDER EMPTYING

Several drugs have recently been investigated for their potential beneficial effect on gallbladder emptying. Daily intravenous administration of CCK in patients on total parenteral nutrition prevents sludge and gallstone formation[68]. Ceruletide, a synthetic CCK analogue, can also stimulate gallbladder emptying. Recently, increased fragment clearance was observed when a single ceruletide infusion was given directly after shock-wave lithotripsy[105].

Cholestyramine is a resin that binds bile salts and thereby interrupts the negative feedback of bile salts on duodenal CCK release. Ingestion of cholestyramine induces a powerful and long-lasting CCK-mediated gallbladder contraction[95,106].

Erythromycin is regarded as a direct motilin-receptor agonist and probably also induces motilin release[107]. Erythromycin reduces fasting and postprandial residual gallbladder volume[108,109]. Currently, several motilin-like compounds, so-called motilides, such as EM-523, are being investigated for their potential prokinetic effect on the gallbladder[110].

The effects of cisapride on postprandial motility are conflicting. Intravenous administration has been shown to improve gallbladder emptying, whereas oral cisapride might reduce postprandial gallbladder emptying[111,112].

Non-steroidal anti-inflammatory drugs have been shown to prevent recurrence of gallstones after dissolution with oral bile salts[113]. This might be due to decreased mucin production or to a prokinetic effect on gallbladder emptying, as has been observed with indomethacin in gallstone patients[114].

Future research into gallbladder motility will increase insight into the role of gallbladder hypomotility in the formation of gallstones. It will also lead

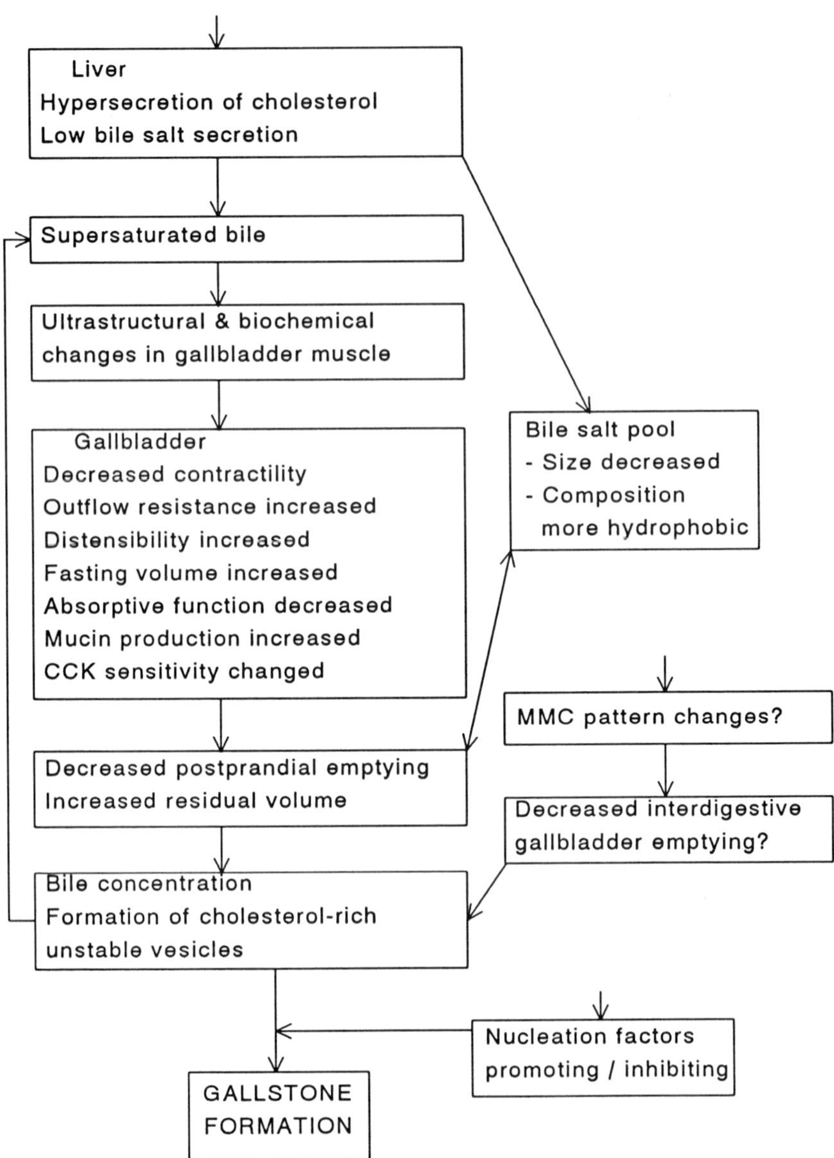

Fig. 4 Role of disordered gallbladder emptying in the pathogenesis of cholesterol gallstones. Note that at least three factors are probably independent: hepatic cholesterol secretion, migrating motor complex (MMC) pattern changes and nucleation factors

to the development of new strategies for the prevention of *de-novo* gallstone formation, especially in selected risk-groups, or prevention of recurrence after successful non-surgical therapy for gallstones.

ACKNOWLEDGEMENTS

This study was supported by The Netherlands Foundation for Medical Research (NWO-MW) grant no. 900-522-106 and by the Royal Netherlands Academy of Arts and Sciences.

References

1. Barbara L, Sama C, Morselli Labate AM. A population study on the prevalence of gallstone disease: the Sirmione study. Hepatology. 1987;7:913–17.
2. Hougaard Jensen K, Jorgensen T. Incidence of gallstones in a Danish population. Gastroenterology. 1991;100:790–4.
3. Meijer WS. Galblaas extirpates in Nederland; frequentie, operatieve sterfte en postoperatieve complicaties (1987–1989). Ned Tijdschr Geneeskd. 1991;135:1688–91.
4. Van Erpecum KJ, van Berge Henegouwen GP, Stoelwinder B, Stolk MFJ, Eggink WF, Govaert WHA. Cholesterol and pigment gallstone disease: comparison of the reliability of three bile tests for differentiation between the two stone types. Scand J Gastroenterol. 1988;23:948–54.
5. Grundy SM, Duane WC, Adler RD, Aron JM, Metzger AL. Biliary lipid outputs in young women with cholesterol gallstones. Metabolism. 1974;23:67–73.
6. Nilsell K, Angelin B, Liljeqvist L, Einarsson K. Biliary lipid output and bile acid kinetics in cholesterol gallstone disease. Evidence for an increased hepatic secretion of cholesterol in Swedish patients. Gastroenterology. 1985;89:287–93.
7. Grundy SM, Metzger AL, Adler RD. Mechanisms of lithogenic bile formation in American Indian women with cholesterol gallstones. J Clin Invest. 1972;51:3026–43.
8. Cohen DE, Leighton LS, Carey MC. Bile salt hydrophobicity controls vesicle secretion rates and transformations in native bile. Am J Physiol. 1992;263:G386–95.
9. Metzger AL, Adler R, Heymsfield S. Diurnal variations in biliary lipid composition. N Engl J Med. 1973;288:333–6.
10. Holzbach RT, Marsh M, Olszewski M, Holan K. Cholesterol solubility in bile. Evidence that supersaturated bile is frequent in healthy man. J Clin Invest. 1973;52:1467–79.
11. Lee SP, Park HZ, Madani H, Kaler EW. Partial characterization of a nonmicellar system of cholesterol solubilization in bile. Am J Physiol. 1987;252:G384.
12. Harvey PRC, Sömjen G, Lichtenberg MS, Petrunka C, Gilat T, Strasberg SM. Nucleation of cholesterol from vesicles isolated from bile of patients with and without cholesterol gallstones. Biochim Biophys Acta. 1987;921:198–204.
13. Lichtenberg D, Ragimova S, Bor A *et al*. Stability of mixed micellar systems made by solubilizing phosphatidylcholine-cholesterol vesicles by bile salts. Hepatology. 1990;12:149S–54S.
14. Halpern Z, Dudley MA, Kibe A, Lynn MP, Breuer AC, Holzbach RT. Rapid vesicle formation and aggregation in abnormal human biles: a time-lapse video-enhanced contrast microscopy study. Gastroenterology. 1986;90:875–85.
15. Sömjen GJ, Gilat T. Contribution of vesicular and micellar carriers to cholesterol transport in human bile. J Lipid Res. 1985;26:699–704.
16. Pattinson NR. Solubilisation of cholesterol in human bile. FEBS Lett. 1985;181:342.
17. Whiting MJ, Watts JM. Cholesterol gallstone pathogenesis: a study of potential nucleating agents for cholesterol crystal formation in bile. Clin Sci. 1985;68:589–96.
18. Holan KR, Holzbach RT, Hermann RE, Cooperman AM, Claffey WJ. Nucleation time: a key factor in the pathogenesis of cholesterol gallstone disease. Gastroenterology. 1979;77:611–17.
19. Van Erpecum KJ, van Berge Henegouwen GP, Stoelwinder B, Schmidt YMG, Willekens FLH. Bile concentration is a key factor for nucleation of cholesterol crystals and cholesterol saturation index in gallbladder bile of gallstone patients. Hepatology. 1990;11:1–6.
20. Neiderhiser DH, Morningstar WA, Roth H. Absorption of lecithin and lysolecithin by the gallbladder. J Lab Clin Med. 1973;82:891–7.
21. Neiderhiser DH, Roth HP. Absorption of cholesterol by the gallbladder. J Lipid Res. 1976;17:117–24.

22. Purdum PP, Shamburek RD, Hylemon PB, Moore EW. Rapid phospholipid transfer across cultured human gallbladder epithelia. Gastroenterology. 1992;102:A871.
23. Kibe A, Holzbach RT, LaRusso NF *et al.* Inhibition of cholesterol crystal formation by apolipoproteins in supersaturated model bile. Science. 1984;255:514–16.
24. Groen AK, Stout JPJ, Drapers JAG, Hoek FJ, Grijm R, Tytgat GNJ. Cholesterol nucleation influencing activity in T-tube bile. Hepatology. 1988;8:347–52.
25. Pattinson NR, Willis KE. Effect of phospholipase C on cholesterol solubilization in model bile: a concanavalin A-binding nucleation-promoting factor from human gallbladder bile. Gastroenterology. 1991;101:1339–44.
26. Harvey PRC, Upadhya GA, Strasberg SM. Immunoglobulins as nucleating proteins in the gallbladder bile of patients with cholesterol gallstones. J Biol Chem. 1992;266:13996–4003.
27. Chijiiwa K, Koga A, Yamasaki T, Shimada K, Noshiro H, Nakayama F. Fibronectin: a possible factor promoting cholesterol monohydrate crystallization in bile. Biochim Biophys Acta. 1991;1086:44–8.
28. Ostrow JD. APF/CBP, an anionic polypeptide in bile and gallstones that may regulate calcium salt and cholesterol precipitation from bile. Hepatology. 1992;16:1493–6.
29. Mok K, Out M, de Bruin M, Goldhoorn B, Tytgat GNJ, Groen AK. An evaluation of the quantitative importance of individual pronucleating proteins in the biliary concanavalin A-binding protein fraction. Gastroenterology. 1992;102:A323.
30. Lee SM, LaMont JT, Carey MC. Role of gallbladder mucus hypersecretion in the evolution of cholesterol gallstones. Studies in the prairie dog. J Clin Invest. 1981;67:1712–23.
31. Smith BF. Human gallbladder mucin binds biliary lipids and promotes cholesterol crystal nucleation in model bile. J Lipid Res. 1987;28:1088–97.
32. Lee SP, Carey MC, LaMont JT. Aspirin prevention of cholesterol gallstone formation in prairie dogs. Science. 1981;211:1429–31.
33. Cohen BI, Mosbach EH, Ayyad N, Yoshii M, McSherry CK. Aspirin does not inhibit cholesterol lithiasis in two established animal models. Gastroenterology. 1991;101:1109–16.
34. Broomfield PH, Chopra R, Sheinbaum RC *et al.* Effects of ursodeoxycholic acid and aspirin on the formation of lithogenic bile and gallstones during loss of weight. N Engl J Med. 1988;319:1567–72.
35. Marks JW, Bonorris GG, Schoenfield LJ. Roles of deoxycholate and arachidonate in pathogenesis of cholesterol gallstones in obese patients during rapid loss of weight. Dig Dis Sci. 1991;36:957–60.
36. van Berge Henegouwen GP, van der Werf SDJ, Ruben AT. Fatty acid composition of phospholipids in bile in man: promoting effect of deoxycholate on arachidonate. Clin Chim Acta. 1987;165:27–37.
37. Lee SP, Nicholls JF. Nature and composition of biliary sludge. Gastroenterology. 1986;90:677–86.
38. Harvey PRC, Rupar CA, Gallinger S, Petrunka CN, Strasberg SM. Quantitative and qualitative comparison of gallbladder mucus glycoprotein from patients with and without gallstones. Gut. 1986;27:374–81.
39. Brenneman DE, Connor WE, Forker EL *et al.* The formation of abnormal bile and cholesterol gallstones from dietary cholesterol in the prairie dog. J Clin Invest. 1972;51:1495–503.
40. Meyer PD, DenBesten L, Gurll NJ. Effects of cholesterol gallstone induction on gallbladder function and bile salt pool size in the prairie dog model. Surgery. 1978;83:599–604.
41. Roslyn JJ, DenBesten L, Thompson JE, Cohen K. Chronic cholelithiasis and decreased bile salt pool size: cause or effect? Am J Surg. 1980;139:119–24.
42. Gurll NJ, Meyer PD, DenBesten L. Effect of cholesterol crystals on gallbladder function in cholelithiasis. Surg Forum. 1977;28:412–13.
43. Doty JE, Pitt HA, Kichenbecker SL, DenBesten L. Impaired gallbladder emptying before gallstone formation in prairie dog. Gastroenterology. 1983;85:168–74.
44. Fridhandler TM, Davison JS, Shaffer EA. Defective gallbladder contractility in the ground squirrel and prairie dog during the early stages of cholesterol gallstone formation. Gastroenterology. 1983;85:830–6.
45. Poston GH, Singh P, Draviam E, Yao CZ, Gomez G, Thompson JC. Early stages of gallstone formation in guinea pig are associated with decreased biliary sensitivity to cholecystokinin. Dig Dis Sci. 1992;37:1236–44.

46. Roslyn J, DenBesten L, Thompson JE, Jr. Effects of periodic emptying of gallbladder on gallbladder function and formation of cholesterol gallstone. Surg Forum. 1979;30:403–4.
47. Roslyn JJ, DenBesten L, Pitt HA, Kuchenbecker SL, Polarek JW. Effects of cholecystokinin on gallbladder stasis and cholesterol gallstone formation. J Surg Res. 1981;30:200–4.
48. Roslyn JJ, Doty J, Pitt HA, Conter RL, DenBesten L. Enhanced gallbladder absorption during gallstone formation: the roles of cholesterol saturated bile and gallbladder stasis. Am J Med Sci. 1986;292:75–80.
49. Conter RL, Roslyn JJ, Porter-Fink V, DenBesten L. Gallbladder absorption increases during early cholesterol gallstone formation. Am J Surg. 1986;151:184–92.
50. Pitt HA, Doty JE, DenBesten L, Kichenbecker SL. Stasis before gallstone formation: Altered gallbladder compliance or cystic duct resistance. Am J Surg. 1982;143:144–9.
51. Conter RL, Washington JL, Liao C, Kauffman GL, Jr. Gallbladder mucosal blood flow increases during early cholesterol gallstone formation. Gastroenterology. 1992;102:1764–70.
52. Li YF, Moody FG, Weisbrodt NW, Zalewsky CA, Coelho JCU, Senninger N. Decrease of contractility of prairie dog gallbladder muscle strips following cholesterol feeding. Surg Forum. 1984;35:224–6.
53. Li YF, Moody FG, Weisbrodt NW *et al.* Gallbladder contractility and mucus secretion after cholesterol feeding in the prairie dog. Surgery. 1986;100:900–4.
54. O'Leary DP, LaMorte WW, Scott TE, Booker ML, Stevenson J. Inhibition of prostaglandin synthesis fails to prevent gallbladder mucin hypersecretion in the cholesterol-fed prairie dog. Gastroenterology. 1991;101:812–20.
55. Marks JW, Bonorris GG, Albers G, Schoenfield LJ. The sequence of biliary events preceding the formation of gallstones in humans. Gastroenterology. 1992;103:566–70
56. Chapman WC, Peterkin GA, LaMorte WW, Williams LFJ. Alterations in biliary motility correlate with increased gallbladder prostaglandin synthesis in early cholelithiasis in prairie dog. Dig Dis Sci. 1989;34:1420–4.
57. Kotwall CA, Clanachan AS, Baer HP, Scott GW. Effects of prostaglandins on motility of gallbladders removed from patients with gallstones. Arch Surg. 1984;119:709–12.
58. Li YF, Weisbrodt NW, Moody FG, Coelho JU, Gouma DJ. Calcium-induced contraction and contractile protein content of gallbladder smooth muscle after high-cholesterol feeding of prairie dogs. Gastroenterology. 1987;92:746–50.
59. Li YF, Bowers RL, Haley-Russell D, Moody FG, Weisbrodt NW. Actin and myosin isoforms in gallbladder smooth muscle following cholesterol feeding in prairie dogs. Gastroenterology. 1990;99:1460–6.
60. Van der Linden W. Emptying of the human gallbladder and predisposition to gallstone formation. Tijdschr Gastroenterol. 1974;17:121–8.
61. Brugge WR, Brand DL, Atkins H, Lane B, Abel WG. Gallbladder dyskinesia in chronic acalculous cholecystitis. Dig Dis Sci. 1986;31:461–7.
62. Friedman GD, Kannel WB, Dawber TR. The epidemiology of gallbladder disease: observations in the Framingham study. J Chron Dis. 1966;19:273–92.
63. Braverman DZ, Johnson ML, Kern F, Jr. Effects of pregnancy and contraceptive steroids on gallbladder function. N Engl J Med. 1980;302:362–4.
64. Singletary BK, Van Thiel DH, Eagon PK. Estrogen and progesterone receptors in human gallbladder. Hepatology. 1986;6:574–8.
65. Maringhini A, Ciambra M, Baccelliere P *et al.* Biliary sludge and gallstones in pregnancy: incidence, risk factors, and natural history. Ann Intern Med. 1993;119:116–20.
66. Roslyn JJ, Pitt HA, Mann LL, Ament ME, DenBesten L. Gallbladder disease in patients on long term parenteral nutrition. Gastroenterology. 1983;84:148–54.
67. Messing B, Bories C, Kunstlinger F, Bernier JJ. Does total parenteral nutrition induce gallbladder sludge formation and lithiasis? Gastroenterology. 1983;84:1012–19.
68. Sitzmann JV, Pitt HA, Steinborn PA, Pasha ZR, Sanders RC. Cholecystokinin prevents parenteral nutrition induced biliary sludge in humans. Surg Gynecol Obstet. 1990;170:25–31.
69. Ho KY, Weissberger AJ, Marbach P, Lazarus L. Therapeutic efficacy of the somatostatin analog SMS 201-995 (Octreotide) in acromegaly. Ann Intern Med. 1990;112:173–81.
70. Lembcke B, Creutzfeldt W, Schleser S, Ebert R, Shaw C, Kooper I. Effect of the somatostatin analogue sandostatin (SMS 201-995) on gastrointestinal, pancreatic and biliary function

and hormone release in normal men. Digestion. 1987;36:108–24.
71. Mitsukawa T, Takemura J, Nishizono F *et al.* Effects of atropine. Am J Gastroenterol. 1989;84:1371–4.
72. Stolk MF, Van Erpecum KJ, Koppeschaar HP *et al.* Postprandial gall bladder motility and hormone release during intermittent and continuous subcutaneous octreotide treatment in acromegaly. Gut. 1993;34:808–13.
73. Cucchiaro G, Branum GD, O'Dorisio T, Meyers WC. Effect of somatostatin and its analogue sandostatin on biliary lipid composition. Gastroenterology. 1990;98:A246.
74. Marks JW, Bonorris GG, Schoenfield LJ. Roles of deoxycholate and arachidonate in pathogenesis of cholesterol gallstones in obese patients during rapid loss of weight. Dig Dis Sci. 1991;36:957–60.
75. Kucio C, Besser P, Jonderko K. Gallbladder motor function in obese versus lean females. Eur J Clin Nutr. 1988;42:121–4.
76. Marzio L, Capone F, Neri M, Mezzetti A, De A, Cuccurullo F. Gallbladder kinetics in obese patients. Effect of a regular meal and low-calorie meal. Dig Dis Sci. 1988;33:4–9.
77. Vezina WC, Paradis RL, Grace DM *et al.* Increased volume and decreased emptying of the gallbladder in large (morbidly obese, tall normal, and muscular normal) people. Gastroenterology. 1990;98:1000–7.
78. Palasciano G, Serio G, Portincasa P *et al.* Gallbladder volume in adults and relationship to age, sex, body mass index and gallstones: a sonographic population study. Am J Gastroenterol. 1992;87:493–7.
79. Palasciano G, Portincasa P, Belfiore A *et al.* Gallbladder volume and emptying in diabetics: the role of neuropathy and obesity. J Intern Med. 1992;231:123–7.
80. Festi D, Orsini M, LiBassi S *et al.* Risk of gallstone formation during rapid weight loss: protective role of gallbladder motility. Gastroenterology. 1992;102:A311.
81. Stone BG, Ansel HJ, Peterson FJ, Gebhard RL. Gallbladder emptying stimuli in obese and normal-weight subjects. Hepatology. 1992;15:795–8.
82. Pomeranz IS, Davison JS, Shaffer EA. The effects of prosthetic gallstones on gallbladder function and bile composition. J Surg Res. 1986;41:47–52.
83. Spengler U, Sackmann M, Sauerbruch T, Holl J, Paumgartner G. Gallbladder motility before and after extracorporeal shock-wave lithotripsy. Gastroenterology. 1989;96:860–3.
84. Berr F, Mayer M, Sackmann M, Sauerbruch T, Holl J, Paumgartner G. Pathogenic factors in early recurrence of cholesterol gallstones. Gastroenterology. 1994;106:215–24.
85. Boyden EA. The effect of natural foods on the distention of the gallbladder with a note on the change in pattern of the mucosa as it passes from distention to collapse. Anat Rec. 1925;30:333.
86. Everson GT, Braverman DZ, Johnson ML, Kern F, Jr. A critical evaluation of real-time ultrasonography for the study of gallbladder volume and contraction. Gastroenterology. 1980;79:40–6.
87. Maudgal DP, Kupfer RM, Zentler-Munro PL, Northfield TC. Postprandial gallbladder emptying in patients with gallstones. Br J Med. 1980;280:141–3.
88. Fisher RS, Stelzer F, Rock E, Malmud LS. Abnormal gallbladder emptying in patients with gallstones. Dig Dis Sci. 1982;27:1019–24.
89. Pomeranz IS, Shaffer EA. Abnormal gallbladder emptying in a subgroup of patients with gallstones. Gastroenterology. 1985;88:787–91.
90. Van Erpecum KJ, van Berge Henegouwen GP, Stolk MFJ, Hopman WPM, Jansen JBMJ, Lamers CBHW. Fasting gallbladder volume, postprandial emptying and cholecystokinin release in gallstone patients and normal subjects. J Hepatol. 1992;14:194–202.
91. Behar J, Lee KY, Thompson WR, Biancani P. Gallbladder contraction in patients with pigment and cholesterol stones. Gastroenterology. 1989;97:1479–84.
92. Portincasa P, Di Ciaula A, Baldassarre G, *et al.* Sonographic and 'in vitro' studies on the role of gallstones, smooth muscle function and gallbladder wall inflammation. J Hepatol. 1994;20:(in press).
93. Kishk SMA, Darweesh RMA, Dodds WJ *et al.* Sonographic evaluation of resting gallbladder volume and postprandial emptying in patients with gallstones. Am J Roentgenol. 1987;148:875–9.
94. Gomez G, Lluis F, Guo Y *et al.* Bile inhibits release of cholecystokinin and neurotensin. Surgery. 1986;100:363–8.

95. Gomez G, Upp JR, Lluis F *et al.* Regulation of the release of cholecystokinin by bile salts in dogs and humans. Gastroenterology. 1988;94:1036–46.

96. Marzio L, Neri M, Capone F *et al.* Gallbladder contraction and its relationship to interdigestive duodenal motor activity in normal human subjects. Dig Dis Sci. 1988;33: 540–4.

97. Stolk MF, Van Erpecum KJ, Smout AJ *et al.* Motor cycles with phase III in antrum are associated with high motilin levels and prolonged gallbladder emptying. Am J Physiol. 1993;264:G596–600.

98. Qvist N, Pedersen SA, Oster-Jorgensen E, Rasmussen L, Hovendal CP, Rasmussen JW. The migrating motor complex and the enterohepatic circulation of bile acids: a scintigraphic study using 75Se-HCAT. J Gastrointest Motil. 1991;3:1–4.

99. van Berge Hengouwen GP, Hofmann AF. Nocturnal gallbladder storage and emptying in gallstone patients and healthy subjects. Gastroenterology. 1978;75:879–85.

100. Lanzini A, Jazrawi RP, Northfield TC. Simultaneous quantitative measurements of absolute gallbladder storage and emptying during fasting and eating in humans. Gastroenterology. 1987;92:852–61.

101. Heaton KW, Austad WI, Lack L, Tyor MP. Enterohepatic circulation of C14-labeled bile salts in disorders of the small bowel. Gastroenterology. 1968;55:5–16.

102. Heaton KW, Read AE. Gallstones in patients with disorders of the terminal ileum and disturbed bile salt metabolism. Br Med J. 1969;3:494–6.

103. Vlahcevic ZR, Bell CC, Buhac I, Farrar JT, Swell L. Diminished bile acid pool size in patients with gallstones. Gastroenterology. 1970;59:165–73.

104. Nilsell K. Bile acid pool size and gallbladder storage capacity in gallstone disease. Scand J Gastroenterol. 1990;25:389–94.

105. Ziegenhagen DJ, Zehnter E, Kruis W, Pohl C. Induced gallbladder contraction accelerates fragment clearance after extracorporeal shockwave lithotripsy. J Gastroenterol Hepatol. 1993;8:406–9.

106. Palasciano G, Portincasa P, Belfiore A, Baldassarre G, Albano O. Opposite effects of cholestyramine and loxiglumide on gallbladder dynamics in humans. Gastroenterology. 1992;102:633–9.

107. Peeters T, Matthijs G, Depoortere I, Cachet T, Hoogmartens J, Vantrappen G. Erythromycin is a motilin receptor agonist. Am J Physiol. 1989;257:G470–4.

108. Catnach SM, Fairclough PD, Trembath RC *et al.* Effect of oral erythromycin on gallbladder motility in normal subjects and subjects with gallstones. Gastroenterology. 1992;102: 2071–6.

109. Jebbink MC, Masclee AA, van der Kleij FG *et al.* Effect of loxiglumide and atropine on erythromycin-induced reduction in gallbladder volume in human subjects. Hepatology. 1992;16:937–42.

110. Depoortere I, Peeters TL, Vantrappen G. The erythromycin derivative EM-523 is a potent motilin agonist in man and in rabbit. Peptides. 1990;11:515–19.

111. Marzio L, DiFelice F, Laico MG, Imbimbo B, Lapenna D, Cuccurullo F. Gallbladder hypokinesia and normal gastric emptying of liquids in patients with dyspeptic symptoms. A double-blind placebo-controlled clinical trial with cisapride. Dig Dis Sci. 1992;37:262–7.

112. Ziegenhagen DJ, Glimm E, Kruis W, Zehnter E. Oral cisapride increases gallbladder volume in volunteers. J Gastrointest Motil. 1992;4:119–23.

113. Hood K, Gleeson D, Ruppin DC, Dowling RH. Prevention of gallstone recurrence by non-steroidal anti-inflammatory drugs. Lancet. 1988;2:1223–5.

114. O'Donnell LJ, Wilson P, Guest P *et al.* Indomethacin and postprandial gallbladder emptying. Lancet. 1992;339:269–71.

115. Strom BL, West SL. The epidemiology of cholesterol gallstone disease. In: Cohen S, Soloway RD, editors. Gallstones. New York: Churchill Livingstone; 1985:1–26.

116. Antero Kesaniemi Y, Koskenvuo M, Vuoristo M, Miettinen TA. Biliary lipid composition in monozygotic and dizygotic pairs of twins. Gut. 1989;30:1750–6.

117. Russo F, Cavallini A, Messa C *et al.* Endogenous sex hormones and cholesterol gallstones: a case-control study in an echographic survey of gallstones. Am J Gastroenterol. 1993;88:712–17.

118. Nervi F, Covarrubias C, Bravo P *et al.* Influence of legume intake on biliary lipids and cholesterol saturation in young Chilean men. Identification of a dietary risk factor for

cholesterol gallstone formation in a highly prevalent area. Gastroenterology. 1989;96: 825–30.
119. Hayes KC, Livingston A, Trautwein EA. Dietary impact on biliary lipids and gallstones. Annu Rev Nutr. 1992;12:299–326.
120. Booker ML, Scott TE, LaMorte WW. Effect of dietary cholesterol on phosphatidylcholines and phosphatidylethanolamines in bile and gallbladder mucosa in the prairie dog. Gastroenterology. 1989;97:1261–7.
121. Chijiiwa K. The effects of ethinylestradiol, a glucose diet and streptozotocin induced diabetes mellitus on gallstone formation and biliary lipid composition in the hamster. Jpn J Surg. 1990;20:567–76.
122. Valdivieso V, Covarrubias C, Siegel F, Cruz F. Pregnancy and cholelithiasis: pathogenesis and natural course of gallstones diagnosed in early puerperium. Hepatology. 1993;17: 1–4.
123. Thijs C, Knipschild P, Leffers P. Pregnancy and gallstone disease: an empiric demonstration of the importance of specification of risk periods. Am J Epidemiol. 1991;134:186–95.
124. Krejs GJ, Orci L, Conlon JM et al. Somatostatinoma syndrome. N Engl J Med. 1979;301:285–92.
125. Nino Murcia M, Burton D, Chang P, Stone J, Perkash I. Gallbladder contractility in patients with spinal cord injuries: a sonographic investigation. Am J Roentgenol. 1990;154:521–4.
126. Janowitz P, Wechsler JG, Kuhn K et al. The relationship between serum lipids, nucleation time, and biliary lipids in patients with gallstones. Clin Invest. 1992;70:430–6.
127. Yang H, Petersen GM, Roth MP, Schoenfield LJ, Marks JW. Risk factors for gallstone formation during rapid loss of weight. Dig Dis Sci. 1992;37:912–18.
128. Thijs C, Knipschild P, Brombacher P. Serum lipids and gallstones: a case–control study. Gastroenterology. 1990;99:843–9.
129. Shiffman ML, Sugerman HJ, Kellum JH, Brewer WH, Moore EW. Gallstones in patients with morbid obesity. Relationship to body weight, weight loss and gallbladder bile cholesterol solubility. Int J Obes. 1993;17:153–8.
130. Andersen T. Liver and gallbladder disease before and after very-low-calorie diets. Am J Clin Nutr. 1992;56:235S–9S.
131. Hopper KD, Landis JR, Meilstrup JW, McCauslin MA, Sechtin AG. The prevalence of asymptomatic gallstones in the general population. Invest Radiol. 1991;26:939–45.
132. Stampfer MJ, Maclure KM, Colditz GA, Manson JE, Willett WC. Risk of symptomatic gallstones in women with severe obesity. Am J Clin Nutr. 1992;55:652–8.
133. Santamaria F, Vajro P, Oggero V et al. Volume and emptying of the gallbladder in patients with cystic fibrosis. J Pediatr Gastroenterol Nutr. 1990;10:303–6.
134. Jebbink MC, Heijerman HG, Masclee AA, Lamers CB. Gallbladder disease in cystic fibrosis. Neth J Med. 1992;41:123–6.
135. Crespo Uriguen M, Perez Lozana JR, Perez Suarez A, Miyar Gonzalez A. [The extraintestinal manifestations of Crohn's disease: our experience]. Rev Esp Enferm Dig. 1991;80:169–72.
136. Lorusso D, Leo S, Mossa A, Misciagna G, Guerra V. Cholelithiasis in inflammatory bowel disease. A case–control study. Dis Colon Rectum. 1990;33:791–4.
137. Kangas E, Lehmusto P, Matikainen M. Gallstones in Crohn's disease. Hepatogastroenterology. 1990;37:83–4.
138. Persson GE, Thulin AJ. Prevalence of gallstone disease in patients with diabetes mellitus. A case–control study. Eur J Surg. 1991;157:579–82.
139. Maurer KR, Everhart JE, Knowler WC, Shawker TH, Roth HP. Risk factors for gallstone disease in the Hispanic populations of the United States. Am J Epidemiol. 1990;131: 836–44.
140. Jorgensen T. Gall stones in a Danish population. Relation to weight, physical activity, smoking, coffee consumption, and diabetes mellitus. Gut. 1989;30:528–34.
141. Hayes PC, Patrick A, Roulston JE et al. Gallstones in diabetes mellitus: prevalence and risk factors. Eur J Gastroenterol Hepatol. 1993;4:55–9.
142. Liddle RA, Goldstein RB, Saxton J. Gallstone formation during weight-reduction dieting. Arch Intern Med. 1989;149:1750–3.
143. Anonymous. Very low-calorie diets. National Task Force on the Prevention and Treatment

of Obesity, National Institutes of Health. JAMA. 1993;270:967–74.
144. Henriksson P, Einarsson K, Eriksson A, Kelter U, Angelin B. Estrogen-induced gallstone formation in males. Relation to changes in serum and biliary lipids during hormonal treatment of prostatic carcinoma. J Clin Invest. 1989;84:811–16.
145. Gilloteaux J, Kosek E, Kelly TR. Sex steroid induction of gallstones in the male Syrian hamster. J Submicrosc Cytol Pathol. 1993;25:157–72.
146. Faloon WW. Hepatobiliary effects of obesity and weight-reducing surgery. Semin Liver Dis. 1988;8:229–36.
147. Rehnberg O, Haglund U. Gallstone disease following antrectomy and gastroduodenostomy with or without vagotomy. Ann Surg. 1985;201:315–18.
148. Cooper J, Geizerova H, Oliver MF. Clofibrate and gallstones. Lancet. 1975;1:1083.
149. Eastman RC, Arakaki RF, Shawker T et al. A prospective examination of octreotide-induced gall-bladder changes in acromegaly. Clin Endocrinol Oxf. 1992;36:265–9.
150. Shi YF, Zhu XF, Harris AG, Zhang JX, Dai Q. Prospective study of the long-term effects of somatostatin analog (octreotide) on gallbladder function and gallstone formation in Chinese acromegalic patients. J Clin Endocrinol Metab. 1993;76:32–7.
151. Dowling RH, Hussaini SH, Murphy GM, Besser GM, Wass JA. Gallstones during octreotide therapy. Metabolism. 1992;41:22–33.

15
Cholesterol crystal morphology is changed by a new subgroup of lectin-bound biliary proteins

N. BUSCH, F. LAMMERT and S. MATERN

INTRODUCTION

The formation of cholesterol gallstones involves multiple steps including secretion of lithogenic bile and nucleation and growth of cholesterol crystals within the gallbladder followed by agglomeration of crystals into mature stones. For cholesterol crystal nucleation and growth to occur at least three primary defects must be present simultaneously[1]:

Cholesterol supersaturation is a necessary precondition to the eventual crystallization of cholesterol. Supersaturation of bile implies that there are more cholesterol molecules in solution than can be carried in simple and mixed micelles of bile at equilibrium[2]. Equilibrium solubility of native bile is defined as the equilibrium solubility of cholesterol in model bile comprising identical total lipid concentration and molar ratios regarding the three main lipids bile salt, phospholipid and cholesterol[3]. With continuous influx of hepatic bile and repeated excretion of concentrated bile following diurnal CCK stimuli, native human gallbladder bile will rarely reach true thermodynamic equilibrium. Therefore *gallbladder hypomotility* is another important primary defect found in gallstone subjects, resulting in prolonged residence times and augmented residual volumes, thus facilitating formation and retention of cholesterol crystals[4,5]. However, supersaturation alone is not sufficient to produce stones, as many normal subjects without crystals or gallstones have gallbladder bile that is highly supersaturated[6]. Based on these observations a new kinetic thermodynamic concept of cholesterol gallstone pathogenesis was introduced, focusing on a *kinetic factor defect* as the third primary defect responsible for gallstone formation. The accelerated nucleation of lithogenic bile was attributed either to factors that promote precipitation of cholesterol from abnormal supersaturated bile in gallstone patients or to a deficiency of factors which inhibit precipitation from equally supersaturated normal biles[7].

CHOLESTEROL NUCLEATION AND CRYSTAL GROWTH

Nucleation, in general terms, refers to the initial step in crystallization, describing the formation of structured aggregates or nuclei from single solute molecules in supersaturated solutions.

Two types of nucleation can be distinguished depending on the degree of supersaturation and the composition of the solute. In highly supersaturated solutions containing only the solute and the solvent, thermodynamic activity is sufficient to overcome the energy barriers for *homogeneous nucleation* to occur. Numerous nuclei form spontaneously, followed by precipitation of multiple small crystals from the solution. This type of nucleation is more common in simple systems such as model solutions. In complex biological systems such as native bile with comparable low degree of supersaturation (typically 100–200%), *heterogeneous nucleation* occurs more commonly. In this process nucleating agents or kinetic factors are required to overcome the energy barriers. These factors *promote* crystallization. Conversely, factors impeding the traversing of these energy barriers *inhibit* crystallization[8].

Nuclei of cholesterol in bile are submicroscopic aggregates of several hundred cholesterol molecules which form and redissolve continuously[9]. When these nuclei reach a certain critical size molecular association rate overcomes dissociation rate, followed by growth into microscopic crystals.

In trying to elucidate the nucleation process on a molecular basis, we summarize in Fig. 1 the current understanding about solubilization of cholesterol in bile at equilibrium[3,10,11]. Biliary phospholipids and cholesterol are found in the canalicular space as unilamellar vesicles whereas most, if not all, bile salts enter as monomers[12]. During passage through the biliary tree and within the gallbladder biliary lipids are concentrated by removal of inorganic electrolytes and water, causing interconversion of cholesterol carriers that finally proceeds to a solution of simple and mixed micelles for unsaturated (CSI < 1) bile at equilibrium (see previous section). When cholesterol exceeds the saturation limit (CSI > 1), the final result in the gallbladder is a mixture of cholesterol-saturated simple and mixed micelles coexisting with a new population of cholesterol-rich vesicles. Based on video-enhanced polarizing light microscopy, the current model for cholesterol nucleation suggests that biliary vesicles must fuse or at least aggregate, forming multilamellar structures for the crystalline cholesterol monohydrate phase to appear[13,14]. Recent studies have shown that the transformation from cholesterol-rich (cholesterol:lecithin ratio ≥2:1) vesicles to plate-like crystals passes through filamentous structures that are most likely the result of crystallization of anhydrous cholesterol, which is hydrated very slowly in model bile. These observations also suggest that, if vesicles in the supersaturated bile systems are not that cholesterol-rich (ratio <2:1), direct crystallization of classic cholesterol monohydrate plates may occur[15].

KINETIC FACTORS OF CHOLESTEROL CRYSTALLIZATION

Since the introduction of the kinetic concept of cholesterol crystallization in bile many factors have been reported to influence cholesterol nucleation

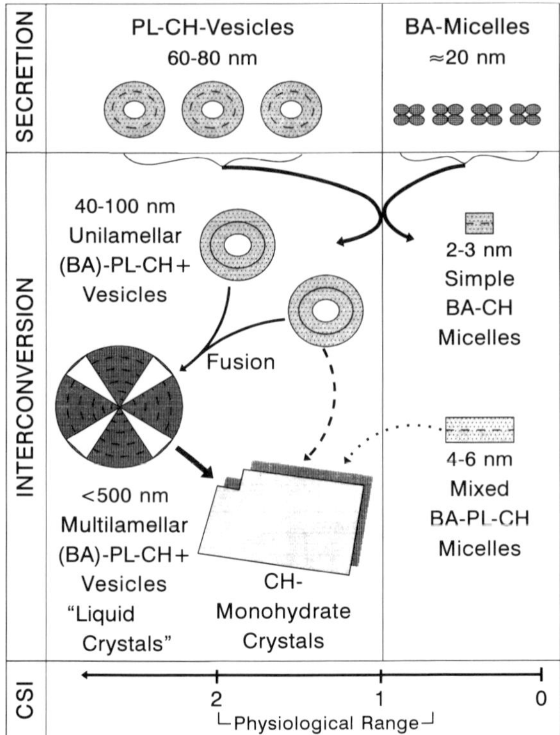

Fig. 1 Schematic representation of cholesterol carriers in bile. Following secretion interconversion of carriers begins within the canalicular space and continues until thermodynamic equilibrium is reached in the gallbladder (for details see text)

and crystal growth. Among the non-protein factors, besides cholesterol supersaturation, biliary lipid composition, hydrophobicity of bile salts, and total lipid concentration as well as elevated concentrations of total calcium ions have been proven to modulate nucleation[13,14,16,17]. Their influences are directly predicated by physical chemistry of charged colloids and by restraints of phase equilibria[17,18]. The influence on nucleation was assessed using the nucleation time assay based on the time of first appearance of cholesterol monohydrate crystals as observed by polarizing light microscopy[7]. This time, better referred to as the crystal detection time, represents a sequence of events including fusion and/or aggregation of vesicles, nucleation and subsequent growth of solid cholesterol crystals to a microscopically detectable size (about 200 nm). In reality the nucleation time represents only one time-point of a crystal growth curve[19]. Experimental determination of the nucleation process itself is precluded because of detection limits.

More than a decade ago evidence was provided that biliary proteins play a major role in cholesterol crystallization[4,20]. Inhibiting activity was shown to be directly attributable to the presence of a crude protein fraction isolated from normal gallbladder bile by cumbersome methods[21]. On the other hand abnormal bile was shown to contain potent pronucleating activity[22]. Total protein concentration in gallbladder bile was found to be significantly higher in cholesterol gallstone patients[23], and very high biliary protein ($>10\,g/l$) was nearly always associated with cholesterol crystals irrespective of the concentrations of total lipids, bile salts and phospholipids[24].

Cholesterol crystallization-promoting proteins

During the past few years several *promoter proteins* have been isolated from human bile. Gallbladder mucin was shown to be an important promoting factor in cholesterol crystallization and stone formation. Purified mucin accelerates cholesterol crystal detection times in model bile at concentrations in the mg/ml range[25,26]. In animal models of cholesterol gallstone disease, hypersecretion of mucus precedes the appearance of cholesterol crystals. The development of a mucin gel on the gallbladder wall and its accumulation in gallbladder sludge is assumed to be of primary importance in accelerating crystal formation and gallstone formation[27]. Since the introduction of lectin affinity chromatography, progress has been made in isolation of non-mucus promoter proteins. Potent promoting activity was found in the biliary protein fraction bound to concanavalin A[28]. The activity has been attributed to a 130 kDa glycoprotein recently identified as aminopeptidase N[29]. Other concanavalin A reactive promoter proteins separated from human bile were identified as immunoglobulins[30], phospholipase C[31], and α_1-acid glycoprotein[32].

Cholesterol crystallization-inhibiting proteins

Apolipoproteins A-I and A-II are present in bile as intact peptides. Because of their known ability to solubilize and transport lipids, the influence of human serum apolipoproteins on cholesterol crystallization was tested in model bile. Apo A-I and A-II at concentrations found in gallbladder bile inhibited nucleation[33]. These studies demonstrated that protein factors may act as inhibitors. The modest effect of apolipoproteins on nucleation times tested in model biles and the lack of differences in concentrations of Apo A-I and A-II between normal and gallstone patients, however, was not sufficient to explain the much longer nucleation times of native normal gallbladder bile[4,34].

Using various lectin affinity chromatography columns mixtures of inhibiting and promoting proteins have been partially purified from normal human gallbladder bile[35]. All lectin-bound biliary protein factors exhibited promoting and inhibiting effects on cholesterol crystal growth, depending on the concentration tested. The concanavalin A reactive fraction proved to be enriched in promoting activity while the *Helix pomatia* reactive fraction was most enriched in inhibiting activity[35]. From the *Helix pomatia*-bound fraction the first specific inhibitor, a $\sim120\,kDa$ glycoprotein with subunits of $58/63\,kDa$, has been isolated from bile[36].

Isolation of inhibiting and promoting proteins from identical model bile suggests that a balance of antagonistic factors is important in cholesterol gallstone formation. In normal bile this balance is in favour of inhibition of cholesterol crystallization. In abnormal bile an imbalance of kinetic factors induced by either a deficiency of inhibitors or an excess of promoters may facilitate nucleation and cholesterol crystal growth[37,38].

CHOLESTEROL CRYSTAL BINDING PROTEINS

Differences in inhibiting activity, being higher for the *Heix pomatia*-bound fraction than determined for the isolated 120 kDa heterodimeric protein, indicate that additional inhibitors must be present in the lectin-bound biliary protein fractions. In trying to identify these proteins we assumed that inhibitors interact with the crystals, thus retarding cholesterol crystallization[39]. If this hypothesis is correct, it should be possible to isolate and identify inhibitor proteins with the aid of the crystals. In addition, crystal morphology should be changed when grown under the influence of the inhibitor proteins.

Biliary proteins were isolated from abnormal human gallbladder bile by affinity chromatography to concanavalin A or lentil lectins. Part of each bound fraction was further purified on a *Helix pomatia* lectin column. Aliquots of each of these four different lectin-bound fractions were added to supersaturated model bile. At the end of crystal growth, as monitored by the growth assay, cholesterol crystals were harvested by filtration, washed with buffer and resolubilized in organic solvent. The proteins bound to the harvested crystals were recovered after removal of cholesterol by diafiltration and ultrafiltration steps. Despite significant differences between the four lectin-bound fractions added to the growth experiment we isolated the same subgroup of crystal-bound proteins as determined by SDS-PAGE. The major protein band represents the known 58/63 kDa heterodimer. In addition, protein bands with molecular weights of about 74, 28 and 16 kDa were identified. Proteins of each band were isolated by preparative SDS-PAGE from the *Helix pomatia*-bound fraction and tested in the crystal growth assay. All four proteins proved to be potent inhibitors of cholesterol crystallization. Resolving the proteins by 2D-electrophoresis, we found in each band isoforms ranging from pH 4.0 to 9.0. Only isoforms with isoelectric points between pH 6.5 and 8.5 bound to cholesterol crystals.

In parallel, aliquots of cholesterol crystals were examined by scanning electron microscopy during crystal growth. Scanning EM images of crystals grown under the influence of effector proteins showed mainly layer growth with parallel lamination, thus producing compact microliths. Without effector proteins polycyclic crystals with multiple screwed and stepwise dislocations were predominant. Microliths consist of irregular concrements and clusters formed by random aggregation of polycyclic crystals[40,41].

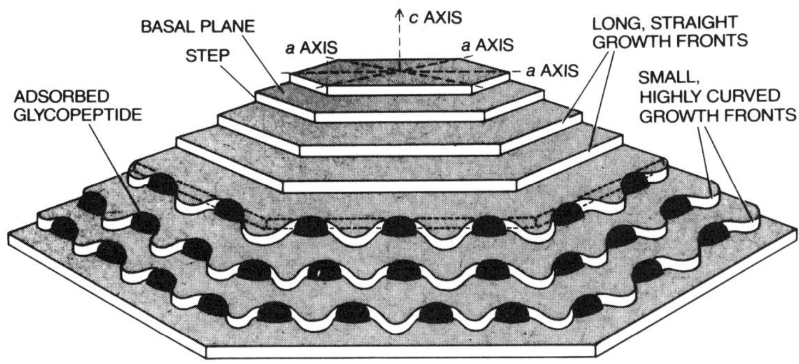

Fig. 2 Schematic of the putative action of 'antifreeze' glycoproteins as an example for crystal growth inhibition by proteins. Glycopeptides absorbed by ice probably impede crystal growth by inhibiting the normal propagation of ice-growth steps, or layers, across the crystal surface. An ice crystal grows when water molecules in the surrounding liquid join at steps on the basal (horizontal) plane of the crystal. Such steps start at the centre of the basal plane and normally grow outward in long, straight-edged fronts (shown as the top layers of the figure). In contrast, steps that meet glycopeptide antifreezes bound to the basal plane of an underlying step divide into many small fronts that become highly curved (lower layers of the figure). Such curved fronts have a high ratio of surface area to volume, a condition that halts their growth if the temperature of the surrounding liquid does not fall. Exactly how the antifreeze molecules bind to an ice crystal is not known. (From DeVries AL, Eastman JT. Antarctic fishes. Sci Am, November 1986, p. 112; with permission)

CONCLUSIONS

Human bile contains antagonistic protein factors promoting or inhibiting cholesterol crystallization, thus playing an imporant role in cholesterol gallstone formation. Evidence has been provided that promoter proteins target vesicle formation and aggregation[42]. On the other hand our results suggest that inhibiting activity is mediated by a new subgroup of lectin-bound biliary proteins binding to cholesterol crystals.

Concerning stone formation in humans other inhibitor proteins have been reported. Nakagawa *et al.* reported a 14 kDa glycoprotein that prevents formation of urinary calcium oxalate nephrolithiasis in healthy persons[43,44]. From human pancreatic calculi a small acidic glycoprotein has been isolated that showed an inhibiting effect on calcium carbonate precipitation[45,46]. Finally, Shimizu *et al.* were able to isolate from cholesterol gallstones a small (< 10 kDa) glycoprotein that tightly bound bile pigment and strongly inhibited precipitation of calcium carbonate *in vitro*[47].

Examples of crystal growth inhibiting glycoproteins are also found in sera of polar fish. These 'antifreeze proteins' prevent formation of ice even in the markedly subfreezing temperatures of the polar seas[48,49]. As illustrated in Fig. 2, it is believed that these glycopeptides absorbed by ice crystals impede crystal growth by inhibiting the regular propagation of ice growth layers across the crystal surface.

This concept probably applies to all crystal growth inhibitors in biomineralization. A growth inhibitor of cholesterol crystals may also attach itself to the most rapidly growing microdomains of a microcrystal (like spiral and edge dislocations) thus changing crystal morphology and retarding cholesterol crystallization.

Acknowledgement

This work was supported by grants Bu 822/1-1 and He 906/18-1 from the Deutsche Forschungsgemeinschaft.

References

1. Carey MC. Formation of cholesterol gallstones: the new paradigms. In: Paumgartner G, Stiehl A, Gerok W, editors. Trends in bile acid research. Dordrecht: Kluwer; 1988:259–81.
2. Carey MC, Cohen DE. Biliary transport of cholesterol in vesicles, micelles and liquid crystals. In: Paumgartner G, Stiehl A, Gerok W, editors. Bile acids and the liver. Lancaster: MTP Press; 1987:287–300.
3. Small DM, Bourges M, Dervichian DG. Ternary and quaternary aqueous systems containing bile salt, lecithin and cholesterol. Nature. 1966;211:816–18.
4. Bèhar J, Lee KY, Thompson WR, Biancani P. Gallbladder contraction in patients with pigment and cholesterol stones. Gastroenterology. 1989;97:1479–84.
5. Van der Werf SDJ, van Berge Henegouwen GP, Palsma DMH, Ruben AT. Motor function of the gallbladder and saturation of duodenal bile. Neth J Med. 1987;30:160–71.
6. Holzbach RT, Marsh M, Olszewski M, Holan KR. Cholesterol solubility in bile. Evidence that supersaturated bile is frequent in healthy man. J Clin Invest. 1973;52:1467–79.
7. Holan KR, Holzbach RT, Hermann RE, Cooperman AM, Claffey WJ. Nucleation time: a key factor in the pathogenesis of cholesterol gallstone disease. Gastroenterology. 1979;77:611–17.
8. Holzbach RT, Busch N. Nucleation and growth of cholesterol crystals. Kinetic determinants in supersaturated bile. Gastroenterol Clin N Am. 1991;20:67–83.
9. Small DM. Cholesterol nucleation and growth in gallstone formation. N Engl J Med. 1989;302:1305–7.
10. Carey MC, Small DM. The physical chemistry of cholesterol solubility in bile. J Clin Invest. 1978;61:988–1036.
11. Carey MC, LaMont JT. Cholesterol gallstone formation. 1. Physical-chemistry of bile and biliary lipid secretion. Prog Liver Dis. 1992;10:139–63.
12. Cohen DE, Carey MC. Physical chemistry of biliary lipids during bile formation. Hepatology. 1990;12:143S–8S.
13. Halpern Z, Dudley MA, Lynn MP, Nader JM, Breuer AC, Holzbach RT. Vesicle aggregation in model systems of supersaturated bile: relation to crystal nucleation and lipid composition of the vesicular phase. J Lipid Res. 1986;27:295–306.
14. Halpern Z, Dudley MA, Kibe A, Lynn MP, Breuer AC, Holzbach RT. Rapid vesicle formation and aggregation in abnormal human bile. Gastroenterology. 1986;90:875–85.
15. Konikoff FM, Chung DS, Donovan JM, Small DM, Carey MC. Filamentous, helical, and tubular microstructures during cholesterol crystallization from bile: Evidence that cholesterol does not nucleate classic monohydrate plates. J Clin Invest. 1992;90:1155–61.
16. Kibe A, Dudley MA, Halpern Z, Lynn MP, Breuer AC, Holzbach RT. Factors affecting cholesterol monohydrate nucleation time in model systems of supersaturated bile. J Lipid Res. 1985;26:1102–11.
17. Donovan JM, Carey MC. Physical-chemical basis of gallstone formation. Gastroenterol Clin N Am. 1991;20:47–66.
18. Cabral DJ, Small DM. Physical chemistry of bile. In: Schulz SG, Forte JG, Rauner BB, editors. Handbook of physiology – the gastrointestinal system. III. Section 6. Baltimore: American Physiological Society; 1989:621–62.
19. Busch N, Tokumo H, Holzbach RT. A sensitive method for determination of cholesterol crystal growth using model solutions of supersaturated bile. J Lipid Res. 1990;31:1903–9.
20. Sedaghat A, Grundy SM. Cholesterol crystals and the formation of cholesterol gallstones.

N Engl J Med. 1980;302:1274–7.

21. Holzbach RT, Kibe A, Thiel E, Howell LH, Marsh M, Hermann RE. Biliary proteins: unique inhibitors of cholesterol crystal nucleation in human gallbladder bile. J Clin Invest. 1984;73:35–45.

22. Burnstein JM, Ilson RG, Petrunka CN, Strasberg SM. Evidence for a potent nucleation factor in gallbladder bile of patients with cholesterol gallstones. Gastroenterology. 1984;85:801–7.

23. Gallinger S, Harvey PRC, Petrunka CN, Ilson RG, Strabserg SM. Biliary proteins and the nucleation defect in cholesterol cholelithiasis. Gastroenterology. 1987;92:867–75.

24. Jüngst D, Lang T, von Ritter C, Paumgartner G. Role of high total protein in gallbladder bile in formation of cholesterol gallstones. Gastroenterology. 1991;100:1724–9.

25. Gallinger S, Taylor RD, Harvey PRC, Strasberg SM. Effect of mucous glycoprotein on nucleation time of human bile. Gastroenterology. 1985;89:648–58.

26. Smith BF. Human gallbladder mucin binds biliary lipids and promotes cholesterol crystal nucleation in model bile. J Lipid Res. 1987;28:1088–97.

27. Lee SP, Maher K, Nichols JF. Origin and fate of biliary sludge. Gastroenterology. 1988;94:170–8.

28. Groen AK, Noordam C, Drapers JAG, Egbers P, Jansen PLM, Tytgat GNJ. Isolation of a potent cholesterol nucleation promoting activity from human gallbladder bile. Hepatology. 1990;11:525–33.

29. Offner GD, Gong D, Afdahl NH. Identification of a 130-kilodalton human biliary Concanavalin A binding protein as aminopeptidase N. Gastroenterology. 1994;106:755–62.

30. Harvey PRC, Upadhya GA, Strasberg SM. Immunoglobulins as nucleating proteins in the gallbladder bile of patients with cholesterol gallstones. J Biol Chem. 1991;266:13996–4003.

31. Pattinson NR, Willis KE. Effect of phospholipase C on cholesterol solubilization in model bile. A Concanavalin A-binding nucleation-promoting factor from human gallbladder bile. Gastroenterology. 1991;101:1339–44.

32. Abei M, Kawczak P, Nuutinen H, Langnas A, Svanvik J, Holzbach RT. Isolation and characterization of a cholesterol crystallization promoter from human bile. Gastroenterology. 1993;104:539–48.

33. Kibe A, Holzbach RT, LaRusso NF, Mao SJT. Inhibition of cholesterol crystal formation by apolipoproteins in supersaturated model bile. Science (Wash, DC). 1984;225:514–16.

34. Sewell RB, Mao SJ, Kawamoto T, LaRusso NF. Apolipoproteins of high, low, and very low density lipoproteins in human bile. J Lipid Res. 1983;24:391–401.

35. Busch N, Matiuck N, Sahlin S, Holzbach RT. Inhibition and promotion of cholesterol crystallization by protein fractions from normal human gallbladder bile. J Lipid Res. 1991;32:695–702.

36. Ohya T, Schwarzendrubè J, Busch N *et al.* A human biliary glycoprotein that inhibits nucleation and growth of cholesterol crystals. Purification and characterization. Gastroenterology. 1993;104:527–38.

37. Paumgartner G, Sauerbruch T. Gallstones – pathogenesis. Lancet. 1991;338:1117–21.

38. Busch N, Matern S. Current concepts in cholesterol gallstone pathogenesis. Eur J Clin Invest. 1991;21:453–60.

39. Busch N, Holzbach RT. Crystal growth-inhibiting proteins in bile. Hepatology. 1990;12:195S–8S.

40. Busch N, Lammert F, Matern S. A subgroup of lectin bound biliary proteins attaches to cholesterol crystals and modifies crystal morphology. Hepatology. 1992;16:A320.

41. Busch N, Lammert F, Marschall HU, Matern S. Isolation of a new potent inhibitor protein of cholesterol crystal growth from human bile. Hepatology. 1993;18:A158.

42. Groen AK, Ottenhoff R, Jansen PLM, van Marle J, Tytgat GNJ. Effect of cholesterol nucleation-promoting activity on cholesterol solubilization in model bile. J Lipid Res. 1989;30:51–8.

43. Nakagawa Y, Abram V, Krezdy FJ, Kaiser ET, Coe FL. Purification and characterization of the principal inhibitor of calcium oxalate monohydrate crystal growth in human urine. J Biol Chem. 1983;258:12594–600.

44. Nakagawa Y, Ahmed M, Hall SL, Deganello S, Coe FL. Isolation from human calcium oxalate renal stones of nephrocalcin, a glycoprotein inhibitor of calcium oxalate crystal growth: evidence that nephrocalcin from patients with calcium oxalate nephrolithiasis is deficient in gamma-carboxyglutamic acid. J Clin Invest. 1987;79:1782–7.

45. De Caro A, Multigner L, Lafont H, Lambardo D, Sarles H. The molecular characteristics of human pancreatic acidic phosphoprotein that inhibits calcium carbonate crystal growth. Biochem J. 1984;222:669–77.
46. Montalto G, Bonicel J, Multigner L, Rovery M, Sarles H, De Caro A. Partial amino acid sequence of human pancreatic stone protein, a novel pancreatic secretory protein. Biochem J. 1986;238:227–32.
47. Shimizu S, Sabsay B, Veis A, Ostrow JD, Rege RV, Dawes LG. Isolation of an acidic protein from cholesterol gallstones, which inhibits precipitation of calcium carbonate *in vitro*. J Clin Invest. 1989;84:1990–6.
48. De Vries AL. Antifreeze peptides and glycopeptides in coldwater fishes. Annu Rev Physiol. 1983;45:245–60.
49. De Vries AL. Antifreeze glycopeptides and peptides: interactions with ice and water. Methods Enzymol. 1986;127:293–303.

16
Cholesterol crystal nucleation in bile: role of protein hydrophobicity*

H. A. AHMED, M. L. PETRONI, M. ABU-HAMIDIYYAH,
R. P. JAZRAWI and T. C. NORTHFIELD

INTRODUCTION

Cholesterol nucleation (appearance of cholesterol monohydrate crystals) has a close relationship to the pathogenesis of cholesterol gallstone disease. It has been shown that human bile contains proteins that can enhance or inhibit cholesterol nucleation. Human gallbladder mucin has been shown to accelerate nucleation in model bile[1]. The number of crystals depends on mucin concentration and incubation time. Human biliary α_1-acid glycoprotein, an extensively glycosylated protein with an isoelectric point of less than 4.1, is reported to have a pronucleator activity which decreases in proportion to successive removal of terminal glycans[2]. A purified heat-labile human mucus glycoprotein accelerates nucleation in human bile. However, its pronucleator activity is not different in gallstone patients from control subjects[3]. A concanavalin-A binding non-mucus glycoprotein from human bile has been shown to have cholesterol nucleation-promoting activity, to induce the transfer of cholesterol and phospholipid from micellar to vesicular phase, and to stimulate cholesterol nucleation from vesicles[4,5]. This protein is rich in glucose and/or mannose, but not N-acetylglucosamine or N-acetylneuraminic acid (sialic acid)[6]. T-Tube hepatic bile contains both nucleation-promoting and -inhibiting activities in concanavalin A-unbound fraction, while the bound fraction has only nucleation-promoting activities[7]. The concanavalin A-bound pronucleating activity is found in gallbladder bile from cholesterol and pigment gallstone patients as well as from control subjects; and it is higher only in bile from patients with multiple cholesterol gallstones[5].

Thus, both pronucleating and antinucleating activities can coexist in the same bile sample. The propensity of a bile sample to nucleate depends on the balance of these promoting and inhibiting activities[6]. Phospholipase C

---

*This review article is based on our paper entitled: Hydrophobic/hydrophilic balance of proteins: a major determinant of cholesterol crystal formation in bile. J Lipid Res. 1994;35:211–19.

has been reported to shorten nucleation time, whereas phospholipase A2 has been shown to prolong it[8,9], though at relatively high concentrations. The effects are not related to phospholipase activity. Phospholipase C enhances the transfer of cholesterol and phospholipid from micellar to vesicular phase. The immunoglobulin molecules IgM and IgA from human bile, as identified by amino acid sequencing and immunostaining of Western blots, are reported to have pronucleator activities[10]. Moreover, activities were higher in bile from cholesterol gallstone patients than from control subjects. An immunoglobulin complex, rather than an immunoglobulin, has also been suggested (though not proven), to be a pronucleator effector. A group of glycoproteins with molecular mass of 52–200 kDa are reported to be associated with biliary vesicles separated by ultracentrifugation and gel filtration. They constitute less than 1% by weight of biliary proteins. When these vesicles (with the associated glycoproteins) were added to supersaturated model bile, a pronucleating effect was demonstrated[11]. The effect was not related to the lipid composition or cholesterol content of the vesicles. Another group of non-mucus glycoproteins with molecular weight of 10, 15, 17, 22, 28 and 208 kDa have also been reported to have pronucleating activities[12]. Western blot analysis confirmed the identity of the 22 and 28 kDa glycoproteins as immunoglobulin Fab fragments. Recently, an aminopeptidase has been reported to promote cholesterol nucleation in bile[13].

Antinucleating proteins have been less extensively studied. Recently, a concanavalin-A bound, 42 kDa lipoprotein has been found to have antinucleating activity[14]. Interestingly, the apolipoproteins A-I and A-II have been shown to inhibit cholesterol crystal formation in model bile[15]. However, their concentrations in bile seem not to differ between normal and gallstone subjects[16].

The mechanism for cholesterol crystal formation in human bile seems to follow a specific pathway, in which cholesterol is transported from micellar to vesicular form, which is the immediate supplier of cholesterol for crystal formation[17–22]. Moreover, the percentage of total gallbladder bile cholesterol carried in the vesicles is significantly higher in gallstone patients than in control subjects[22]. The nucleation time is related to vesicular cholesterol concentration. It would be logical for pronucleators to enhance this transfer, and for antinucleators to inhibit or even reverse it.

We hypothesized that the nucleation phenomenon could be non-specific, related to the overall physicochemical characteristics of biliary proteins. We therefore studied the effect of a group of non-specific proteins on cholesterol crystal formation in two model biles, with different cholesterol saturation indices (CSI).

MODEL BILE PREPARATION

Two model biles were prepared according to Kibe et al.[23], substituting Tris-HCl 25 mmol/l, pH 7.4 (37°C), containing 145 mmol/l sodium chloride, 5 mmol/l calcium chloride and 3 mmol/l sodium azide for the Hepes buffer and adjusting the total lipids to 200 g/l (to be diluted 1 : 1 in buffer at the

Table 1 Secondary structure of the proteins used (percentages)[37-40]

Protein coil	a-*Helix*	b-*Pleated sheets*	*Random*
Concanavalin-A	0	72	28
Albumin (bovine)	66	3	31
Chymotrypsin	4	86	10
Chymotrypsinogen	9	36	55
Myoglobin	77	2	21
IgA		Mostly b-sheets	
IgG		Mostly b-sheets	
IgM		Mostly b-sheets	
Apo A-I	70	10	20
Apo A-II	69	11	20
Apo B	25	37	38

time of use). The final concentrations of phosphatidylcholine, cholesterol and sodium taurocholate were 79, 29 and 235 mmol/l, to give a final CSI of 1.2; and 72, 37, 220 mmol/l to give a final CSI of 1.5, respectively[24]. All model bile samples were initially isotropic (crystal-free) on microscopic examination (400 ×) under polarized light using a heating stage (37°C). Under these experimental conditions the nucleation time of model bile was 7 days for the bile with CSI = 1.2, and 5 days for the bile with CSI = 1.5.

NUCLEATION TIME DETERMINATION

Cholesterol nucleation time was determined in model bile as previously described[25] by daily checking of a 10 μl sample for the appearance of cholesterol monohydrate crystals. Samples that did not nucleate by 21 days were arbitrarily considered to have a nucleation time of 22 days. The effect on nucleation time of non-specific proteins (Table 1) at different concentrations (Figs 1 and 2) was checked in six samples for each protein. The model bile was mixed 1:1 with buffer containing double the desired concentration of each of the proteins studied. The effect on crystal promotion or inhibition was expressed as a percentage of nucleation time of control.

HYDROPHOBIC INTERACTION CHROMATOGRAPHY

The hydrophobicity index for the various proteins was determined by measuring their retention time on a phenyl-agarose column[26]. The protein (2 mg) was loaded on 5.0 ml of phenyl-agarose and eluted using ammonium sulphate gradient (2.00–10.10 mol/l in 0.01–0.05 mol/l sodium phosphate, pH 7). Proteins were ranked according to their elution volume.

Gel-permeation chromatography

Micelles and vesicles in model bile were separated by gel-permeation chromatography as described[27]. Aliquots of 150 mCi of [³H]cholesterol and

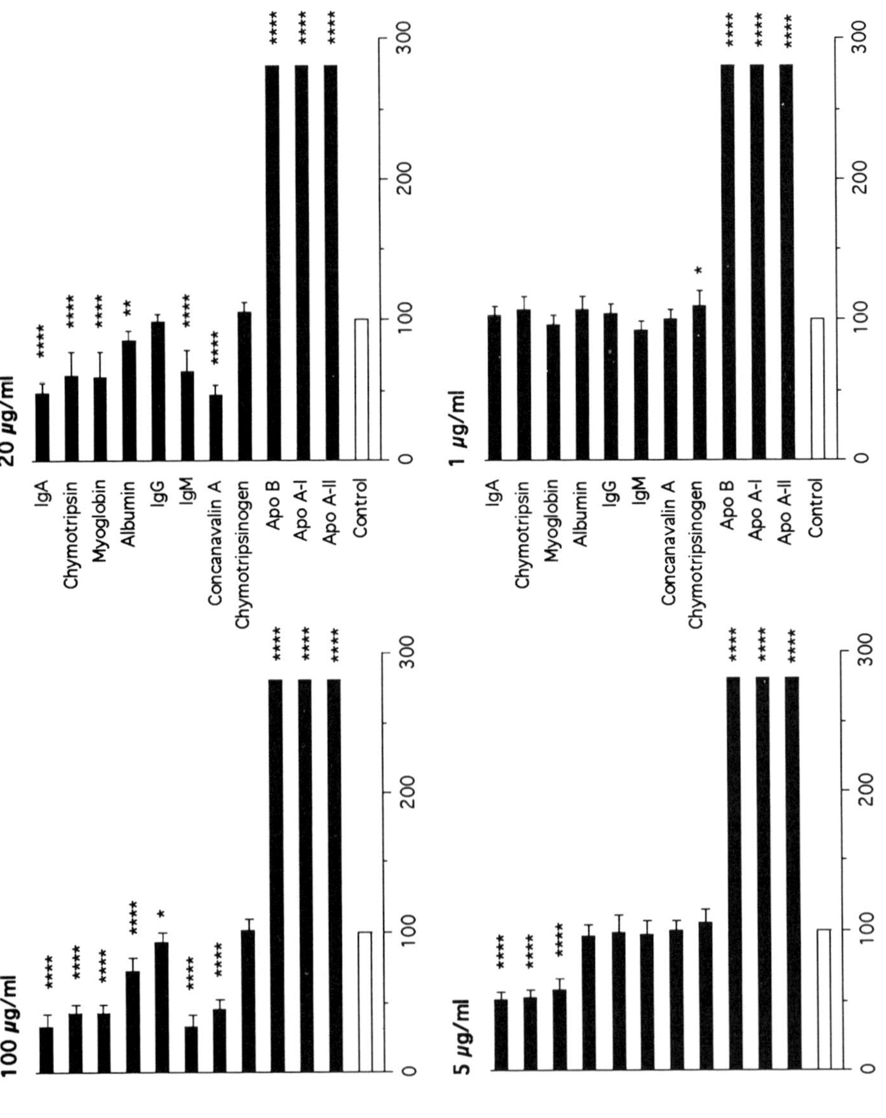

Fig. 1 Effect of non-specific proteins on cholesterol nucleation in model bile with CSI = 1.2. Results expressed as percentage of control: pronucleators had values less than 100%, while antinucleators had values more than 100%. Statistical significance levels (vs control) are expressed as follows: $*p < 0.05$, $**p < 0.01$, $***p < 0.005$; $****p < 0.001$

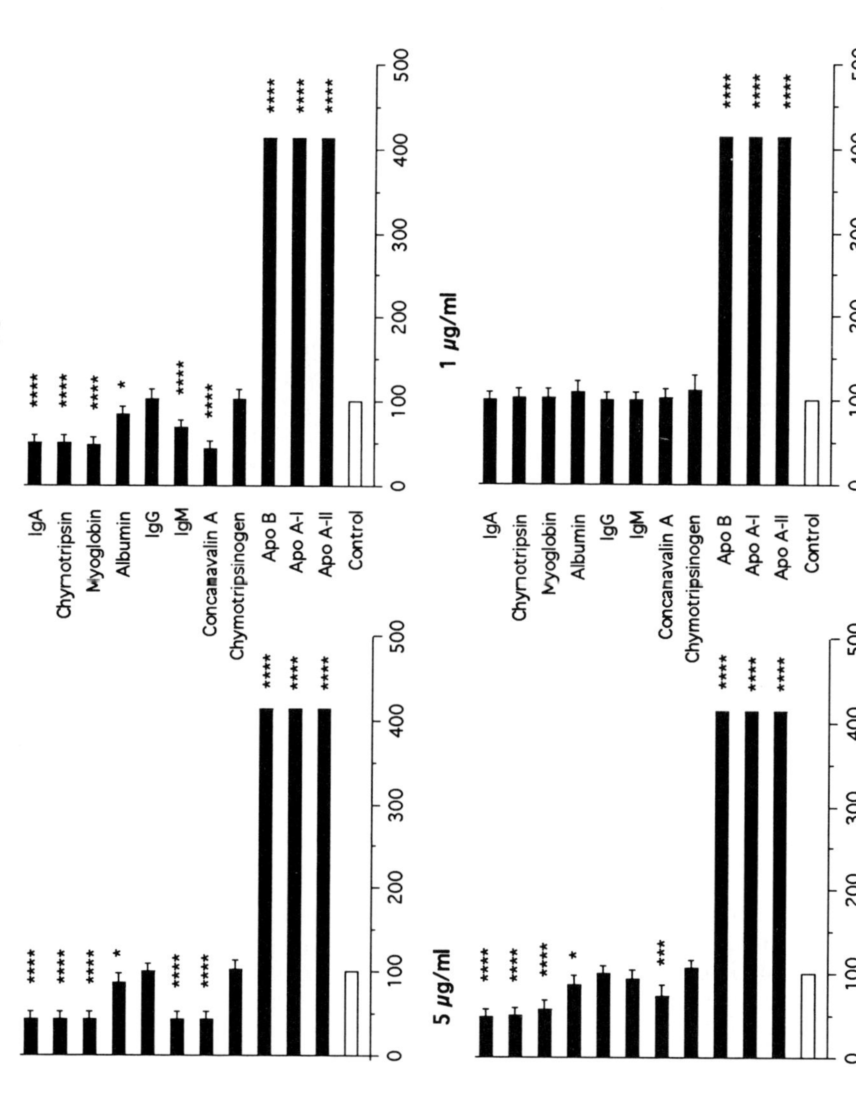

Fig. 2 Effect of non-specific proteins on cholesterol nucleation in model bile with CSI = 1.5. Results expressed as percentage of control: pronucleators had values less than 100%, while antinucleators had values more than 100%. Statistical significance levels (vs control) are expressed as follows: $*p < 0.05$, $**p < 0.01$; $***p < 0.005$; $****p < 0.001$

Table 2 Hydrophobic/hydrophilic rank of non-specific proteins (retention on phenyl-agarose)

Protein	Elution volume (ml)
IgA	30
Chymotrypsin	30
Myoglobin	40
Concanavalin-A	47
Albumin	50
IgG	50
IgM	56
Chymotrypsinogen	60
Apo B	76
Apo A-I	86
Apo A-II	89

100 mCi of $[^{14}C]$phosphatidylcholine were added to biliary lipids at the time of model bile preparation. The model bile (with or without proteins) was incubated at 37°C and 0.5 ml aliquots were taken out at time zero and after 2, 7 and 30 days to be fractionated by gel filtration chromatography on Sepharose 6B. Fractions (3 ml) were collected and 50 ml aliquots were counted for the DPM from $[^{3}H]$cholesterol and $[^{14}C]$phosphatidylcholine. The vesicular and micellar cholesterol distribution was expressed as percentage area under the curve.

Statistical analysis

Results were expressed as mean $\pm$ SEM. Correlation coefficients were calculated using Spearman's rank correlation (R_s). Nucleation times were expressed as a percentage of control values and the unpaired Student's t-test was used to compare the different proteins. Differences were considered significant for a p value of <0.05. Area under the curve was used to calculate percentage cholesterol distribution in the vesicular and micellar fractions.

RESULTS AND DISCUSSION

Our results concerning the effect of proteins on cholesterol crystal formation in the two model bile preparations studied (Figs 1 and 2) are consistent with the hypothesis that the activity of proteins as pro- or antinucleators is a non-specific phenomenon related to the physicochemical properties of the proteins rather than a specific, enzyme-substrate-like mechanism. Interestingly, Pattinson *et al.* subjected native biliary proteins to pronase digestion and reported that this had no effect on nucleation time in gallbladder bile from cholesterol gallstone patients, non-gallstone patients and common bile duct bile from cholesterol gallstone patients[28]. These results might seem to argue against the importance of proteins in general for cholesterol nucleation in bile. However, according to these authors, not all biliary proteins were hydrolysed, and it could be argued that either the pro- or antinucleating proteins are pronase-resistant (and this has already been demonstrated for some pronucleating proteins[7]), or that an effect on nucleation time could be produced by a very small protein concentration. Furthermore, since pronase is an endopeptidase, its action will not result in complete digestion of proteins, but will convert them into shorter peptides, as shown by the excellent electrophoretic pattern in the report. These peptides can still be quantitatively, and possibly also qualitatively, different if the original protein families (pronase substrates) were also different. The shorter peptides seem to retain the overall pro- or antinucleating effect of their original larger protein families. We think, therefore, that the results in this report argue against a specific effect for proteins on nucleation time, rather than against a non-specific effect.

The proteins we studied were different in their hydrophobic indices as measured by retention on phenyl-agarose and also in their secondary structure. Myoglobin, chymotrypsin and IgA were the most potent pronucleators, while the apolipoproteins A-I, A-II and B were clearly antinucleators under the experimental conditions. Other proteins showed less pronounced pronucleating or antinucleating activities. The effect of proteins on cholesterol nucleation time was similar in both model bile preparations, despite the different CSI used, the only exception being two of the intermediate-rank proteins (albumin and concanavalin-A) which were more active at the higher CSI, for which they showed a significant pronucleating effect down to a concentration of 5 μg/ml.

These pro- or antinucleating effects of the proteins studied did not seem to relate to their secondary structure (Table 1). Myoglobin (77% a-helix) and chymotrypsin ($> 80\%$ b-pleated sheets) were both potent pronucleators, while all three apolipoproteins (which differed in their secondary structures) were effective antinucleators.

The proteins were also examined with regard to the relationship between their individual hydrophobicity and their effect on cholesterol nucleation time. The proteins were ranked according to their retention on a hydrophobic ligand column (phenyl-agarose). This procedure, in contrast to reverse-phase HPLC, does not entail the use of organic solvents, so that the proteins are kept in their intact native state[29]. The data obtained are more reliable than the calculated hydrophobic indices, which do not take into account the folded nature of the protein structure and assume that values predicted from amino acid hydrophobicity can be extrapolated to protein hydrophobicity[30,31]. We found that the more hydrophobic proteins (apolipoprotein A-I, A-II and B) inhibited, while the more hydrophilic proteins (chymotrypsin, myoglobin and IgA) enhanced the process of cholesterol nucleation in model bile. Intermediate-rank proteins for effect on nucleation time were also intermediate on the hydrophobic scale (Fig. 3). These results were largely consistent for both model bile preparations studied.

As is evident from the results using albumin and concanavalin-A, a protein could be a potent pronucleator at a relatively high concentration, but lose this property at a lower concentration (Fig. 1), as if an effective increase in the hydrophobicity occurs. It has been shown that hydrophobic interactions between some proteins (β-lactoglobulin, bovine and human serum albumin,

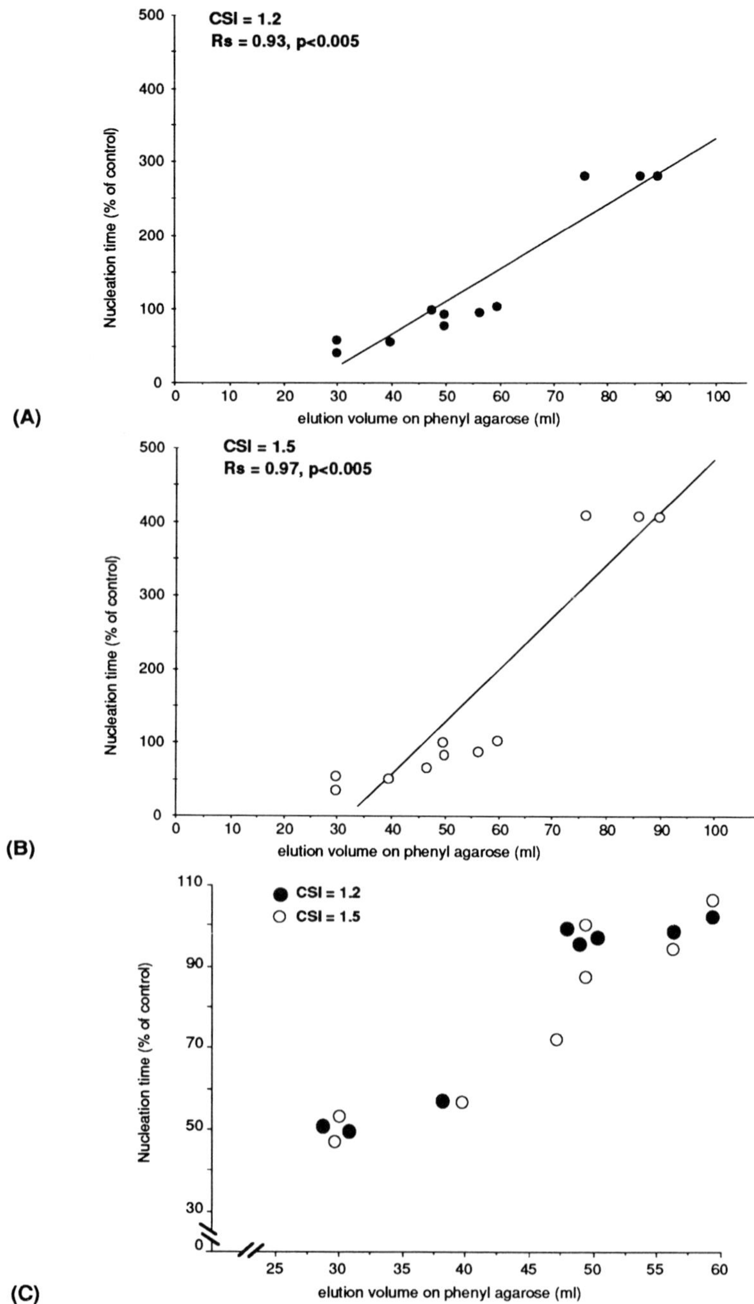

Fig. 3 Correlation of nucleation time (percentage of control) in model bile having CSI = 1.2 (**A**) and 1.5 (**B**) for a protein concentration of 5 μg/ml with the elution volume (ml) of proteins from phenyl-agarose column as an index of protein hydrophobicity. Section (**C**) shows the same correlations omitting the arbitrary values for apolipoproteins. R_s indicates Spearman's rank correlation coefficient

human transferrin, lysozyme) and long-chain alcohols (C_{8-12}) are increased on protein dilution[32,33]. This might explain the loss of pronucleating activity at the low concentrations studied. Alternatively, a critical protein concentration might be required to demonstrate the pronucleator effect under the experimental conditions. On the other hand, with apolipoprotein dilution, the absolute concentration of the protein decreases, but also the degree of self-association decreases, thus exposing more hydrophobic surfaces originally used in self-association[34]. These effects are likely to counterbalance each other, thus preserving the antinucleating effect of the apolipoproteins studied at the lowest concentrations used.

Most workers in the area agree that cholesterol is present in bile mainly in micellar and vesicular forms, with the latter working as the immediate supplier of cholesterol for crystal formation. Pronucleating proteins are expected to enhance the transfer of cholesterol from the more stable form (micelles) into the less stable form (vesicles), while the antinucleating proteins inhibit or possibly reverse this process. In our experiments (Fig. 4, Table 3), the pronucleating protein (myoglobin) enhanced the transfer of cholesterol from micellar to vesicular form to a greater extent compared to albumin and control bile, while the antinucleating protein (apolipoprotein A-I) reversed this process. Earlier work from Groen et al.[4], using a density-gradient centrifugation technique carried out at a single time interval (48 h), suggested that the concanavalin-A-bound fraction of bile from cholesterol gallstone patients increases the amount of vesicular cholesterol and phospholipid, and also induces nucleation of cholesterol from the vesicular fraction. More recently, Ginanni Corradini et al.[35] showed an inverse correlation between the amount of native gallbladder bile proteins (in both cholesterol gallstone patients and controls) and the cholesterol nucleation of both whole bile and isolated micellar fractions. Using a similar technique to the one we used, they also showed that native biliary proteins induce phasing out and redistribution of micellar cholesterol and lecithin towards vesicles.

The effect of myoglobin, albumin and apolipoprotein A-I on the cholesterol: phospholipid molar ratio in vesicular and micellar fractions from model bile (CSI = 1.2) was studied. With myoglobin the vesicular cholesterol: phospholipid ratio increased rapidly over the first 2 days of incubation and stayed stationary thereafter, while with albumin and control bile the increase occurred over the first 7 days. With apolipoprotein A-I the vesicular cholesterol: phospholipid ratio increased to a smaller extent and apparently over the whole 30 days of study. Since cholesterol was shown to be transferred from micellar to vesicular form with myoglobin, albumin and control bile, the increase in cholesterol: phospholipid ratio can be explained by increased vesicular cholesterol content. With apolipoprotein A-I the cholesterol was shown to be transferred from the vesicular to the micellar form; so the small increase in the vesicular cholesterol: phospholipid ratio is likely to be due to faster transfer of phospholipid from the vesicles to the micelles. However, this needs to be further investigated. The overall recovery of cholesterol in both micellar and vesicular phases dropped from 95% at day 2 for all the samples studied to about 80% at 7 days for control bile and with albumin. With myoglobin the recovery dropped to 65% at 7 days, while with

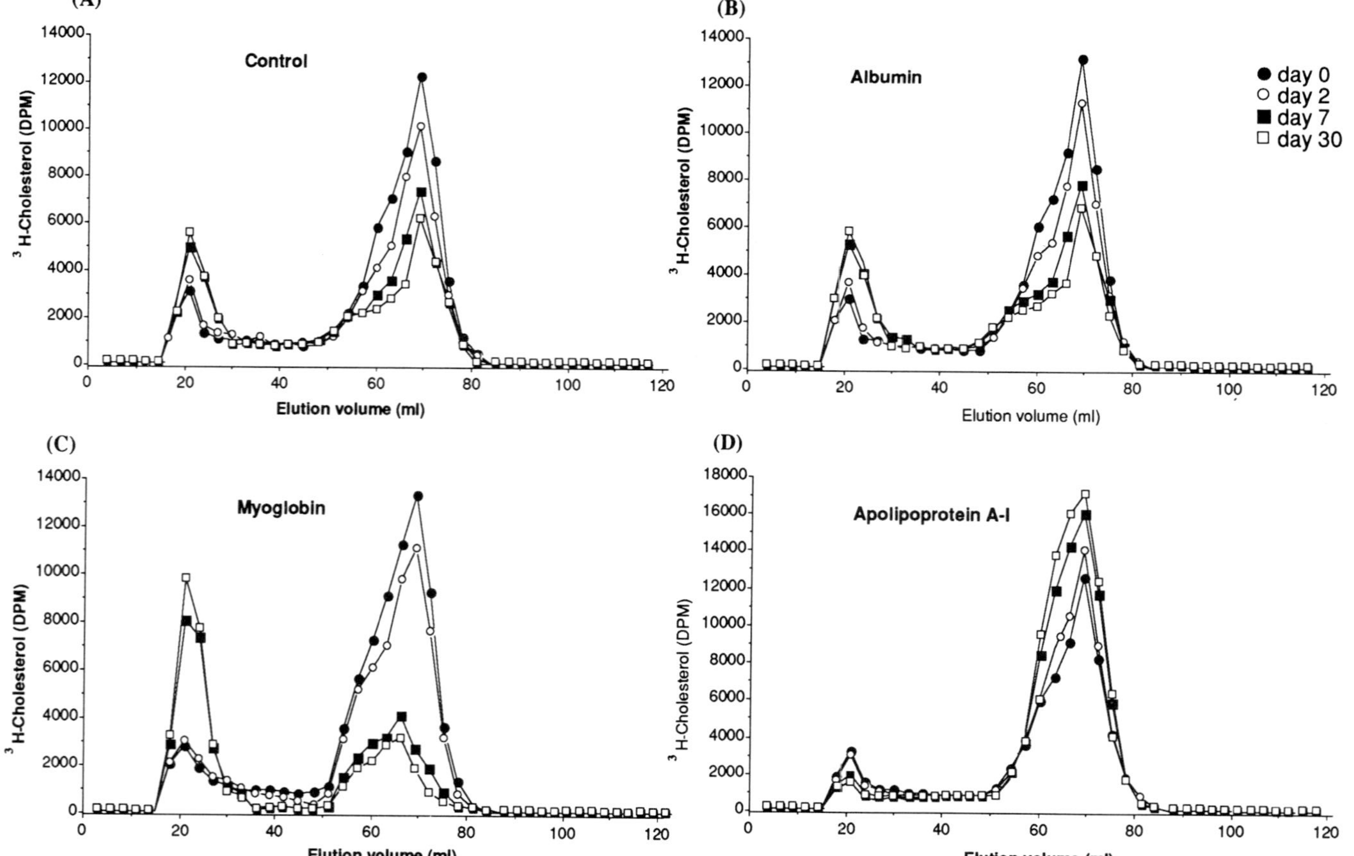

Fig. 4 Separation of vesicular and micellar phases in model bile (CSI = 1.2) on Sepharose 6-B after 0, 2, 7 and 30 days of incubation for control, albumin, myoglobin and apolipoprotein A-I. The experiment has been performed once for each protein at the specified times using a protein concentration of $20\,\mu g/ml$. Myoglobin enhanced the transfer of cholesterol from vesicles to micelles to a greater extent than albumin and control, while apolipoprotein

Table 3 Effect of proteins on vesicular:micellar cholesterol distribution in model bile at CSI = 1.2 (protein concentration of 20 μg/ml)

Incubation time (days)	Control	Albumin	Myoglobin	Apolipoprotein A-I
0	0.19	0.19	0.19	0.19
2	0.27	0.24	0.23	0.16
7	0.47	0.47	1.09	0.10
30	0.54	0.56	1.57	0.08

Table 4 Effect of proteins on the cholesterol:phospholipid molar ratio in vesicular (V) and micellar (M) fractions in model bile (CSI = 1.2)

Incubation time (days)	Control		Albumin		Myoglobin		Apolipoprotein A-I	
	V	M	V	M	V	M	V	M
0	2.1	0.54	2.1	0.54	2.1	0.54	2.1	0.54
2	2.7	0.49	2.9	0.46	3.3	0.31	2.4	0.52
7	3.3	0.40	3.2	0.37	3.4	0.32	2.3	0.50
30	3.2	0.33	3.3	0.30	3.2	0.30	2.6	0.51

apolipoprotein A-I the recovery stayed virtually unchanged at 95%. The drop in cholesterol recovery clearly parallels the pro- or antinucleating activities of the proteins studied. The micellar cholesterol:phospholipid ratio was decreasing throughout the time-course of the experiment for myoglobin, albumin and control bile (Table 4); though the drop was quicker for myoglobin. With apolipoprotein A-I there was a little decrease over the time-course of the experiment, though to a much smaller extent than with the other proteins and control bile. It has already been shown that apolipoproteins are essential for the stability of lipid aggregates in plasma lipoproteins[36]. Thus, it could be speculated that the hydrophobic antinucleating proteins, possibly through co-solubilization at the micellar–water interphase, increase the micellar hydrophobic domain and hence the cholesterol-carrying capacity. They can also possibly act as cholesterol carriers themselves. On the other hand, the hydrophilic pronucleating proteins not only fail to stabilize the micellar aggregates, but may also help vesicular aggregation (a prerequisite for cholesterol nucleation) through electrostatic interactions between their carbohydrate chains, since most pronucleating proteins in bile were shown to be glycoproteins.

In conclusion, our *in-vitro* experiments are consistent with the hypothesis that the effect of proteins on cholesterol nucleation in supersaturated model bile is non-specific and related to the individual protein hydrophobicity. This effect is mediated through alteration of the transfer of cholesterol from micellar to vesicular form. One can speculate that, *in vivo*, the overall hydrophobic/hydrophilic balance of biliary proteins would control the vesicular:micellar cholesterol equilibrium. If the overall balance shifts towards predominant hydrophobicity, cholesterol crystal formation is likely to occur, provided that the absolute and relative concentration of biliary lipids and other factors (e.g. gallbladder emptying) permit this event. On the other hand, if the balance shifts towards predominant hydrophobicity, cholesterol crystal formation is not likely to occur even in the presence of supersaturation.

References

1. Levy PF, Smith BF, LaMont JT. Human gallbladder mucin accelerates nucleation of cholesterol in artificial bile. Gastroenterology. 1984;87:270–5.
2. Abei M, Nuutinen H, Kawaczak P, Schwarzendrube J, Pillay SP, Holzbach T. Identification of human biliary α1-acid glycoprotein as a cholesterol crystallisation promoter. Gastroenterology. 1994;106:231–8.
3. Gallinger S, Taylor RD, Harvey PRC, Petrunka CN, Strasberg SM. Effect of mucous glycoprotein on nucleation time of human bile. Gastroenterology. 1985;89:648–58.
4. Groen AK, Ottenhoff R, Jansen PLM, van Marle J, Tytgat GNJ. Effect of cholesterol nucleation-promoting activity on cholesterol solubilisation in model bile. J Lipid Res. 1989;30:51–8.
5. Groen AK, Noordam CN, Drapers JAG, Egbers P, Jansen PLM, Tytgat GNJ. Isolation of a potent cholesterol nucleation-promoting activity from human gallbladder bile: role in the pathogenesis of gallstone disease. Hepatology. 1990;11:525–33.
6. Robert P, Harvey C, Upadhhya A, Toth JL, Strasberg SM. Lectin binding characteristics of a cholesterol nucleation promoting protein. Clin Chim Acta. 1989;185:185–90.
7. Groen AK, Stout JPJ, Drapers JAG, Hoek FJ, Grijm R, Tytgat GNJ. Cholesterol nucleation influencing activity in T-tube bile. Hepatology. 1988;8:347–52.
8. Groen AK, Noordam C, Drapers JAG, Egbers P, Hoek FJ, Tytgat GNJ. An appraisal of the role of biliary phospholipases in the pathogenesis of gallstone disease. Biochim Biophys Acta. 1989;1006:179–82.
9. Pattinson NR, Willis KE. Effect of phospholipase C on cholesterol solubilisation in model bile. A concanavalin A-binding nucleation promoting factor from human gallbladder bile. Gastroenterology. 1991;101:1339–44.
10. Harvey PRC, Upadhya GA, Strasberg SM. Immunoglobulins as nucleating proteins in the gallbladder bile of patients with cholesterol gallstones. J Biol Chem. 1991;266:13996–4003.
11. Miquel JF, Rigotti A, Rojas E, Brandan E, Nervi F. Isolation and purification of human vesicles with potent cholesterol-nucleation-promoting activity. Clin Sci. 1992;82:175–80.
12. Lipsett PA, Hildreth J, Kaufman HS, Lillemoe KD, Pitt HA. Human gallstones contain pronucleating nonmucin glycoproteins that are immunoglobulins. Ann Surg. 1994;219:25–33.
13. Nunez L, Amigo L, Rigotti A *et al.* Cholesterol crystallisation-promoting activity of aminopeptidase-N isolated from the vesicular carrier of biliary lipids. FEBS Lett. 1993;329:84–8.
14. Holzbach RT, Schwarzendrube J, Ohya T, Abei M, Busch N. Different biliary glycoproteins have opposing inhibiting or promoting effects on cholesterol crystallisation in gallstone pathogenesis. Meeting on pathochemistry, pathophysiology and pathomechanics of the biliary system. Bologna (Italy), 19–22 March 1992. Abstract book, p. 8.
15. Kibe A, Holzbach RT, LaRusso NF, Mao SJT. Inhibition of cholesterol crystal formation by apolipoproteins in supersaturated model bile. Science. 1984;225:514–16.
16. Sewell RB, Mao SJT, Kawamoto T, LaRusso NF. Apolipoproteins of high, low, and very low density lipoproteins in human bile. J Lipid Res. 1983;24:391–401.
17. Peled Y, Halpern Z, Eitan B, Goldman G, Konikoff F, Gilat T. Biliary micellar cholesterol nucleates via the vesicular pathway. Biochim Biophys Acta. 1989;1003:246–9.
18. Lee SP, Park HZ, Madani H, Kaler EW. Partial characterisation of a nonmicellar system of cholesterol solubilisation in bile. Am J Physiol. 1987;252:G374–83.
19. Halpern Z, Dudley MA, Kibe A, Lynn MP, Breuer AC, Holzbach RT. Vesicle aggregation in model systems of supersaturated bile: relation to crystal nucleation and lipid composition in the vesicular phase. J Lipid Res. 1986;27:295–306.
20. Harvey PRC, Somjen GJ, Lichtenberg SM, Petrunka CN, Gilat T, Strasberg CM. Nucleation of cholesterol from vesicles isolated from bile of patients with or without cholesterol

gallstones. Biochim Biophys Acta. 1987;921:198–204.
21. Peled Y, Halpern Z, Baruch R, Goldman G, Gilat T. Cholesterol nucleation from its carriers in human bile. Hepatology. 1988;8:914–18.
22. Schriever CE, Jungst D. Association between cholesterol-phospholipid vesicles and cholesterol crystals in human gallbladder bile. Hepatology. 1989;9:541–6.
23. Kibe A, Dudley MA, Halpern Z, Lynn MP, Breuer AC, Holzbach RT. Factors affecting cholesterol monohydrate crystal nucleation time in model system of supersaturated bile. J Lipid Res. 1985;26:1102–11.
24. Carey MC. Critical tables for calculating the cholesterol saturation of model bile. J Lipid Res. 1978;19:945–55.
25. Holan KR, Holzbach RT, Hermann RE, Cooperman AM, Claffey WJ. Nucleation time: a key factor in the pathogenesis of cholesterol gallstone disease. Gastroenterology. 1979;77:611–17.
26. Chicz RM, Regnier FE. High-performance liquid chromatography: effective protein purification by various chromatographic modes. In Deutscher MP, editor. Methods in enzymology, vol. 182. London: Academic Press, Harcourt Brace Jovanovich, 1990:409–14.
27. Somjen GJ, Gilat T. Contribution of vesicular and micellar carriers to cholesterol transport in human bile. J Lipid Res. 1985;26:699–704.
28. Pattinson NR, Willis KE. Nucleation of cholesterol crystals from native bile and the effect of protein hydrolysis. J Lipid Res. 1991;32:215–21.
29. Regnier FE. High-performance liquid chromatography of biopolymers. Science. 1983;222:245–52.
30. Kyte J, Doolittle RF. A simple method for displaying the hydropathic character of a protein. J Mol Biol. 1982;157:105–32.
31. Rose GD, Geselowitz AR, Lesser GJ, Lee RH, Zehfus MH. Hydrophobicity of amino acid residues in globular proteins. Science. 1985;229:834–8.
32. Abu-Hamdiyyah M, Kumari K. General anesthetic agents and the conformation of proteins. 2. Strengthening of hydrophobic interaction in β-lactoglobulin and the cutoff effect in anesthetic potency. Langmuir. 1989;7:81–8.
33. Abu-Hamdiyyah M. General anesthetic agents and the conformation of proteins. 4. Strengthening of hydrophobic interaction in bovine and human serum albumins, in human transferrin and in lysozyme by 1-alkanols and the cutoff effect in anesthetic potency. Langmuir. 1991;7:81–8.
34. Donovan JM, Brenedek GB, Carey MC. Self-association of human apolipoproteins A-I and A-II and interactions of apolipoprotein A-I with bile salts. Quasi-elastic light scattering studies. Biochemistry. 1987;26:8116–25.
35. Ginanni Corradini S, Alvaro D, Giacomelli L, Cedola M, Angelico M. Differential pattern of lipid–protein association in fast and slow cholesterol nucleating human gallbladder biles: implications for cholesterol nucleation from biliary lipid carriers. Biochim Biophys Acta. 1991;1086:125–33.
36. Pownall HJ, Massey JB, Sparrow JT, Gotto AM. Lipid–protein interactions and lipoprotein reassembly. In: Gotto AM, Jr, editor. Plasma lipoproteins. Amsterdam: Elsevier; 1987: 95–127.
37. LaRusso NF. Proteins in bile: how they get there and what they do. Am J Physiol. 1984;247:G199–205.
38. Levitt M, Chotia C. Structural patterns in globular proteins. Nature. 1976;261:552–8.
39. Schiffer M, Girling RL, Ely KR, Edmundson AB. Structure of α 1-type Bence-Jones protein at 3.5 Å resolution. Biochemistry. 1973;12:4620–31.
40. Epp O, Colman P, Fehlhammer H, Bode W, Schiffer M, Huber R. Crystals and molecular structure of a dimer composed of the variable portions of the Bence-Jones protein REI. Eur J Biochem. 1974;45:513–24.

17
Nutrition-associated cholestasis

P. B. SOETERS

INTRODUCTION

Intrahepatic cholestasis, occurring in severely ill patients, has often been ascribed to parenteral nutrition. Clinical observation, however, allows us to conclude that along with parenteral nutrition several other factors, alone or in concert, are responsible for the occurrence of intrahepatic cholestasis.

At one extreme, sepsis not primarily originating in the abdomen (for instance pneumococci pneumonia) may cause cholestasis *in the absence* of parenteral nutrition; at the other extreme, cholestasis may subside despite ongoing parenteral nutrition, for instance when a defunctionalized part of the distal small bowel is refunctionalized.

PATHOGENETIC FACTORS

Parenteral nutrition has been shown to diminish bile flow in dogs compared to postabsorptive controls. Nevertheless patients receiving long-term parenteral nutrition without sepsis or abdominal catastrophe do not develop overt cholestasis. Only very modest increases in γ-GT and AF do occur, if care is taken that patients are not overfed, do not receive more than 6 g glucose/kg per day and receive a well-tested and safe lipid emulsion. Some lipid emulsions, however, do cause, even in metabolically stable patients, a rapid (within 2–3 weeks) and severe cholestasis, sometimes accompanied by rises in transaminases as a sign of liver cell death.

The mechanisms involved appear to be related to deficient lipid clearance leading to steatosis, hypertriglyceridaemia, hyperphospholipidaemia and ultimately cholestasis. In severe and long-standing cholestasis fibrosis and cirrhosis may develop. Similar mechanisms may play a contributing role during sepsis, where lipid clearance has been shown to be compromised.

Besides purely nutritional factors there are also metabolic factors which contribute to intrahepatic cholestasis. Sepsis, a disturbed enterohepatic circulation with a diminished bile acid pool, lack of bile in the gut lumen, endotoxin resorption, depletion, and bacterial overgrowth – all seem to play a contributing role in the compromised excretion of bile by the liver. Whether there is one final common pathway is not certain. It is very likely, however, that toxic substances (for instance endotoxin resorbed from the gut) interfere directly or indirectly with the excretion of bile across the canalicular membrane.

All the proposed factors described are to some degree supported by experimental evidence, allowing study of every single factor separately. In the clinical situation this is difficult if not impossible. It is evident, however, that in most instances intrahepatic cholestasis is caused by a combination of factors.

MORBIDITY

Mild parenteral nutrition-associated intrahepatic cholestasis is a self-limiting disorder. In severe cases, and especially in paediatric patients, cirrhosis and liver failure may ensue. When the severity of cholestasis lies within these two extremes it is not certain what the functional consequences are with regard to specific liver function (clotting, synthesis of albumin and other proteins, etc.).

TREATMENT

The fact that there is a sliding scale should prompt us to treat cholestasis. Treatment should be tailored to the causative factors present in the individual patient, and may include: treatment of sepsis, restoration of intestinal continuity, refunctionalization of the gut in cases where there is a defunctionalized mucous small bowel stoma, treatment of bacterial growth, restoration of the bile acid pool, or bile flow to the intestine.

18
Cholestatic liver diseases in children

C. COLOMBO

INTRODUCTION

The great majority of paediatric cholestatic disorders are recognized during the first year of life because of jaundice with conjugated hyperbilirubinaemia. A significant proportion of these children will develop chronic liver disease, and will require liver transplantation[1,2].

The propensity of the infant to develop cholestasis in the presence of a wide variety of insults can be at least in part attributed to developmental immaturity of the liver, with particular regard to hepatic excretory function, which has been well documented by a series of experimental data[3]. A state of physiological cholestasis in early life is now recognized as characteristic of normal development. The best evidence of this immaturity in the human infant is provided by the pattern of serum bile acid concentrations, which are increased throughout the first year of life and attain normal adult values only at 3–4 years of age[4].

Several factors contribute to physiological cholestasis during development and these include quantitative and qualitative differences of bile acid synthesis, inefficient hepatic bile acid uptake, decreased hepatocellular secretion and ileal absorption of bile acids. The bile acid pool, synthetic rate and intraluminal bile acid concentrations are decreased in premature and full-term infants; in addition, a series of bile acids are produced by the immature liver, that are not normally found in the adult, indicating the existence of alternative pathways in bile acid synthesis in early life[5,6]. These synthetic pathways are also activated under cholestatic conditions later in life.

DIFFERENT FORMS OF CHOLESTASIS IN INFANCY

Cholestasis in infancy is caused by a heterogeneous group of disorders, which cause either extrahepatic cholestasis due to mechanical obstruction or intrahepatic cholestasis due to a functional disturbance of choleresis (Table 1). The intrahepatic disorders include congenital infections, specific metabolic diseases, familial intrahepatic cholestatic syndromes, endocrine

Table 1 Disorders associated with cholestasis in infancy

Intrahepatic	Extrahepatic
Infections, sepsis	Biliary atresia
Inborn errors of metabolism	Choledochal cyst
Familial syndromes	Choledocholithiasis
Vanishing bile duct syndromes	Anatomical abnormalities of the biliary tree
Chromosome anomalies	Bile/mucus plug
Drugs/parenteral nutrition	Sclerosing cholangitis
Endocrine/metabolic abnormalities	

and chromosomal abnormalities, toxic insults during sepsis or total parenteral nutrition. The vanishing bile duct syndromes can be recognized in early life and may be syndromic (in Alagille syndrome, paucity of intrahepatic bile ducts is variably associated with cardiovascular anomalies, a distinctive facial appearance, vertebral anomalies, and posterior embryotoxon), or non-syndromic, either idiopathic or associated with specific metabolic, infectious, or immunological disorders[7].

Biliary atresia is the main form of extrahepatic cholestasis in infancy and accounts for almost 50% of cases of neonatal liver diseases, but there are also other conditions, such as choledochal cysts or lithiasis, spontaneous perforation or stenosis of the common bile duct, and neonatal sclerosing cholangitis[8].

Although the clinical course of all these disorders may be highly heterogeneous, there is a considerable degree of overlap in clinical presentation and biochemical characteristics of intra- and extrahepatic cholestatic conditions in infancy. Indeed, most neonatal liver diseases present in a similar way, with jaundice, pruritus, variable degrees of lipid retention, fat malabsorption and growth retardation.

From the analysis of the larger published series of neonatal cholestasis, it has become evident that cryptogenic forms are predominant in infancy[9]. In fact, a specific treatable medical disease, such as galactosaemia, sepsis, or hypothyroidism, is responsible for cholestasis in less than 20% of cases; up to 10% are attributable to α_1-antitrypsin deficiency and around 5% to familial intrahepatic cholestatic syndromes. The most frequent disorders are 'idiopathic' neonatal hepatitis and extrahepatic biliary atresia, which can be recognized in up to 70% of infants. The term 'idiopathic obstructive cholangiopathies' has been proposed to indicate the spectrum of chronic cholestatic conditions of unknown aetiology in infancy, which include extrahepatic biliary atresia, neonatal sclerosing cholangitis, intrahepatic duct hypoplasia or paucity and neonatal idiopathic hepatitis. These conditions have been estimated to occur in a combined frequency of approximately one in 2000–3000 live births and are characterized by ongoing destruction of interlobular and/or extrahepatic bile ducts with progression to cirrhosis. Evolution from one form to the other has been well documented, thus suggesting the existence of a common pathogenetic insult, leading to progressive inflammation at various levels of the hepatobiliary tract; however this hypothesis remains to be proven[10].

Therefore, pathogenetic definition of cases of idiopathic cholestasis is a

Table 2 Treatable causes of neonatal cholestasis

Congenital infectious hepatitis	Herpes simplex virus
	Cytomegalovirus
	Syphilis
	Listeria monocytogenes
	Tuberculosis
	Toxoplasmosis
Metabolic diseases	Galactosaemia
	Hereditary tyrosinaemia
	Hereditary fructose intolerance
	Inborn errors of bile acid synthesis
	Cystic fibrosis
Endocrine diseases	Hypothyroidism/hypopituitarism
Toxic insults	Drugs, bacterial endotoxins, TPN
Anatomical lesions	Extrahepatic biliary atresia
	Choledochal cyst, spontaneous perforation
	Inspissated bile/stones in common bile duct

major challenge. In recent years, specific defects in bile acid synthesis[11] and in microfilament and organelle function[12] have been identified as specific entities among paediatric cholestatic liver diseases, particularly in cases with a pattern of intrafamilial recurrence and, in the future, congenital deficiency of bile acid transport proteins may eventually be discovered in a few patients with undefined cholestatic syndromes.

In children with the recently identified inborn errors of bile acid synthesis involving the steroid nucleus[11], the clinical presentation is often indistinguishable from other neonatal cholestatic syndromes. Histological findings are also non-specific and consistent with idiopathic neonatal hepatitis. Early diagnosis is of major importance since in these children oral bile acid therapy has been reported to be life-saving[11]. The absence of elevated serum bile acid concentrations, often with normal values of GGT, in an infant with cholestasis is highly suggestive[13]. Analysis of urinary bile acids by FAB-MS can demonstrate characteristic spectra of intermediates of bile acid synthesis[11,13].

EVALUATION OF INFANTS WITH CHOLESTASIS

There are several important goals in the evaluation of infants with cholestasis. First of all, specific infective, metabolic, and endocrine diseases susceptible of medical treatment must be identified and adequately treated (Table 2).

Differentiation of intrahepatic from extrahepatic cholestasis is an equally important goal: in fact, extrahepatic disorders, particularly biliary atresia, require early surgical intervention for optimal outcome. The probability of a successful Kasai portoenterostomy for biliary atresia improves if the infant is younger than 2 months at the time of surgery[14].

Therefore, in the diagnostic work-up of the infant with cholestasis a series of tests are usually performed in order to exclude infectious, metabolic and endocrine causes of cholestasis as well as to establish patency of the extrahepatic biliary tree. No biochemical test has been so far identified which can provide discriminant information. In contrast, the simple observation of stool colour is generally useful for this purpose, since the finding of persistently alcoholic stool is highly suggestive of extrahepatic obstruction, which will be confirmed by hepatobiliary scintigraphy, percutaneous liver biopsy, and eventually laparotomy and intraoperative cholangiography[1].

Liver biopsy, if correctly interpreted by an expert pathologist, provides the most reliable diagnostic information and permits the correct diagnosis in 90–95% of cases. The occurrence of portal fibrosis, bile duct proliferation and intraportal bile plugs is significantly more frequent in children with extrahepatic cholestasis.

TREATMENT OF CHOLESTATIC LIVER DISEASES IN CHILDHOOD

There is no specific treatment for most children with the progressive forms of intrahepatic cholestasis and for those with progressive cirrhosis, despite surgical intervention for extrahepatic biliary atresia.

In children with end-stage liver disease, liver transplantation remains the only therapeutic option for long-term survival[15]. In the future, another form of definitive therapy may be available for certain metabolic disorders: gene therapy for CF associated liver disease has been shown to be feasible in the experimental animal[16].

In children with chronic cholestasis, long-standing reduction of bile flow produces medical and nutritional consequences which have a negative impact on the quality of life. The establishment of empirical therapeutic regimens directed to enhance bile flow and to contrast the consequences of chronic cholestasis is therefore of major importance[17].

During cholestasis, retention of constituents of bile may result in jaundice, pruritus and xanthomatosis; reduced intraluminal bile acid concentrations cause malabsorption and malnutrition. Finally intrahepatic accumulation of hepatotoxic compounds is considered important in the progression of fibrosis and cirrhosis.

A few therapeutic strategies have been proposed in the attempt to limit the progression of liver damage. Colchicine has been employed in the attempt to limit fibrogenesis, but the results of treatment have been disappointing[18]. Oral bile acid therapy is presently under evaluation[19-39].

Ursodeoxycholic acid treatment in paediatric cholestatic disease

A possible pathogenetic mechanism of liver damage in cholestatic liver diseases is the intracellular accumulation of detergent endogenous bile acids, which may damage cell membranes, induce oxygen radical formation or increase intracellular calcium[19]. In the assumption that replacement of these compounds with a non-toxic bile acid may be beneficial, UDCA therapy has

Table 3 Effects of ursodeoxycholic acid treatment in children with intrahepatic cholestasis

Author	Type of study	No. of cases	Pruritus	Hepatic function	Liver enzymes cholesterolaemia
Balistreri 1993[20]	Open	31 Alagille 27 Byler	+		+
Narkewicz 1992[21]	Open	7 Alagille	+	–	+
Paradis 1993[22]	Placebo-controlled, cross-over	8 Alagille 14 Byler 13 Indian cirrhosis	–	–	+

Table 4 Effects of ursodeoxycholic acid treatment in children with extrahepatic biliary atresia

Author	Type of study	No. of patients	Survival OLTX	Nutritional status	Pruritus	Hepatic function	Bilirubin, liver enzymes
Ullrich 1987[23]	Open	2		+			+
Nittono 1989[24]	Open	6		+			+
Balistreri 1992[20]	RCT	29	–	+	+		+
Paradis 1993[22]	Placebo-controlled, cross-over	11			–	–	+

RCT: Randomized controlled trial

been proposed as a therapeutic strategy of chronic cholestasis also in infants and children. The effects of UDCA have been explored in children with extrahepatic biliary atresia, Alagille syndrome, Byler disease, North American Indian cholestasis, TPN associated cholestasis and liver disease associated with cystic fibrosis[20–39]. Data regarding neonatal cholestatic liver diseases have been so far reported mostly in abstract form.

Evaluation of treatment efficacy in paediatric cholestasis is problematical, due to the fact that all these disorders are quite rare, with limited number of patients enrolled in each study. Higher doses of UDCA compared to those employed in adults (up to $45\,\mathrm{mg\,kg^{-1}\,day^{-1}}$) have been used in paediatric patients to obtain clinical and biochemical responses. In infants this may be explained not only by immaturity of the enterohepatic circulation, but also by age-related differences in cell membrane composition and fluidity[2,3]. In CF patients with liver disease, doses higher than $20\,\mathrm{mg\,kg^{-1}\,day^{-1}}$ are needed to compensate for poor intestinal absorption[33].

The striking improvement of serum liver enzyme levels reported in adult patients with chronic cholestatic liver diseases has also been observed in the paediatric population (Tables 3 and 4). Sudden deterioration of liver function has been reported in a few small infants with severe cholestasis of different aetiology[26].

Two open studies[20,21] and one cross-over placebo-controlled study[22] have been carried out in children with intrahepatic cholestatic syndromes (Table 3): biochemical improvement was associated with a marked decrease in plasma cholesterol levels during UDCA administration. There was no improvement in hepatic function, assessed by caffeine clearance, galactose elimination capacity and hepatobiliary scintigraphy[21,22], although the period of observation might have been too short. Improvement in pruritus, reported by the two pilot studies[20,21], was not observed in the placebo-controlled trial[22].

Table 4 summarizes the results of studies on UDCA treatment in children with biliary atresia[20,22-24]. A randomized placebo-controlled trial in 29 children[20] has confirmed the beneficial effects of UDCA treatment on liver biochemistry and growth rate observed by open studies; however, it has also shown that UDCA treatment does not influence the outcome of the disease in terms of survival and need for transplantation. The effects on pruritus are still controversial and need to be confirmed by proper studies.

Ursodeoxycholic acid treatment in liver disease associated with cystic fibrosis

According to recent studies, CF-associated liver disease may be considered the first example of inherited disease characterized by an exclusively ductular secretory insufficiency resulting from a specific defect of bile duct cells[39]. Obstruction of bile ductules by inspissated biliary secretions in CF patients may in fact result from the defect of CFTR (cystic fibrosis transmembrane regulator), a cAMP-dependent chloride channel located in the apical membrane of epithelial cells[40,41]. It has been recently shown that bile duct cells are the unique site of CFTR gene expression at the hepatobiliary level; therefore the biliary tract epithelium is affected similarly to secretory epithelial cells in airways and pancreas.

In CF patients, dysfunction of CFTR-associated chloride channel in the apical membrane of bile duct cells would impair chloride efflux, a process which is considered of key importance in generating negative intraluminal potential, paracellular movement of sodium and water, and thus dilution of bile. The actual lack of CFTR in bile ducts of patients with liver disease associated to CF remains to be proven, but it is quite probable that this will be done in the near future.

Liver disease associated with CF is considered one of the more appropriate indications for UDCA therapy. In these patients, UDCA administration may reduce the viscosity of bile and also displace detergent endogenous bile acids, which are retained during cholestasis.

A series of uncontrolled studies have reported the effects of UDCA treatment on different parameters in CF-associated liver disease (Table 5)[27-39]. All studies have reported positive effects of UDCA treatment on serum liver enzyme levels, with a consistent and sustained improvement in biochemical indices related to cytolysis and cholestasis[27-39].

Beneficial effects on quantitative liver function (hepatic excretory function and microsomal reserve) were reported after short-term treatment with

Table 5 Pilot studies on UDCA for CF-associated liver disease

Authors	No. of patients	Dose (mg kg^{-1} day^{-1})	Duration (months)	Parameters evaluated
Colombo 1990[27]	9	10–15*	6	Liver biochemistry Fat absorption Bile acid metabolism
Cotting 1990[28]	9	15–20	6	Liver biochemistry Quantitative liver function Nutritional status
Galabert 1992[30]	22	10–20*	12	Liver biochemistry Fat absorption
Colombo 1992[32]	13	15–20	12	Liver biochemistry Hepatic excretory function
Lindblad 1993[36]	10	10–15	24	Liver biochemistry Histology

*With taurine supplementation

Table 6 UDCA for CF-associated liver disease: controlled trials

Authors	Design	No. of patients	Dose (mg kg^{-1} day^{-1})	Duration (months)	Parameters evaluated
Bittner 1991[37]	Placebo-controlled	38	10	6	Liver biochemistry
O'Brien 1992[38]	Randomized UDCA vs no treatment	12	20	6	Liver biochemistry ^{99}Tc-HIDA scintigraphy Indocyanine green
Colombo 1993[39]	Placebo-controlled	55	15	12	Liver biochemistry Schwachman score Fat absorption Nutritional status

UDCA, but were not consistently maintained[28,31,34]. By means of hepato-biliary scintigraphy improvement in hepatic excretory function and biliary drainage were documented, particularly in CF patients treated at an early stage of the disease[32]. Data on the effects of treatment on liver histology are at present preliminary: a study from Sweden in a limited number of patients has reported only a marginal improvement in inflammation and fibrosis after 2 years of treatment with UDCA[36]. From the available data it seems unlikely that patients with advanced liver disease and portal hypertension might benefit from UDCA therapy, although the nutritional effects of UDCA have been observed only in more compromised CF patients[28].

With regard to double-blind evaluation of UDCA efficacy, two randomized placebo-controlled studies[37,39] and a randomized study comparing the effects of a 6-month period on UDCA versus no treatment in a limited number of patients[38] have confirmed the positive effects of treatment on serum liver enzymes (Table 6).

In the multicentre double-blind trial carried out in Italy[39], 55 patients from 12 CF centres were randomly assigned to receive for 1 year either UDCA (10 to 20 mg/kg b.w. daily) or placebo. In view of the fact that taurine deficiency is often present in CF patients[42], taurine (20–40 mg/kg b.w. daily) or a second placebo were randomly added double-blind to patients in both groups. A significant improvement in liver biochemistry was observed in the two groups of patients treated with UDCA, with or without taurine.

The Schwachman score, a clinical score widely used in the follow-up of CF patients, remained unchanged in the two groups of patients treated with UDCA for 1 year, whereas it deteriorated in the two groups which did not receive UDCA, suggesting a positive effect of treatment on the general conditions of CF patients. Finally, patients treated with taurine, with or without UDCA, showed a trend towards a reduction in fat malabsorption and also a significant increase in serum prealbumin levels. Therefore, during chronic UDCA administration, taurine supplementation may be indicated in patients with severe pancreatic insufficiency and poor nutritional status.

CONCLUSIONS

Overall the results of UDCA therapy in paediatric cholestatic liver diseases are promising; however, the long-term effects of treatment are still poorly defined and it is not known whether treatment has any effect on prognosis. In view of the life-long need for treatment of most paediatric cholestatic conditions, cost–effectiveness should be evaluated by proper long-term studies with clinically relevant end-points.

REFERENCES

1. Balistreri WF. Neonatal cholestasis – medical progress. J Pediatr. 1985;106:171–84.
2. Watkins JB. Neonatal cholestasis: developmental aspects and current concepts. Sem Liver Dis. 1993;13:276–88.
3. Suchy FJ, Bucuvalas JC, Novak DA. Determinants of bile formation during development: ontogeny of hepatic bile acid metabolism and transport. Sem Liver Dis. 1987;7:77–84.
4. Barbara L, Lazzari R, Roda A *et al.* Serum bile acids in newborns and children. Pediatr Res. 1980;14:1222–5.
5. Colombo C, Zuliani G, Ronchi M, Breidenstein J, Setchell KDR. Biliary bile acid composition of the human fetus in early gestation. Pediatr Res. 1987;21:197–200.
6. Setchell KDR, Dumaswala R, Colombo C, Ronchi M. Hepatic bile acid metabolism during early development revealed from the analysis of human fetal gallbladder bile. J Biol Chem. 1988;263:16637–44.
7. Woolf GM, Vierling JM. Disappearing intrahepatic bile ducts: the syndromes and their mechanisms. Sem Liver Dis. 1993;13:261–75.
8. Amedee-Manesme O, Bernard O, Brunelle F *et al.* Sclerosing cholangitis with neonatal onset. J Pediatr. 1987;11:225–9.
9. Balistreri WF. Neonatal cholestasis: lessons from the past, issues for the future. Sem Liver Dis. 1987;7:61–6.
10. Landing BH. Considerations of the pathogenesis of neonatal hepatitis, biliary atresia and choledochal cyst: the concept of infantile obstructive cholangiopathy. Prog Pediatr Surg. 1974;6:113–39.
11. Setchell KDR. Disorders of bile acid synthesis. In: Walker WA, Durie PR, Hamilton JR, Walker-Smith JA, Watkins JB, editors. Pediatric gastrointestinal diseases. Pathophysiology, diagnosis and management, Vol. 2. Toronto and Philadelphia: BC Decker; 1991:992–1013.
12. Weber A, Tuchweber B, Yousef I *et al.* Severe familial cholestasis in North American Indian children: a clinical model of microfilament dysfunction? Gastroenterology. 1981;81:653–62.
13. Setchell KDR, Piccoli DA, O'Connell NC, Jacquemin E, Bernard O. Progressive intrahepatic

cholestasis with normal γ-glutamyltransferase is highly associated with the β-hydroxysteroid dehydrogenase/isomerase deficiency, an inborn error of bile acid synthesis – a new category of metabolic liver disease. Hepatology. 1993;18:178A (488) (Abstract).

14. Mieli-Vergani G, Howard ER, Portmann B, Mowat AP. Late referral for biliary atresia – missed opportunities for effective surgery. Lancet. 1989;1:421–3.

15. Whitington PF, Balistreri WF. Liver transplantation in pediatrics; indications, contraindications and pretransplant management. J Pediatr. 1991;118:169–77.

16. Yang Y, Raper SE, Cohn JA, Engelhardt JF, Wilson JM. An approach for treating the hepatobiliary disease of cystic fibrosis by somatic gene transfer. Proc Natl Acad Sci USA. 1993;90:4601–5.

17. Sokol RJ. Medical management of the infant or child with chronic liver disease. Sem Liver Dis. 1987;7:155–67.

18. Collins JC, Morecki R, McPhillips J, Gartner LM. Colchicine treatment of pediatric chronic cholestatic liver disease. In: Lentze MJ, Reichen J, editors. Paediatric cholestasis. Novel approaches to treatment. Dordrecht: Kluwer Academic Publishers; 1992:305–8.

19. Heuman DM. Hepatoprotective properties of ursodeoxycholic acid (editorial). Gastroenterology. 1993;104:1865–70.

20. Balistreri WF, Setchell KDR, Ryckman FC. Bile acid therapy in pediatric liver disease. In: Paumgartner G, Stiehl A, Gerok W, editors. Bile acids and the hepatobiliary system – from basic science to clinical practice. Dordrecht: Kluwer Academic Publishers; 1993:271–82.

21. Narkewicz MR, Sokol RJ, Smith D, Gregory C, Lear JL. Ursodeoxycholic acid does not improve quantitative tests of hepatic function in children with intrahepatic cholestasis despite clinical improvement. Hepatology. 1992;16:258A (853) (Abstract).

22. Paradis K, El Arab N, Yousef I, Lacaille F, Schreiber R, Levy E, Rasquin-Weber A. Use of ursodeoxycholic acid in children with cholestatic liver disease. Hepatology. 1993;18:301A (978) (Abstract).

23. Ullrich D, Rating D, Schroter W. Treatment with ursodeoxycholic acid renders children with biliary atresia suitable for liver transplantation. Lancet. 1987;2:1234 (letter).

24. Nittono H, Tokita A, Hayashi M, Watanabe T, Obinata K, Nakatsu N, Miyano T. Ursodeoxycholic acid therapy in the treatment of biliary atresia. Biomed Pharmacother. 1989;43:37–41.

25. Cocjin J, Vanderhal A, Sehgal S, Rosenthal P. Ursodeoxycholic acid therapy for total parenteral nutrition-associated cholestasis in the neonate. Pediatr Res. 1993;29:301A (1788) (Abstract).

26. Paradis K, Weber A. Sudden liver deterioration in infants receiving ursodeoxycholic acid. Gastroenterology. 1992;102:A866 (Abstract).

27. Colombo C, Setchell KDR, Podda M, Crosignani A, Roda A, Curcio L, Giunta A. The effects of ursodeoxycholic acid therapy in liver disease associated with cystic fibrosis. J Pediatr. 1990;117:482–9.

28. Cotting J, Lentze M, Reichen J. Effects of ursodeoxycholic acid treatment on nutrition and liver function in patients with cystic fibrosis and longstanding cholestasis. Gut. 1990;31:918–21.

29. Nakagawa M, Colombo C, Setchell KDR. Comprehensive study of the biliary bile acid composition of the patients with cystic fibrosis and associated liver disease before and after ursodeoxycholic acid administration. Hepatology. 1990;12:322–34.

30. Galabert C, Montet JC, Lengrand D, Lecuire A, Sotta C, Figarella C, Chazalette JP. Effects of ursodeoxycholic acid on liver function in patients with cystic fibrosis and chronic cholestasis. J Pediatr. 1992;121:138–41.

31. Reichen J, Paumgartner G, Cotting J, Lentze MJ. Effect of long-term ursodeoxycholate on liver function, nutritional state and serum bile acids in cystic fibrosis with long-standing cholestasis. In: Paumgartner G, Stiehl A, Gerok W, editors. Bile acids as therapeutic agents – from basic science to clinical practice. Dordrecht: Kluwer Academic Publishers; 1991:335–44.

32. Colombo C, Castellani MR, Balistreri WF, Seregni E, Assaisso ML, Giunta A. Scintigraphic documentation of an improvement in hepatobiliary excretory function after treatment with ursodeoxycholic acid in patients with cystic fibrosis and associated liver disease. Hepatology. 1992;15:677–84.

33. Colombo C, Crosignani A, Assaisso ML *et al.* Ursodeoxycholic acid therapy in cystic

fibrosis associated liver disease: a dose-response study. Hepatology. 1992;16:924–30.

34. Cotting J, Dufour JF, Lentze MJ, Paumgartner G, Reichen J. Ursodeoxycholate in the treatment of cholestasis in cystic fibrosis: a 2-year experience and review of the literature. In: Lentze MJ, Reichen J, editors. Paediatric cholestasis: novel approaches to treatment. Dordrecht: Kluwer Academic Publishers; 1992:345–54.

35. Colombo C, Crosignani A, Bertolini E, Assaisso ML, Bettinardi N, Apostolo MG, Giunta A. Ursodeoxycholic acid treatment in hepatobiliary complications of cystic fibrosis. In: Paumgartner S, Stiehl A, Gerok W, editors. Bile acids and the hepatobiliary system – from basic science to clinical practice. Dordrecht: Kluwer Academic Publishers; 1992:283–8.

36. Lindblad A, Strandvik B. Long-term study of the effect of ursodeoxycholic acid on liver morphology and liver function in patients with cystic fibrosis (Abstract). Proceedings of the 18th European Cystic Fibrosis Conference 1993;89.

37. Bittner P, Posselt HG, Sailer T et al. The effect of treatment with ursodeoxycholic acid in cystic fibrosis and hepatopathy: results of a placebo-controlled study. In: Paumgartner G, Stiehl A, Gerok W, editors. Bile acids as therapeutic agents – From basic science to clinical practice. Dordrecht: Kluwer Academic Publishers; 1991:345–8.

38. O'Brien S, Fitzgerald MX, Hegarty JE. A controlled trial of ursodeoxycholic acid treatment in cystic fibrosis-related liver disease. Eur J Gastroenterol Hepatol. 1992;4:857–63.

39. Colombo C, Podda M, Battezzati PM et al. Ursodeoxycholic acid for cystic fibrosis-associated liver disease: final report of a multicenter trial (Abstract). Hepatology. 1993;18:142A (342).

40. Cohn JA, Strong TV, Picciotto MR, Nairn AC, Collins FS, Fitz JG. Localization of the cystic fibrosis transmembrane conductance regulator in human bile duct epithelial cells. Gastroenterology. 1993;105:1857–64.

41. Fitz JG, Basavappa S, McGill J, Melhus O, Cohn JA. Regulation of membrane chloride currents in rat bile duct epithelial cells. J Clin Invest. 1993;91:319–28.

42. Anonymous. Taurine supplementation in cystic fibrosis. Nutr Rev. 1988;46:257–8.

19
Inborn errors of bile acid synthesis: a new category of metabolic liver disease

K. D. R. SETCHELL

INTRODUCTION

In recent years, methods based upon the application of fast atom bombardment-ionization mass spectrometry (FAB-MS) have been developed for the rapid screening of urine samples for the presence of bile acid conjugates[1]. Using this approach it is possible to define whether urinary bile acid excretion is elevated, and consequently to assess the degree of cholestasis. Furthermore, since the mass spectrum reveals the molecular weights of the bile acids present, this qualitative profile permits the elucidation of derangements in bile acid synthesis and metabolism[2-4].

In liver disease, serum and urinary bile acid concentrations are often elevated, and prior to the advent of the above techniques it was difficult to determine if these changes were primary or secondary to the cholestasis. By the application of FAB-MS, two new inborn errors in bile acid synthesis were identified that are clinically manifest as progressive intrahepatic cholestasis. These metabolic defects (Fig. 1), a 3β-hydroxy-C_{27}-steroid dehydrogenase/isomerase deficiency[5] and a Δ^4-3-oxosteroid-5β-reductase deficiency[6], involve the enzymes that catalyse the reactions involved in altering the steroid nucleus in the pathway for primary bile acid synthesis from cholesterol[7].

BIOCHEMICAL AND CLINICAL PRESENTATION OF INBORN ERRORS IN BILE ACID SYNTHESIS

The biochemical presentation of these defects feature: (a) a lack of, or markedly diminished synthesis of the primary bile acids, cholic and chenodeoxycholic acids; (b) excessive production and subsequent accumulation of precursors in the pathway proximal to the enzyme defect; (c) synthesis of

Metabolic defects in bile acid synthesis

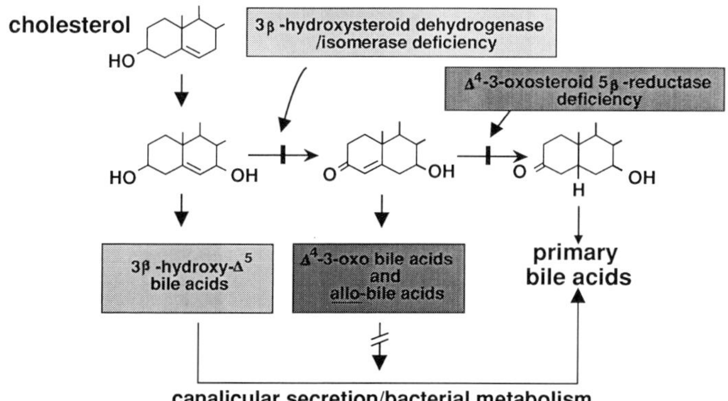

Fig. 1 Biochemical pathway for primary bile acid synthesis from cholesterol depicting the changes to the steroid nucleus and the sites of inborn errors in bile acid synthesis

atypical bile acids that retain the AB-ring structure of the sterol precursors which are the substrates for the deficient enzyme and conjugation of these unique bile acids; (4) elimination of these conjugated hydrophilic metabolites via renal excretion, which becomes the major route of hepatic clearance.

Clinical presentation of both the 3β-hydroxy-C_{27}-steroid dehydrogenase/ isomerase deficiency and the Δ^4-3-oxosteroid-5β-reductase deficiency has been variable, with the latter defect presenting significantly earlier in life, while the 3β-hydroxy-C_{27}-steroid dehydrogenase/isomerase deficiency has been found to account for an increasing number of patients presenting with late-onset idiopathic liver disease[8,9].

In a number of these cases the early presentation was a state of significant fat-soluble vitamin malabsorption, with serum liver enzymes being normal. The age-related differences between the two inborn errors may be related to the extent of canalicular secretion of the atypical metabolites. It is probable that the 3β-hydroxy bile acids, which are selectively sulphated, undergo a more efficient canalicular secretion and therefore enter the intestine to be metabolized further by bacterial 3β-hydroxysteroid dehydrogenases[10] to cholic and chenodeoxycholic acids. This is supported by the finding of low but significant concentrations of primary bile acids in the bile of patients with the 3β-hydroxy-C_{27}-steroid dehydrogenase/isomerase deficiency. On the other hand, patients with the Δ^4-3-oxosteroid-5β-reductase deficiency do not secrete 3-oxo-Δ^4 bile acids in bile[6], presumably because of their poor solubility, or limited specificity for the canalicular transport proteins.

Clinically and histologically, patients with these defects show typical features of cholestatic liver disease. Elevations in serum transaminases accompanied by a conjugated hyperbilirubinaemia are usual; however, a normal γ-glutamyltranspeptidase is a common – although it should be stressed, not exclusive – feature of these progressive intrahepatic cholangiopathies[8,9,11]. In particular, this clinical feature appears highly (Fig. 2)

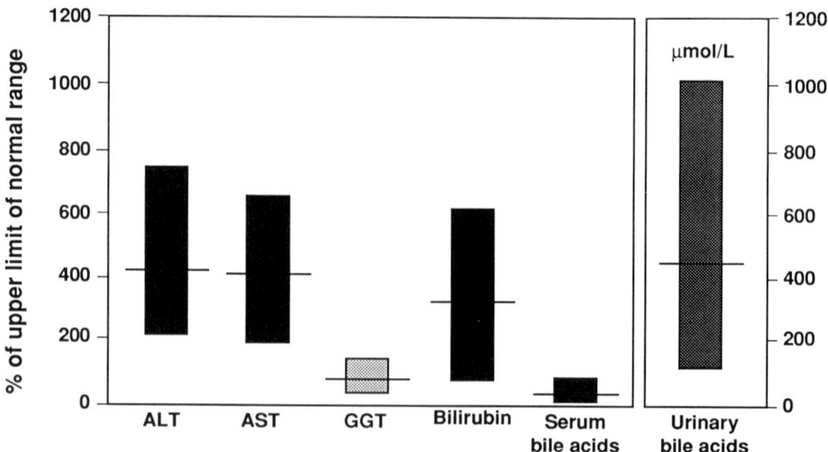

Fig. 2 Summary of biochemical presentations of patients ($n = 15$) with a 3β-hydroxy-C_{27}-steroid dehydrogenase/isomerase deficiency

associated with the 3β-hydroxy-C_{27}-steroid dehydrogenase/isomerase deficiency. Although not routinely included in the clinical work-up, serum bile acid concentrations when measured by routine immunoassays or enzyme assays are normal or undetectable, because the unique bile acid metabolites synthesized in these defects do not cross-react in routine assays. Byler's disease[12] is a clinical entity exhibiting normal serum γ-glutamyltranspeptidase levels; however, differential diagnosis is possible from serum or urinary bile acid measurements, because patients with Byler's disease contrastingly have high levels of primary bile acids. Diagnosis or suspicion of a possible inborn error in bile acid synthesis is thus facilitated by the inclusion of serum γ-glutamyltranspeptidase and bile acid measurements in the clinical work-up of patients with idiopathic cholestasis.

TREATMENT

Early diagnosis of these defects is important, because effective treatment is possible by the administration of primary bile acids. Administration of cholic acid (50–75 mg/day) is accompanied by significant down-regulation in the synthesis of the atypical bile acids[11,13]. Our experience to date indicates that, providing cirrhosis is not advanced and synthetic function is not severely compromised, a normalization in serum liver enzymes, resolution of jaundice, and an improvement in liver histology is attained with primary bile acid therapy[11,13,14] and the need for liver transplantation, the only alternative treatment, can be avoided.

References

1. Sjövall J, Lawson AM, Setchell KDR. Mass spectrometry of bile acids. In: Law JH, Rilling HC, editors. Methods in enzymology, vol. III. London: Academic Press; 1985:63–113.

2. Setchell KDR, Street JM. Inborn errors of bile acid synthesis. Semin Liver Dis. 1987;7: 85–99.
3. Setchell KDR. Disorders of bile acid synthesis. In: Walker WA, Durie PR, Hamilton JR, Walker-Smith JA, Watkins JA, editors. Pediatric gastrointestinal disease, pathophysiology, diagnosis, management, vol. 2. Toronto/Philadelphia: Decker; 1990:992–1013.
4. Setchell KDR, O'Connell NC. Bile acid biosynthesis. In: Suchy FJ, editor. Liver disease in children. St. Louis, MO: Mosby; 1994:835–51.
5. Clayton P, Leonard JV, Lawson AM, Setchell KDR, Andersson S, Egestad B, Sjövall J. Familial giant cell hepatitis associated with synthesis of $3\beta,7\alpha$-dihydroxy- and $3\beta,7\alpha,12\alpha$-trihydroxy-5-cholenoic acids. J Clin Invest. 1987;79:1031–8.
6. Setchell KDR, Suchy FJ, Welsh MB, Zimmer-Nechemias L, Heubi J, Balistreri WF. Δ^4-3-Oxosteroid 5β-reductase deficiency described in identical twins with neonatal hepatitis – a new inborn error in bile acid synthesis. J Clin Invest. 1988;82:2148–57.
7. Russell D, Setchell KDR. Bile acid biosynthesis. Biochemistry. 1993;31:20:4737–49.
8. Setchell KDR, Flick R, Watkins JB, Piccoli D. Chronic hepatitis in a 10 year old due to an inborn error in bile acid synthesis – diagnosis and treatment with oral bile acid. Gastroenterology. 1990;98:A631 (abstr.).
9. Jacquemin E, Setchell KDR, O'Connell NC, Estrada A, Maggiore G, Schmitz J, Hadchouel M, Bernard O. 3β-Hydroxy-C_{27}-steroid-dehydrogenase/isomerase deficiency in children: a new cause of progressive familial intrahepatic cholestasis. J Pediatr. 1994 (Submitted).
10. Hylemon PB. Metabolism of bile acids in intestinal microflora. In: Danielsson H, Sjövall J, editors. Sterols and bile acids. Amsterdam/New York/Oxford: Elsevier; 1985;331–4.
11. Setchell KDR, Balistreri WF, Piccoli DA, Clerici C. Oral bile acid therapy in the treatment of inborn errors in bile acid synthesis associated with liver disease. In: Paumgartner G, Stiehl A, Gerok W, editors. Bile acids as therapeutic agents, from basic science to clinical practice. Dordrecht/Boston/London: Kluwer; 1990:367–73.
12. Clayton RJ, Iber FL, Ruebner BH, McKusick VA. Byler's disease: fatal intrahepatic cholestasis in an Amish kindred. Am J Dis Child. 1969;117:112–24.
13. Ichimiya H, Nazer H, Gunmasekaran T, Clayton P, Sjövall J. Treatment of chronic liver disease caused by 3β-hydroxy-Δ^5-C_{27}-steroid dehydrogenase deficiency with chenodeoxycholic acid. Arch Dis Childh. 1990;65:1121–4.
14. Daugherty CC, Setchell KDR, Heubi JE, Balistreri WF. Resolution of hepatic biopsy alterations in 3 siblings with bile acid treatment of an inborn error of bile acid metabolism (Δ^4-3-oxosteroid-5β-reductase deficiency). Hepatology. 1993;18:1096–101.

Section IV
Ductopenic diseases: pathophysiology and treatment

20
Pathology of ductopenia with a particular reference to primary biliary cirrhosis and liver allograft rejection

B. C. PORTMANN

INTRODUCTION

The term 'ductopenia' in the liver refers to a reduced number of interlobular bile ducts demonstrated histologically[1]. The change may be progressive and lead to a complete disappearance of these structures – vanishing bile duct syndrome – such as observed in chronic or subacute rejection of the liver allograft[2]. First described in primary biliary cirrhosis (PBC)[3] an involvement of the interlobular bile ducts as prime targets of tissue injury has now been recognized in a number of different liver conditions of varied aetiology[4]. Peculiar to the interlobular bile ducts is their unique arterial blood supply, compared with the dual venous and arterial supply of the liver parenchyma[5]. In addition, they often show an enhanced or aberrant expression of class I and II major histocompatibility antigens, presumably via increased cytokine production by activated T cells in many inflammatory processes[6]. Damage to the small bile ducts may be reversible, without notable loss of ducts in acute and chronic hepatitis, in particular that due to hepatitis C virus, some drug reactions, acute (cellular) rejection of liver allografts and acute graft-versus-host disease (GVHD). Conversely, the lesion may be destructive, leading to a significant loss of the interlobular bile ducts, in a range of conditions – so-called vanishing bile duct or ductopenic syndromes (see Table 1). Whereas ductopenia is the hallmark of disorders such as PBC, chronic allograft rejection and chronic GVHD, in others (exemplified by primary or secondary sclerosing cholangitis) ductopenia is facultative, and may occur in isolation (small duct disease) or, more often, in association with sclerosing cholangitis of the major bile ducts. These conditions further differ with regard to the early pathological changes leading to ductopenia, their rate of progression, fibrogenic tendency and their aetiopathogenic mechanisms, which in many

Table 1 Liver disorders associated with ductopenia

Neonates and children
Extrahepatic biliary atresia*
Paucity of the interlobular bile ducts
  Syndromic (Alagille's syndrome) and non-syndromic (α-antitrypsin deficiency, bile acid defects, idiopathic)
Sclerosing cholangitis*
  Primary, with or without ulcerative colitis; perinatal onset
  Acquired (immunodeficiency, Langerhans cell histiocytosis)

Adults
Primary biliary cirrhosis
  Autoimmune cholangitis
  Sarcoidosis
*Sclerosing cholangitis**
  Primary or idiopathic: with or without ulcerative colitis
  Acquired: (a) opportunistic (primary or secondary immunodeficiency – AIDS)*; (b) ischaemic (liver allograft, arterial cytotoxic infusion)*; (c) toxic (ruptured or treated hydatid cyst)*
Idiopathic adulthood ductopenia
Hepatic allograft rejection
Graft versus host disease
Suppurative cholangitis, usually with biliary obstruction*
Miscellaneous (Hodgkin's disease, drug)

---

*Extrahepatic bile ducts additionally and/or preferentially affected

instances remain obscure[4]. Both in children and adults, destruction and loss of bile ducts is often, but not invariably, followed by a progressive portal–portal bridging fibrosis and the eventual development of a biliary cirrhosis. Thus, in their later stages, these various diseases share many pathological features, which in turn closely resemble the changes observed in secondary biliary cirrhosis. In this account the pathology of the long-recognized ductopenia of PBC is contrasted with that of chronic allograft rejection.

PRIMARY BILIARY CIRRHOSIS

Primary biliary cirrhosis (PBC) can be considered as the model ductopenic syndrome. The term 'chronic non-suppurative destructive cholangitis'[7] more accurately describes the early lesions which are said to affect the interlobular bile ducts 40–80 μm in diameter[8], larger branches becoming involved later. The actual size of the diseased ducts may be difficult to estimate, as they tend to enlarge following rupture of their basement membranes, but it is generally accepted that the smallest branches tend to disappear first[9]. Epithelioid cell granulomas intimately related to damaged bile ducts comprise the most distinctive lesion (Fig. 1a). Bile duct epithelium swelling and stratification with an irregular luminal border, increased eosinophilia of individual cells, basement membrane disruption and infiltration by lymphocytes surrounded by cytoplasmic vacuoles all suggest a PBC, but to some extent overlap with early stages of other ductopenic disorders (Fig. 1b). Characteristic bile duct lesions with or without granuloma formation are segmental within the duct system, and might therefore not be sampled by biopsy needles. A chronic portal inflammation with a predominance of

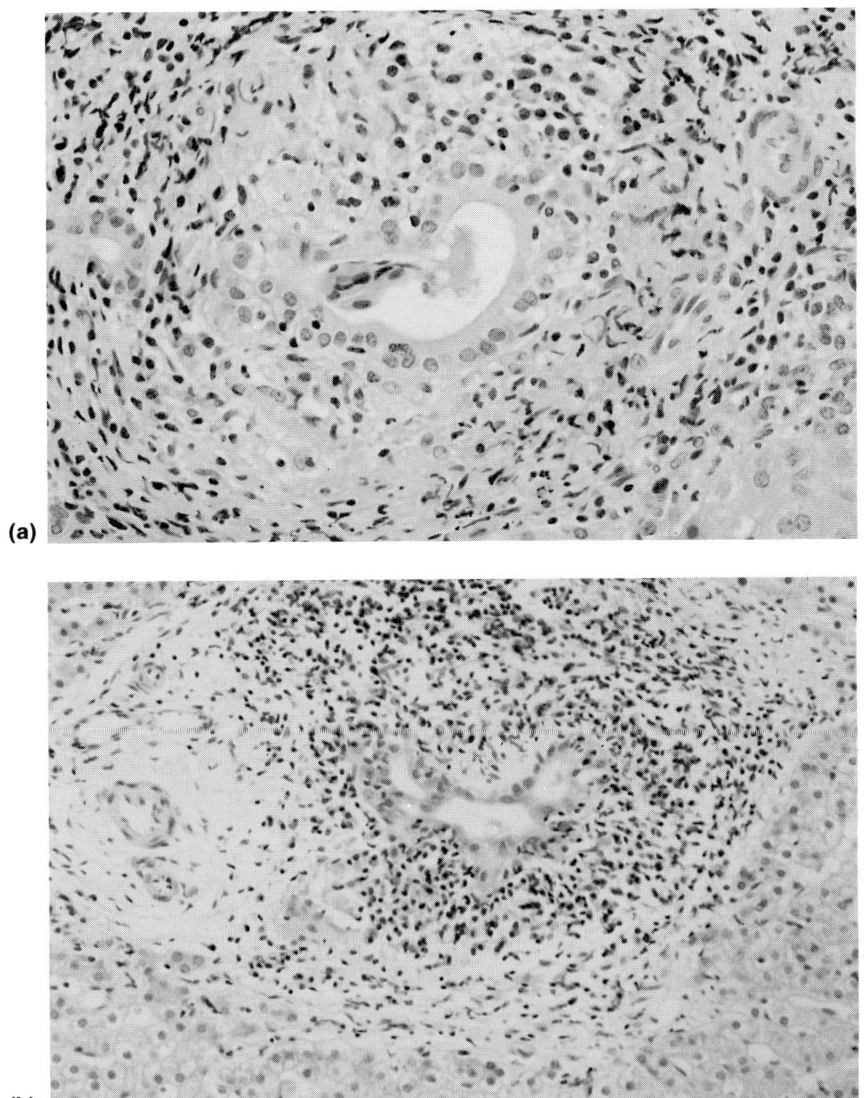

Fig. 1   Florid bile duct lesion in early primary biliary cirrhosis. (**a**) A dilated interlobular bile duct with disrupted basement membrane is surrounded by an epithelioid cell granulomatous infiltrate (H&E). (**b**) Predominantly lymphocytes are intimately related to, and focally infiltrate, a distorted bile duct. Note the relatively intact parenchymal limiting plate (H&E)

lymphocytes which may form aggregates – and may include germinal centres, epithelioid macrophages, plasma cells and eosinophils with variable infiltration of duct branches – is therefore more common in routine histology. In stage 1 the lesion is confined within the portal boundaries and ductopenia, as evidenced by hepatic arterial branches unaccompanied by a bile duct, is usually absent or mild[9].

The similarity of the bile duct damage in PBC to that observed in GVHD[10] and liver allograft rejection[11] has been used as a circumstantial support to the bile duct destruction being immunologically mediated. Immunochemical studies have demonstrated enhanced expression on bile duct epithelium of MHC class I antigens[12] and aberrant expression of MHC class II antigens[13,14], the latter also found in primary sclerosing cholangitis, in extrahepatic obstruction and other forms of chronic liver disease[6,15]. Cytotoxic T-cells constitute the main cell infiltrating the bile ducts[16,17], which not surprisingly show an increased expression of intercellular adhesion molecule 1[18]. Recently, a molecule cross-reacting with the mitochondrial pyruvate dehydrogenase complex-E2, the main component reacting with mitochondrial antibodies, has been shown to be expressed on biliary epithelial cells in PBC patients[19,20].

Disease progression

From this initial stage there is a marked individual variation in the rate of progression of the disease, though sooner or later the lesion extends to the parenchymal limiting plates (stage 2) in the form of *classic* (lymphocytic) and/or *biliary* piecemeal necrosis[21] (Fig. 2a). The former is supposed to represent an extension of the necro-inflammatory process to involve the liver cells, possibly as part of the same immunological process which affects the duct system; this may closely resemble the changes of a chronic active hepatitis which often enters the differential diagnosis at this stage. In contrast, biliary piecemeal necrosis is more likely to result from the 'toxic' effect of bile retention, which occurs proximal to the damaged and disappearing bile ducts. This is characterized by cholate-static changes and copper-associated protein load of periportal hepatocytes, which become dissociated by a loose fibrous tissue. This contrasts sharply with the hard collagen of the original portal tract. Seemingly sprouting and proliferating bile ductules occur at the periphery of the portal areas, which to a variable extent result from actual cholangiolar proliferation and/or from ductular metaplasia of acinar zone 1 hepatocytes. The change may be prominent and, when associated with numerous neutrophils (so-called cholangiolitis), it may reflect a more rapidly progressive and fibrogenic lesion[21] (Fig. 2b). Both reactive ductules and periportal cholate-stasis seem to stimulate the progressive fibrous expansion of the portal areas with subsequent formation of radiating, porto-portal bridging septa (stage 3) and the eventual development of a biliary type cirrhosis (stage 4). The gradual fibrous expansion of the portal tracts with the formation of septa lined by biliary piecemeal necrosis, marginal ductular reaction, copper accumulation and later bilirubinostasis are all features attributable to the effects of a prolonged impairment of bile excretion, and therefore shared by other ductopenic syndromes. Thus the morphological distinction between PBC and other disorders, in particular primary sclerosing

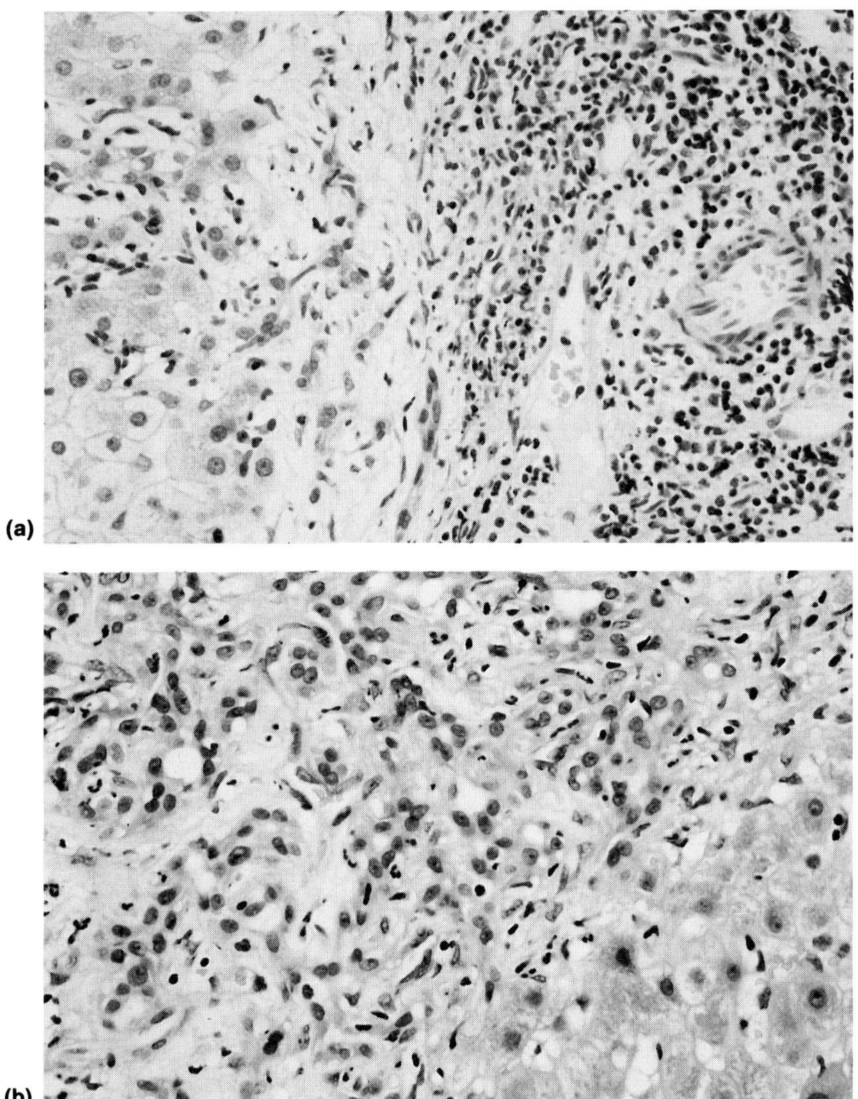

Fig. 2 Biliary piecemeal necrosis in stage 2 PBC. (a) The markedly inflamed and ductopenic portal tract (right part of the field) is expanded to the left by loose connective tissue which dissociates the parenchymal limiting plate (H&E). (b) Particularly severe ductular reaction set in a fibrous matrix which shows only sparse neutrophils (H&E)

cholangitis, may become difficult from stage 2 onwards, when characteristic bile duct changes are no longer to be seen[22].

PBC-like syndromes

As mentioned above, there is some histological overlap between PBC and chronic active hepatitis (CAH), particularly in stages 1–2, and this may present a problem of differentiation in approximately 15% of specimens from large biopsy series[4]. In only a few instances does the overlap extend to the clinical and serological data, CAH/PBC mixed type[23].

The term 'autoimmune cholangitis' has been applied to a group of patients whose liver lesion closely resembles that of PBC, but whose serum is antimitochondrial antibody-negative and often contains high titres of anti-nuclear antibodies[24]. Sarcoidosis may present overlapping features with PBC, and in a few patients both diseases seem to have coexisted[25]. Various drugs have been associated with a cholestatic type of reaction which, when prolonged, may mimic the clinical syndrome and serum biochemical abnormalities of PBC. Progressive duct loss is increasingly recognized in this situation[26], but a granulomatous destructive cholangitis indistinguishable from the lesion of PBC is exceptionally recorded[27].

DUCTOPENIA IN THE LIVER ALLOGRAFT

The first successful liver transplant in man is backdated to 1963[28], but it was not until the late 1970s that the interlobular bile ducts were recognized as targets of the immune attack in allograft rejection[29–31]. As mentioned above, similarities have been emphasized at an ultrastructural level between the duct lesion of PBC and allograft rejection[11], but there are many more differences to be found between the two conditions.

Acute (cellular) rejection (AR)

The interlobular bile ducts, together with the vascular endothelia, are main targets of the immune attack in AR. Inflammation is predominantly portal, and in that respect may resemble the florid stage of PBC, but large lymphocytes, blast cells and eosinophils are more prominent than in PBC; granulomas are not observed; and portal endotheliitis or venulitis is more striking in AR[31–33]. The bile-duct epithelium exhibits variable degrees of nuclear crowding, irregularity and hyperchromatism with cytoplasmic vacuolation, pleomorphism and eosinophilic transformation (Fig. 3a). The small duct branches are often overrun by inflammatory cells, their outlines become indistinct, but destruction is generally not a feature; clusters of neutrophils may be present within their lumen, simulating a suppurative cholangitis, but in this setting this usually reflects a more severe degree of rejection rather than ascending infection. At this stage neutrophils are present in large numbers in the bile, and bile culture remains sterile[34].

Immunochemistry shows that most of the lymphocytes in and around the bile ducts are CD8[+] and, to a lesser extent, CD4[+] T cells[35,36]. Acute cellular rejection modified by the standard immunosuppression is rarely severe, but when it is, duct loss and perivenular hepatocyte damage and loss may become

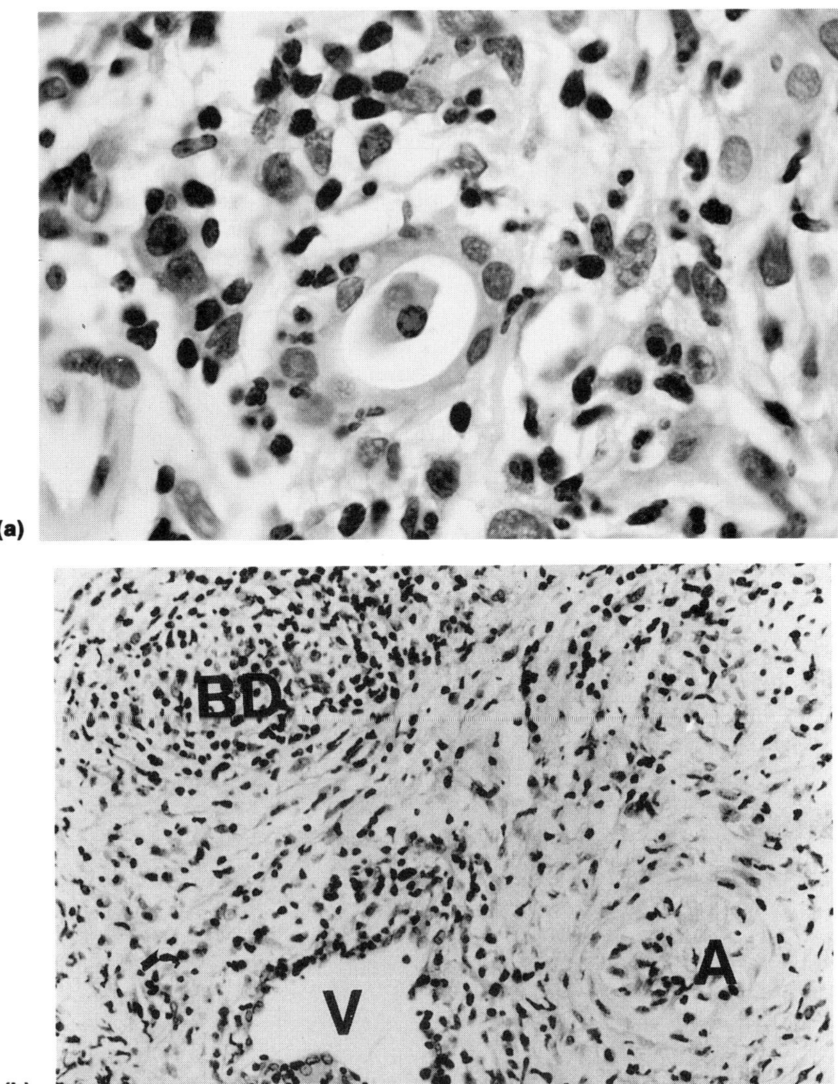

Fig. 3   (a) Bile duct damage in acute cellular rejection; note the presence of immunoblasts with large nucleolated nuclei in the surrounding cell infiltrate (H&E). (b) Accelerated allograft rejection showing cellular portal infiltrate reinforced at the site of a vanished bile duct (BD), venular endotheliitis (V) and obliterative foam cell arteritis A (H&E)

conspicuous. In most instances resolution of the changes will follow a course of high-dose steroids. Occasionally, severe acute rejection has been shown to progress to severe ductopenia with graft loss within 2 months of surgery – acute vanishing bile duct syndrome[37] – a situation in which the changes of both acute cellular and chronic vascular rejection coexist (Fig. 3b).

Chronic (ductopenic) rejection (CR)

CR usually presents between 2 and 12 months after transplantation[38], following one or several episodes of acute, not necessarily severe, rejection – more rarely insidiously over a period of months without documented episode of acute rejection. When fully developed the lesion of CR, such as seen in explanted allografts at re-transplantation, is characterized by severe ductopenia and foam cell obliterative arteriopathy. These two cardinal features, which occur in various combinations, are accepted as the morphological definition of CR[39–41], earlier named 'vanishing bile duct syndrome'[2,42]. 'Ductopenic rejection' was later proposed, a term which, being time-independent, would include the occasional cases which present as early as 20 days after transplantation[37,43].

Unlike acute cellular rejection, CR remains a diagnostic problem due to the inconsistency, insidious development, and uneven distribution of the early histological changes. On sequential biopsy specimens a progression from cellular rejection to CR can be evidenced in some, but not all, cases[44]. Early changes which suggest CR comprise a variable association of the following:

1. Light portal inflammation and oedema with damage to the small interlobular bile ducts in the form of epithelial distortion, nuclear pyknosis and focal disappearance.
2. Perivenular hepatocyte drop-out, with sinusoidal congestion and minimal inflammatory reaction; such a lesion is possibly related to ischaemia and may anticipate the existence of foam cell arteriopathy which usually affects larger arteries than the ones sampled by biopsy needles.
3. Canalicular cholestasis in acinar zone 3 with feathery degeneration and a distinctive absence of periportal ductular reaction.

The further course is characterized by a progressive disappearance of the interlobular bile ducts, primarily the small ($<60\,\mu$m) branches, with a concomitant attenuation of the portal cell infiltrate (Fig. 4a), leaving behind a few sparse mixed inflammatory cells and occasionally a small aggregate of lymphocytes. At this stage a terminal portal axis devoid of bile ducts may be difficult to identify as portal tract, and there may be an apparent paucity of portal tracts. The distribution of the cholestasis around hepatic venules may indirectly help to locate abortive portal tracts due to their adjacent cholestasis-free parenchyma (Fig. 4b). The degree of ductopenia is estimated by counting the ratio of portal tracts without identifiable ducts to the total number of portal tracts present in the specimen. Arbitrarily 10 or more portal tracts devoid of ducts out of 20 examined has been considered diagnostic[1]. This often requires sequential biopsy specimens, which in turn may provide conflicting results due to the uneven distribution of the lesion. Interestingly, and perhaps a corollary of the lack of ductular proliferation, periportal fibrosis is minimal in chronic rejection, at least during the period of observation to graft failure. However, conspicuous perivenular fibrosis may occur with central–central, later central–portal, bridging septa. In rare cases periportal ductular proliferation does occur in early biopsy, followed

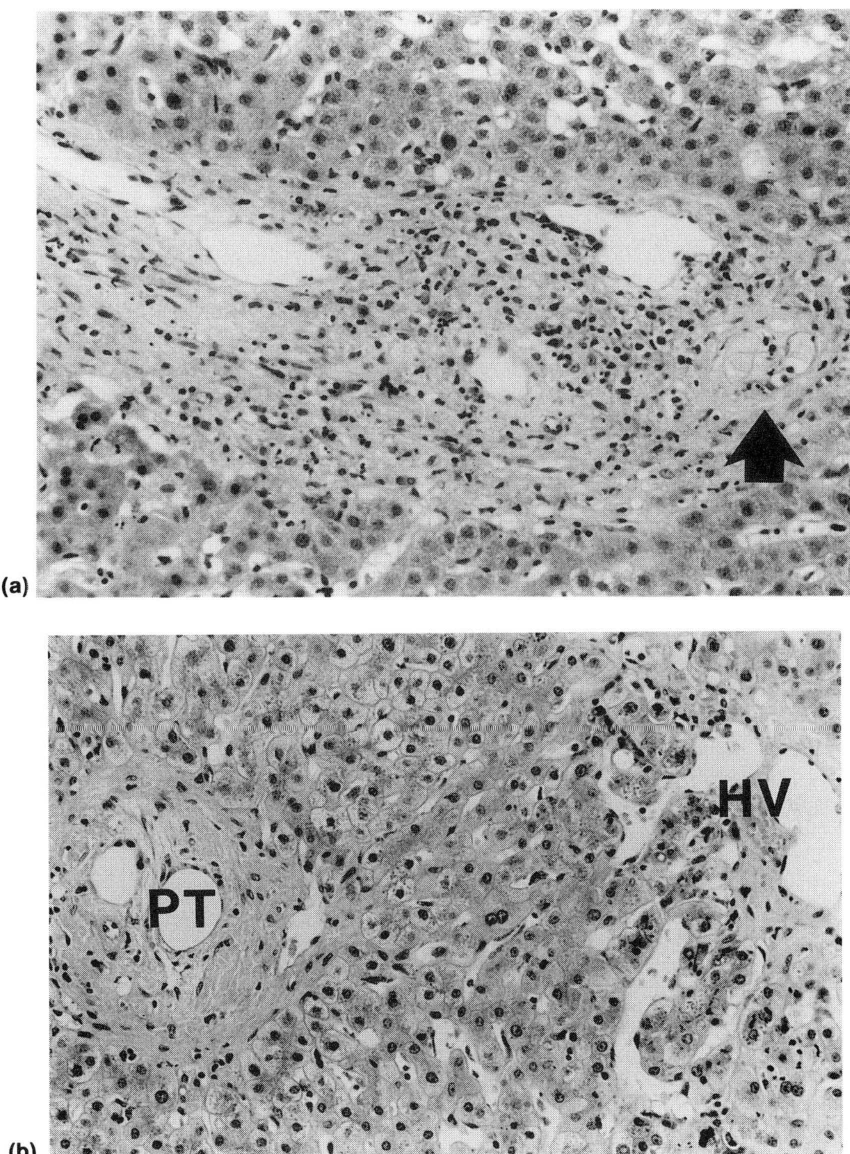

Fig. 4 Chronic allograft rejection. (a) The portal tract, which is devoid of bile duct, shows a light infiltration of mixed inflammatory cells. A small arterial branch occluded by foamy macrophages is arrowed (H&E). (b) Later stage showing a ductopenic portal tract with inconspicuous inflammation or fibrosis and absence of ductular proliferation (PT); there is cholestasis and plate disarray around a seemingly reduplicated hepatic venule (HV) (H&E)

by some degree of periportal fibrosis. These cases usually have an associated, probably ischaemic, cholangitis with stricture, cholangiodestruction and/or cholangitis of the major bile ducts. In that respect non-rejection ischaemic cholangitis constitutes the main differential diagnosis of CR in biopsy material.

Foamy macrophages are often seen in small portal areas of CR cases, and orcein elastic staining may reveal their location within a vascular lumen. More rarely, a small artery showing typical intimal deposition of foam cells is included in the biopsy specimen. Using histometric analysis, Oguma et al.[45] have demonstrated a loss of portal arterioles, less than 35 μm in diameter. More recently, immunohistochemical staining for capillary endothelium using El.5, CD31 and EL-4 antibodies in allograft specimens has revealed a marked reduction of microvascular structures in acute cellular rejection (1.1 ± 0.6) ($n = 25$) and in CR (0.65 ± 0.9) ($n = 15$) compared with normal liver (3.8 ± 0.7) ($n = 11$). Furthermore, an estimation of the number of microvascular structures per bile duct demonstrated that the destruction of portal microvasculature components preceded bile duct loss[46].

Outcome of CR

CR used to be regarded as a progressive and irreversible loss of the intrahepatic bile ducts not responsive to immunosuppressive therapy, the majority of cases requiring graft replacement within a few months to 1 year of transplantation. Two reports, however, have described clinical and histological improvement or resolution in respectively three and six patients whose graft histology had met the criteria of chronic rejection[47,48]. Furthermore, several uncontrolled studies suggest that the drug FK506, in addition to being beneficial in cases of intractable rejection, may have arrested the progress of ductopenic rejection in 50% or more of chronic rejection cases[49–51]. These observations, our experience of a few incomplete or protracted cases of CR, together with an isolated patient who presented 8 years after transplantation[52], suggest that the lesion spectrum of CR is probably broader than originally appreciated.

PBC in the liver allograft

Our initial report of PBC recurrence in the allograft[53] has been the subject of considerable controversy in the literature[54]. Due to the frequently persistent antimitochondrial antibodies, irrespective of a liver lesion, and the rejection process being focused on the small bile ducts, stringent criteria (such as the presence of granulomas) will be required to conclude that a liver lesion may represent PBC recurrence. Features of granulomatous destructive cholangitis, indistinguishable from that of PBC, have now been reported by a few other groups[55–57], usually between 2 and 5 years post-transplant. In repeat biopsies the changes have shown a slow (if any) tendency to progress, a stage 3 disease having been exceptionally recorded[56,58] at between 5 and

10 years. The apparent discrepancy between the various studies may reflect differences in the diagnostic criteria used, in the size of biopsy specimens (considering the patchy distribution of the bile duct lesions at an early stage), and in the immunosuppressive regimens. In that respect it may be important to note that the majority of the patients in our centre, and in the other large published study[56], were on very little or no steroid treatment at the time of recurrence[59], similar to the two patients on FK506 we have reported recently and in whom an accelerated rate of recurrence was observed[60].

SUMMARY AND CONCLUSIONS

Morphological observations in PBC and liver allograft rejection support the view that a T-cell-mediated attack, primarily directed at the small interlobular bile ducts, less than $100\,\mu m$ in diameter, forms the basis of the initial injury in both conditions. The precise antigen(s) to which the patients become sensitized remains to be demonstrated, though an expression of mitochondrial pyruvate dehydrogenase complex-E2 components on biliary cells in PBC, enhanced expression and likely disparity of class I molecules in allograft and an aberrant expression of class II molecules in both PBC and allograft rejection, might prove to be relevant as initiating factors. Further progression of the two conditions is quite different. In PBC there is an extension of the necro-inflammatory process, possibly of the same nature as that responsible for the duct damage, to the periportal parenchyma; cholangiodestruction runs a slow, at times fluctuating, course over many years, whereas periportal and periseptal parenchymal damage secondary to chronic cholate-stasis and the associated ductular reaction seem to play major roles in fibrogenesis and eventual cirrhotic transformation. In contrast, cholangiodestruction of 'chronic' rejection often runs a subacute course, a prominent, acute-type cholestasis affecting acinar zone 3 is associated, the portal inflammation rapidly subsides, and both ductular reaction and fibrous tissue deposition are inconspicuous or mild. Several factors have been proposed to explain these unique features of ductopenic rejection, among them the severe ischaemia due to the associated obliterative arteriopathy, additional involvement of a humoral mechanism, and/or a concomitant cytomegalovirus infection[61,62].

A better understanding of the mechanism of tissue damage at the various stages of evolution of both PBC and CR may help to explain variable responses following the different forms of treatment.

References

1. Ludwig J. Terminology of hepatic allograft rejection (glossary). Semin Liver Dis. 1992;12: 89–92.
2. Portmann B, Neuberger J, Williams R. Intrahepatic bile duct lesions. In: Calne RY, editor. Liver transplantation. London: Grune & Stratton; 1983:279–87.
3. Dauphinee JA, Sinclair JC. Primary biliary cirrhosis. Can Med Assoc J. 1949;61:1–6.
4. Portmann BC, MacSween RNM. Diseases of the intrahepatic bile ducts. In: MacSween RNM, Anthony PP, Scheuer PJ, Burt AD, Portmann BC, editors. Pathology of the liver, 3rd edn. Edinburgh: Churchill Livingstone; 1994:(in press).

5. Burkel WE. The fine structure of the terminal branches of the hepatic arterial system of the rat. Anat Rec. 1970;167:329–49.
6. Van den Oord JJ, Sciot P, Desmet VJ. Expression of MHC products by normal and abnormal bile duct epithelium. J Hepatol. 1986;3:310–17.
7. Rubin E, Schaffner F, Popper H. Primary biliary cirrhosis. Chronic non-suppurative destructive cholangitis. Am J Pathol. 1965;46:387–407.
8. Yamada S, Howe S, Scheuer PJ. Three-dimensional reconstruction of biliary pathways in primary biliary cirrhosis: a computer-assisted study. J Pathol. 1987;152:317–23.
9. Nakanuma Y, Ohta G. Histometric and serial section observation of the intrahepatic bile ducts in primary biliary cirrhosis. Gastroenterology. 1979;76:1326–32.
10. Bernuau D, Feldmann G, Degott C, Gisselbrecht C. Ultrastructural lesions of bile ducts in primary biliary cirrhosis. A comparison with the lesions observed in graft versus host disease. Hum Pathol. 1981;12:782–93.
11. Fennell RH. Ductular damage in liver transplant rejection. Its similarity to that of primary biliary cirrhosis and graft-versus-host disease. In: Sommers SC, Rosen PP, editors. Pathology Annual, 16, Pt 2. New York: Appleton-Century-Crofts; 1981:289–94.
12. Nagafuchi Y, Scheuer PJ. Hepatic β_2-microglobulin distribution in primary biliary cirrhosis. J Hepatol. 1986;2:73–80.
13. Ballardini G, Mirakian R, Bianchi FB, Pisi E, Doniach D, Botazzo GF. Aberrant expression of HLA-DR antigens on bile duct epithelium in primary biliary cirrhosis: relevance to pathogenesis. Lancet. 1984;2:1009–13.
14. Spengler U, Pape GR, Hoffman RM et al. Differential expression of MHC class II subregion products on bile duct epithelial cells and hepatocytes in patients with primary biliary cirrhosis. Hepatology. 1988;8:459–62.
15. Chapman RW, Kelly PMA, Heryet A, Jewell DP, Fleming KA. Expression of HLA-DR antigens on bile duct epithelium in primary sclerosing cholangitis. Gut. 1988;29:870–7.
16. Yamada G, Hyodo I, Tobe K et al. Ultrastructure and immunocytochemical analysis of lymphocytes infiltrating bile duct epithelia in primary biliary cirrhosis. Hepatology. 1986;6:385–91.
17. Krams SM, Van de Water J, Coppel RL et al. Analysis of hepatic T lymphocyte and immunoglobulin deposits in patients with primary biliary cirrhosis. Hepatology. 1990;12:306–13.
18. Adams DH, Hubscher SG, Shaw J et al. Increased expression of intercellular adhesion molecule 1 on bile ducts in primary biliary cirrhosis and primary sclerosing cholangitis. Hepatology. 1991;14:426–31.
19. Joplin R, Lindsay JG, Johnson GD, Stain A, Neuberger J. Membrane dihydrolipoamide acetyltransferase (E2) on human biliary epithelial cells in primary biliary cirrhosis. Lancet. 1992;339:93–4.
20. Van de Water J, Turchany JJ, Leung PSC et al. Molecular mimicry in primary biliary cirrhosis. Evidence for epithelial expression of a molecule cross-reactive with pyruvate dehydrogenase complex-E2. J Clin Invest. 1993;91:2653–64.
21. Portmann B, Popper H, Neuberger J, Williams R. Sequential and diagnostic features in primary biliary cirrhosis, based on serial histologic study in 209 patients. Gastroenterology. 1985;88:1777–90.
22. Wiesner RH, LaRusso NF, Ludwig J, Dickson ER. Comparison of the clinicopathologic features of primary sclerosing cholangitis and primary biliary cirrhosis. Gastroenterology. 1985;88:108–14.
23. Berg PA, Klein R. Autoantibody patterns in primary biliary cirrhosis. In: Krawitt EL, Wiesner RH, editors. Autoimmune liver diseases. New York: Raven Press; 1991:123–42.
24. Michieletti P, Wanless IR, Katz A et al. Antimitochondrial antibody negative primary biliary cirrhosis: a distinct syndrome of autoimmune cholangitis. Gut. 1994;35:260–5.
25. Fagan EA, Moore-Gillon JC, Turner-Warwick M. Multi-organ granulomas and mitochondrial antibodies. N Engl J Med. 1983;308:572–5.
26. Degott C, Feldmann G, Larrey D. Drug-induced prolonged cholestasis in adults: a histological semiquantitative study demonstrating progressive ductopenia. Hepatology. 1992;15:244–51.
27. McMaster KR, Henniger GR. Drug induced granulomatous hepatitis. Lab Invest. 1981;44:61–73.

28. Starzl TE, Marchioro TL, von Kaula KN, Hermann G, Brittain RS, Waddell WR. Homotransplantation of the liver in humans. Surg Gynecol Obstet. 1963;117:659–76.
29. Calne RY, McMaster P, Portmann B, Wall WJ, Williams R. Observations on preservation, bile drainage and rejection in 64 human orthotopic liver allografts. Ann Surg. 1977;186:282–90.
30. Portmann B, Williams R. Histopathology of the transplanted liver. In: Williams R, Cantoni L, editors. Recenti progressi in epatologia. Milan: Casa Editrice Ambrosiana; 1979:369–81.
31. Snover DC, Sibley RK, Freese DK et al. Orthotopic liver transplantation: a pathological study of 63 serial liver biopsies from 17 patients with special reference to the diagnostic features and natural history of rejection. Hepatology. 1984;4:1212–22.
32. Demetris AJ, Lasky S, Van Thiel DH, Starzl TE, Dekker A. Pathology of hepatic transplantation. A review of 62 adult allograft recipients immunosuppressed with a cyclosporin/steroid regimen. Am J Pathol. 1985;118:151–61.
33. Wight DGD, Portmann B. Pathology of liver transplantation. In: Calne Sir Roy, editor. Liver transplantation, 2nd edn. London: Grune & Stratton; 1987:385–435.
34. Adams DH, Burnett D, Stockley RA, Elias E. Pattern of leucocyte chemotaxis to bile after liver transplantation. Gastroenterology. 1989;97:433–8.
35. Perkins JD, Wiesner RH, Banks PM, LaRusso NF, Ludwig J, Krom RAF. Immunohistologic labelling as indicator of liver allograft rejection. Transplantation. 1987;43:105–8.
36. McCaughan GW, Davies JS, Waugh JA et al. A quantiative analysis of T lymphocyte populations in human liver allografts undergoing rejection: The use of monoclonal antibodies and double immunolabeling. Hepatology. 1991;12:1305–13.
37. Ludwig J, Wiesner RH, Batts KP, Perkins JD, Krom RAF. The acute vanishing bile duct syndrome (Acute irreversible rejection) after orthotopic liver transplantation. Hepatology. 1987;7:476–83.
38. Van Hoek B, Wiesner R, Krom R et al. Severe ductopenic rejection following liver transplantation: incidence, time of onset, risk factors, treatment and outcome. Semin Liver Dis. 1992;12:41–50.
39. Grond J, Gouw AS, Poppema S, Sloof MJH, Gips CH. Chronic rejection in liver transplant: a histopathologic analysis of failed graft and antecedent liver biopsies. Transplant Proc. 1983;18:128–35.
40. Freese DK, Snover DC, Sharp HL, Gross CR, Savick SK, Payne WD. Chronic rejection after liver transplantation: a study of clinical, histological and immunological features. Hepatology. 1991;13:882–91.
41. Wiesner RH, Ludwig J, van Hoek B, Krom RAF. Current concept in cell-mediated hepatic allograft rejection leading to ductopenia and liver failure. Hepatology. 1991;14:721–9.
42. Pirsch JD, Kalayoglu M, Hafez GR, D'Alessandro AM, Sollinger HW, Belzer FO. Evidence that the vanishing-bile duct syndrome is vanishing. Transplantation. 1990;49:1015–18.
43. Hübscher S. Histological findings in liver allograft rejection – new insights into the pathogenesis of hepatocellular damage in liver allografts. Histopathology. 1991;18:377–83.
44. Vierling JM, Fennell RH. Histopathology of early and late human hepatic allograft rejection: evidence of progressive destruction of interlobular bile ducts. Hepatology. 1985;5:1076–85.
45. Oguma S, Belle S, Starzl TE, Demetris AJ. A histometric analysis of chronically rejected human liver allografts: insights into the mechanism of bile duct loss: direct immunologic and ischaemic factors. Hepatology. 1989;9:204–9.
46. Matsumoto Y, McCaughan GW, Painter DM, Bishop A. Evidence that portal tract microvascular destruction precedes bile duct loss in human liver allograft rejection. Transplantation. 1993;56:69–75.
47. Noack KB, Wiesner RH, Batts K, van Hoek B, Ludwig J. Severe ductopenic rejection with features of vanishing bile duct syndrome: clinical, biochemical, and histologic evidence for spontaneous resolution. Transplant Proc. 1991;23:1448–51.
48. Hübscher SG, Buckels JAC, Elias E, McMaster P, Neuberger J. Vanishing bile-duct syndrome following liver transplantation – is it reversible? Transplantation. 1991;51:1004–10.
49. Demetris AJ, Fung JJ, Todo S et al. Pathologic observations in human allograft recipients treated with FK506. Transplant Proc. 1990;22:25–34.
50. Shaw BW, Markin R, Stratta R, Lagnas A, Donovan J, Sorrell M. FK 506 for rescue treatment of acute and chronic rejection in liver allograft recipients. Transplant Proc. 1991;23:2994–5.

51. McDiarmid SV, Klintmalm GB, Busuttil RW. FK506 conversion for intractable rejection of the liver allograft. Transplant Int. 1993;6:305–12.
52. Lerut J, Zimmermann A, Gertsch P, Preisig R, Blumgart LH. Chronic rejection and extrahepatic biliary obstruction 8 years after orthotopic liver transplantation using the gallbladder conduit technique. HPB Surg. 1991;5:17–22.
53. Neuberger JM, Portmann B, MacDougall B et al. Recurrence of primary biliary cirrhosis after liver transplantation. N Engl J Med. 1982;306:1–4.
54. Haagsma EB, Manns M, Klein R et al. Subtypes of antimitochondrial antibodies in primary biliary cirrhosis before and after liver transplantation. Hepatology. 1987;7:129–33.
55. Dietze O, Vogel W, Margreiter R. Primary biliary cirrhosis after liver transplantation. Transplant Proc. 1990;22:1501–2.
56. Hubscher SG, Elias E, Buckels JAC et al. Primary biliary cirrhosis: histological evidence of disease recurrence after liver transplantation. J Hepatol. 1993;18:173–84.
57. Balan V, Batts KP, Porayo MK, Krom RAF, Ludwig J, Wiesner RH. Histologic evidence for recurrence of primary biliary cirrhosis after liver transplantation. Hepatology. 1992;18:1392–8.
58. Polson R, Portmann B, Neuberger JM et al. Evidence for disease recurrence after liver transplantation for primary biliary cirrhosis. Gastroenterology. 1989;97:715–25.
59. Portmann B, Neuberger JM. Recurrence of primary disease following liver transplantation. In: Williams R, Portmann B, Tan K-C, editors. The practice of liver transplantation. London: Churchill Livingstone; 1994 (In press).
60. Wong PYN, Portmann B, O'Grady J et al. Recurrence of primary biliary cirrhosis after liver transplantation following FK506-based immunosuppression. J Hepatol. 1993;17: 284–7.
61. O'Grady JG, Alexander GJM, Sutherland S et al. Cytomegalovirus infection and donor/ recipient HLA antigens: interdependent co-factors in pathogenesis of vanishing bile duct syndrome after transplantation. Lancet. 1988;2:302–5.
62. Wright TL. Cytomegalovirus infection and vanishing bile duct syndrome: culprit or innocent bystander? (Editorial). Hepatology. 1992;16:494–6.

21
Immunological aspects of cholestatic liver disease

M. F. BASSENDINE, D. E. J. JONES, M. P. LEON, J. KIRBY,
J. M. PALMER, S. J. YEAMAN and A. G. DIAMOND

INTRODUCTION

Although the aetiologies of the autoimmune cholestatic liver diseases primary biliary cirrhosis and primary sclerosing cholangitis remain unclear, aspects of their immunopathology are becoming increasingly well characterized. In this chapter we will discuss the immunogenetics of these conditions, the nature of the autoantigens and possible mechanisms of antigen presentation.

IMMUNOGENETICS

Immunogenetic factors appear to play a role in the two major ductopenic chronic liver diseases, primary biliary cirrhosis (PBC) and primary sclerosing cholangitis (PSC). In PBC familial clustering is well documented, with the disease occurring in siblings, mothers and daughters, and fathers and daughters[1]. This early anecdotal evidence has been verified by two epidemiological studies in the North of England[2] and North America[3], in which the prevalence for PBC in family members was found to be 2.4% and 4.3% respectively.

Many 'autoimmune' conditions such as insulin-dependent diabetes mellitus, systemic lupus erythematosus and coeliac disease have been shown to have strong associations with the major histocompatibility complex (MHC) antigens encoded by genes on the short arm of chromosome 6. The MHC or human leukocyte antigen (HLA) complex is highly polymorphic, and understanding of its complexity is complicated by frequent changes in the nomenclature[4]. HLA typing was previously performed serologically, but now that the molecular structure of the MHC is much better understood, HLA genotyping can be performed using molecular biology techniques. These methods have been developed initially for the class II region, especially the DR locus, and it has been shown that molecular biology techniques are superior to phenotyping methods both in terms of specificity and sensitivity[5].

In PBC there have been two large genotyping studies in British patients examining HLA class II status. Underhill and colleagues studied both DR and DQ frequencies and found an increase in DR8 and the DQ allele DQB1*0402; the two alleles exhibit linkage disequilibrium suggesting a disease haplotype[6]. A similar study in a less ethnically diverse population confirmed the association with DR8; in 130 patients 18.5% were DR8 compared to 9.2% of 363 healthy local controls (relative risk = 2.0, $p < 0.005$)[7]. A smaller Danish study (23 PBC patients) also used the genotyping method and found no difference in the frequency of DR8[8], but the result must be interpreted with caution in view of the study size. Four previous phenotyping studies have also suggested an association with DR8, in particular the only other large study published to date, where a six-fold increase in the frequency of DR8 was found in 114 Caucasian PBC patients compared with 171 controls[9]. Recently two polymorphic genes (*TAP1* and *TAP2*), located within the class II region and thought to encode membrane transporter molecules responsible for endogenous antigen presentation to the immune system, have been studied in PBC patients[10]. Although no disease association was found, linkage disequilibrium between the DR8 allele and a polymorphism within *TAP1* was identified, which may be important, if only in the DR8 positive patients. A recent genotyping study looking at DP allele frequency in a Japanese population has demonstrated a strong association between DPB1*0501 expression and PBC[11]. MHC class III association in PBC is less well studied, and genotyping of this region less well developed. One study[12] of 25 PBC patients found an excess of C4A*Q0 alleles and a relative risk of 183.8 for individuals carrying both DR8 and C4A*Q0.

In PSC a number of small early studies based on serological phenotyping suggested an association with the HLA B8 DR3 haplotype. This haplotype is associated with a number of organ-specific autoimmune diseases (e.g. lupoid chronic active hepatitis), and provides strong supporting evidence that immunological factors may be important in the pathogenesis of PSC. These results were confirmed and extended by a larger study in 81 PSC patients, with a frequency of the HLA A1 B8 DR3 haplotype of 40% in PSC patients compared with 12% in controls[13]. When all the DR3-positive individuals were eliminated a significant association with DR2 was found: 25 (69%) of 36 remaining patients being DR2-positive compared with 27 (34%) of 79 DR3-negative controls. PSC patients who were DR3-positive were first seen at a significantly younger age than those who were DR2-positive. Another small phenotyping study in PSC found a remarkable association with DRw52a, with 100% of 29 PSC patients being DRw52a-positive compared to 35% of controls[14]. In a subsequent genotyping study from King's College Hospital in London, DRw52a, encoded by DRB3*0101, was the allele most strongly associated with PSC, although only found in 55% of patients[15]. Among the DRB3*0101 (DRw52a)-negative patients DRB5*0101 was found in 53%. This genotyping study is consistent with the secondary association of PSC with DR2 since DRB5*0101, together with DRB1*1501, encodes the serological determinants of DR2. Interestingly both

DRB3*0101 and DRB5*0101 encode for a leucine residue at position 38 of the DR β-chain which is located in the floor of the peptide-binding groove of the DR molecule. This led to the hypothesis that the hydrophobicity of leucine at position 38 of the DR β-chain could influence the binding and hence presentation to T-cells of certain antigenic peptides, and hence be responsible for conferring susceptibility to PSC. However, only 28% of PSC patients in their study were in this category, so this immunogenetic predisposition may be important, but is not essential for the development of PSC.

CELLULAR ASPECTS OF THE IMMUNE RESPONSE

The key interaction in the induction of the immune response is that between the CD4+ T 'helper' cell and the antigen-presenting cell (APC). CD4+ T-cells recognize antigenic peptides bound to MHC class II molecules and can assist the induction of several effector mechanisms including antibody production by B-cells and cytotoxicity mediated by CD8+ T-cells. MHC molecules are membrane-bound glycoproteins which are heterodimeric, consisting of α and β chains, and which present peptides of varying length (8–20 amino-acids) to CD4+ T-cells. The T-cell receptor on the lymphocyte surface recognizes the peptide, which is bound in a groove on the outer surface of the MHC molecule, in the context of several MHC residues. This allows for antigen-specificity and MHC restriction. Induction of the immune response, however, requires more than MHC presentation of peptide to a responding T-cell. In addition cell adhesion molecules mediate a physical interaction between APC and T-cell, and chemical signals in the form of cytokines are secreted. One major co-stimulatory pathway involves B7 (CD80) on the APC surface binding to CD28 on the T-cell (Fig. 1A). B7 is a member of the immunoglobulin gene superfamily; it is a type 1 transmembrane glycoprotein with two immunoglobulin-like extracellular domains. B7 inter-action with CD28 appears to be a major co-stimulatory pathway for interleukin-2 (IL-2) production. Normally CD8+ T-cells do not make enough IL-2 to support their own expansion, being dependent on IL-2 secreted by CD4+ T-cells for help.

The stages of active bile duct destruction in PBC are accompanied by an infiltration of T-cells into the portal tract, suggesting a possible role for them in biliary epithelial cell damage. Many studies have looked at the phenotypes of these infiltrating cells using both immunohistochemistry of tissue sections and FACS analysis of tissue-derived cells. Several conclusions can be drawn: the infiltrate consists of lymphocytes and other mononuclear cells, with the lymphocytes forming a majority[16]. The lymphocytes are mostly $\alpha/\beta+$ T-cells with some B and natural killer (NK) cells[17]. The ratio of CD4+ to CD8+ T-cells seems to vary, and is to some extent dependent on the stage of the disease. HLA-DR expression, a marker of activation, is seen on around one-third of CD4+ T cells[17]. Within the portal tract CD8+ cells have been found adjacent to the biliary epithelial cells[18]. Increased numbers of T-cells, similar in number and type to PBC, have also been found in the portal tract

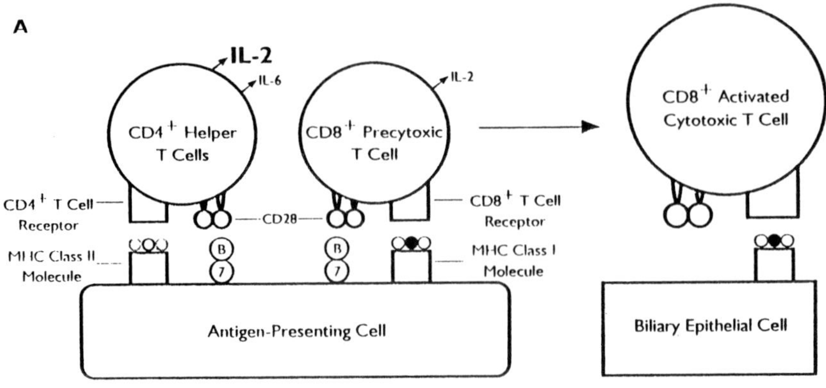

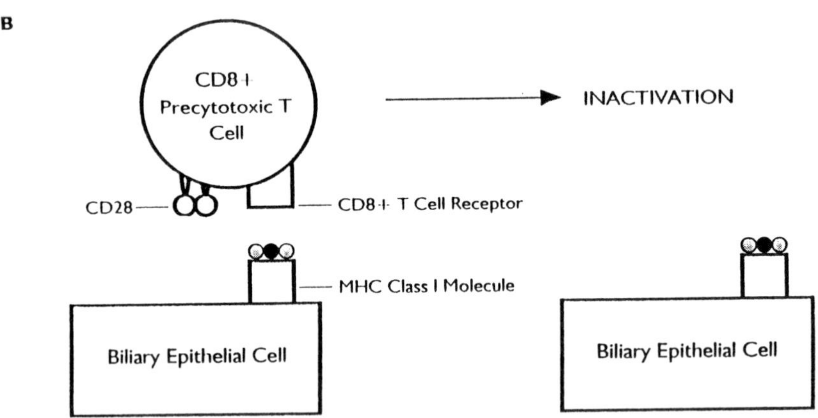

Fig. 1 **A**: Activation of CD8+ cytotoxic T-cells by antigen-presenting cells, involving co-stimulation via B7/CD28 and augmented IL-2 production. **B**: Lack of co-stimulation by biliary epithelial cells, in the absence of IL-2 production, may induce T-cell anergy

in PSC when compared to controls[19]. Such evidence suggests that CD8+ cytotoxic T-cells play a significant role in bile duct damage. In addition the biliary epithelial cells express MHC class I and the cellular adhesion molecules necessary for cytotoxic cell adherence[20].

BILE DUCT EXPRESSION OF MOLECULES INVOLVED IN T-CELL ACTIVATION

Intra- and extrahepatic bile ducts in normal subjects do not express HLA class II molecules, although HLA class I (HLA-A, B, C) antigens are expressed on normal biliary epithelia[21]. However, a number of immunohistochemical studies have shown that intrahepatic bile ducts in patients with both PBC and PSC express HLA-DR antigens. The pattern of class II expression is

Table 1 Levels of HLA class II and B7 expressed by resting and stimulated biliary epithelial cells (BEC) and an EBV-transformed B-cell line

Cell line	Class II MHC	B7 (CD80)	Negative control
Resting BEC	6394 ± 538	8896 ± 925	8934 ± 1381
Stimulated BEC	$3 \times 10^5 \pm 10^3$*	8396 ± 777	7511 ± 1251
EBV line	2×10^5*	64682*	3396

*$p < 0.05$

variable, with not all portal tracts demonstrating it, and in PBC it is not limited to those tracts with the marked mononuclear cell infiltrate[22]. Class II expression on biliary epithelium is not limited to PBC and PSC, however, being found on the bile ducts of patients with extrahepatic biliary obstruction[23]. Despite the fact that HLA class II on biliary epithelium is not specific to PBC and PSC, it has been proposed that such aberrant expression could allow biliary epithelial cells (BEC) to present autoantigens to CD4+ autoreactive T-cells, thereby initiating or exacerbating the autoimmune response. However, it is unclear whether BEC can express the necessary co-stimulatory signals, such as B7, which are required for T-cell activation. We have recently studied the expression of B7 on biliary epithelial cells *in vitro*. Cultured biliary epithelial cells were separated from liver by an immunoprecipitation method[24]. The expression of both MHC class II molecules and B7 was examined under resting conditions and after activation by incubation with the pro-inflammatory cytokines, interferon-γ and TNF-α. Antigen quantification was performed by flow microfluorimetry. An EBV transformed B cell line (able to efficiently present antigen) was used as a positive control for both antigens. The results are expressed as molecules of equivalent FITC (directly proportional to the number of antigen molecules) (Table 1). We have demonstrated that B7 expression is seen neither on the resting BEC nor, in contrast to MHC class II, after cytokine activation. The failure of BEC to express B7 *in vitro* argues against a role for these cells in autoantigen presentation, at least in the initial breakdown of self-tolerance. As BEC appear unable to provide a co-stimulatory signal via B7 it will be important to determine whether antigen presentation by class II-positive BEC in the absence of this co-stimulatory signal can induce peripheral tolerance; this may be a potentially important physiological protective mechanism against destruction of BEC (Fig. 1B). However, when CD4+ T-cell help is present activated CD8+ cytotoxic T-cells can kill BEC that are not expressing B7 because co-stimulation is not required for cytotoxic effector function.

AUTOANTIGENS

Until recently there has been little data available regarding antigen-specificity of T-cells in PBC and PSC, but some progress is now being made in PBC following identification and characterization of the major mitochondrial autoantigens. The usefulness of antimitochondrial antibodies (AMA) as serological markers in PBC has been well documented, and in view of this close association between AMA and PBC much research has focused on determining the nature of the autoantigens. The major PBC-specific antigen, termed M2, was shown by Berg and colleagues to be associated with the inner mitochondrial membrane and to consist of several antigenic determinants (M2a, b, c, d and e). The identity of the M2 non-organ-, non-species-specific autoantigens remained elusive until 1988 when two groups independently showed that the 70 kDa M2a antigen that had been cloned by Gershwin and colleagues in 1987[25] was the E2 component of pyruvate dehydrogenase complex (PDC)[26,27]. It rapidly became clear that the other M2 antigenic determinants visualized on immunoblotting were all components of the 2-oxoacid dehydrogenase multienzyme complexes located in mammalian mitochondria[16]. Following identification of PDC-E2 as the major autoantigen, analysis of the main immunodominant region (MIR) on that polypeptide recognized by AMA has been carried out using PDC-E2 from a variety of sources. Work from our laboratory initially used limited tryptic digestion of bovine heart PDC-E2, which cleaves the polypeptide into two well-defined fragments, followed by immunoblotting of PBC patients' sera, and showed that the MIR lies within the lipoyl domains[28]. The importance of the lipoyl domains was further supported by work using wild-type and mutant forms of PDC-E2 from *E. coli*[29]. More recently Quinn *et al.* used recombinant human inner lipoyl domains with defined lipoate contents, and found that PBC sera have both higher titre and higher affinity against the lipoyl domains bearing the covalently attached lipoic acid co-factor than against the identical, but un-lipoylated, domain[30].

Autoantibody responses have been described in PSC, but the antigen-specificity of such responses is less well characterized than those in PBC. Using an immunoperoxidase technique on isolated neutrophils Snook *et al.* described an anti-neutrophil nuclear antibody (ANNA) in 84% of 32 patients with PSC[31]. The antigen recognized by this PSC-specific ANNA has not yet been identified. Circulating anti-colon antibodies have been described in 62.5% of PSC patients with ulcerative colitis (UC) as compared to 17% of patients with UC alone[32].

Although autoantibodies in PBC have proved useful tools in the identification of potential autoantigens, there is little evidence currently available to suggest that they play a direct role in biliary epithelial cell damage. The presence of a marked activated T-cell infiltrate in the portal tracts at the time of biliary epithelial cell damage, together with the up-regulation of BEC markers thought to be under the control of cytokines secreted by T-cells, suggests that T-cell mediated mechanisms play a significant role in the pathogenesis of PBC. We have demonstrated that T-cells specific for bovine PDC-E2/X are present in the peripheral circulation in the majority of PBC patients, but in only a minority of controls[33]. Moreover, the T-cell response to PDC-E2/X is most marked in patients with early-stage disease. Our findings appear to suggest that T-cell responses to PDC-E2/X are associated with the early active stages of PBC. One possible explanation of our data is that they represent a xenoantigeneic response to bovine PDC components to which most people have had dietary exposure. We have recently characterized for the first time T-cell responses to human PDC and its constituent components E1, E2/X and E3. Human PDC was isolated from heart muscle obtained from explanted organs at cardiac allograft[34]. We demonstrated that autoreactive T-cells specific for human PDC are present in both PBC patients and controls[35], and confirmed that a T-cell proliferative response to PDC-E2/X is seen in the majority of PBC patients (16/28 stimulation index > 2.5) but is largely absent from controls (5/32 SI > 2.5, $p < 0.005$). It has previously been demonstrated that T-cells specific for recombinant human PDC-E2 overexpressed in *E. coli* are present in the mononuclear cell infiltrate in late-stage disease[36]. Taken together these findings suggest that T-cell responses to E2 may have a role to play in the immunological attack on biliary epithelial cells. Further characterization of this T-cell response to autoantigen in PBC will help us to understand the pathogenesis of this condition. In addition greater understanding of the mechanism(s) of breakdown of self-tolerance to PDC-E2/X which is associated with PBC may allow us to develop new approaches to therapy. In animal models of autoimmunity, for example non-obese diabetic mice, tolerization to the autoantigen can prevent development of the autoimmune disease[37,38]. By analogy it may be that a radical new immunotherapy for PBC could be developed in which antigen-specific T-cell tolerance could be induced in the early stages of the disease, possibly by the oral administration of antigen.

References

1. Gregory WL, Bassendine MF. Genetic factors in primary biliary cirrhosis. J Hepatol. 1994; 20:689–92.
2. James OFW, Myszor M. Epidemiology and genetics of primary biliary cirrhosis. In: Popper H, Schaffner F, editors. Progress in liver disease, vol. 9. Philadelphia: Saunders; 1990: 523–36.
3. Back N, Schaffner F. Familial primary biliary cirrhosis. J Hepatol. 1994;20:698–701.
4. Bodmer JG, March SGE, Albert ED *et al.* Nomenclature for factors of the HLA system. Vox Sang. 1992;63:142–57.
5. Mytilineos J, Scherer S, Opelz G. Comparison of RFLP-DRβ and serological HLA-DR typing in 1500 individuals. Transplantation. 1990;50:870–3.
6. Underhill JA, Donaldson PT, Bray GP, Doherty DG, Portmann BC, Williams R. Genetic analysis in a large series of patients with primary biliary cirrhosis reveals an increased frequency of HLA DRw8 and DQB1*0402. Hepatology. 1992;16:604–8.
7. Gregory WL, Mehal W, Dunn AN *et al.* Primary biliary cirrhosis: contribution of HLA class II allele DR 8. Q J Med. 1993;86:393–9.
8. Morling N, Dalhoff K, Fugger L *et al.* DNA polymorphisms of the HLA class II genes in primary biliary cirrhosis. Immunogenetics. 1992;35:112–16.
9. Gores GJ, Moore SB, Fisher LD, Powell FC, Dickson ER. Primary biliary cirrhosis: association with class II major histocompatibility antigens. Hepatology. 1987;7:889–92.
10. Gregory WL, Daly AK, Dunn AN *et al.* Analysis of HLA class II encoded antigen processing genes TAP 1 and TAP 2 in primary biliary cirrhosis. Q J Med. 1994;87:237–44.
11. Seki T, Kiyosawa K, Ota M *et al.* Association of primary biliary cirrhosis with human leukocyte antigen DPB1*0501 in Japanese patients. Hepatology. 1993;18:73–8.
12. Manns MP, Bremm A, Schneider PM *et al.* HLA DRw8 and complement C4 deficiency as risk factors in primary biliary cirrhosis. Gastroenterology. 1991;101:1367–73.
13. Donaldson PT, Farrant JM, Wilkinson ML, Hayllar K, Portmann BC, Williams R. Dual association of HLA DR2 and DR3 with primary sclerosing cholangitis. Hepatology. 1991;13:129–33.
14. Prockazka EJ, Terasaki PI, MinSik Park DVM, Goldstein LI, Busuttil RW. Association

of primary sclerosing cholangitis with HLA DRw52a. N Engl J Med. 1990;322:1842–4.
15. Farrant JM, Doherty DG, Donaldson PT *et al.* Amino acid substitutions at position 38 of the DR β polypeptide confer susceptibility to and protection from primary sclerosing cholangitis. Hepatology. 1992;16:390–5.
16. Jones DEJ, Gregory WL, Bassendine MF. Primary biliary cirrhosis. In: Thomas HC, Waters JP, editors. Immunology and liver disease. Lancaster: Kluwer; 1993:121–41.
17. Bjorkland A, Festin R, Mendel-Hartvig I, Nyberg A, Loof L, Totterman T. Blood and liver infiltrating lymphocytes in primary biliary cirrhosis: increase in activated T and natural killer cells and recruitment of primed memory T-cells. Hepatology. 1991;13:1106–11.
18. Yamada G, Hyodo I, Tobe K *et al.* Ultrastructural immunocytochemical analysis of lymphocytes infiltrating bile duct epithelia in primary biliary cirrhosis. Hepatology. 1986;3:385–91.
19. Snook JA, Chapman RW, Sachdev GK, Heryet A, Kelly PM, Fleming KA. Peripheral blood and portal tract lymphocyte populations in primary sclerosing cholangitis. J Hepatol. 1989;9:36–41.
20. Adams DH, Hubscher SG, Shaw J *et al.* Increased expression of ICAM-1 on bile ducts in primary biliary cirrhosis and primary sclerosing cholangitis. Hepatology. 1991;14:426–31.
21. Van den Oord JJ, Sciot R, Desmet VJ. Expression of MHC products by normal and abnormal bile duct epithelium. J Hepatol. 1987;3:310–17.
22. Nakanuma Y, Kono N. Expression of HLA-DR antigen on the inter-lobular bile ducts in primary biliary cirrhosis and other hepatobiliary diseases: an immunohistochemical study. Hum Pathol. 1991;22:431–6.
23. Chapman RW, Kelly P, Heryet A, Jewell DP, Fleming KA. Expression of HLA-DR antigens on bile duct epithelium in primary sclerosing cholangitis. Gut. 1988;29:422–7.
24. Joplin R, Strain AJ, Neuberger J. Immuno-isolation and culture of biliary epithelial cells from normal human liver. In Vit Cell Dev Biol. 1989;25:1189–92.
25. Gershwin ME, Mackay IR, Sturgess A, Coppel RL. Identification and specificity of a cDNA encoding the 70 kDa mitochondrial antigen recognised in primary biliary cirrhosis. J Immunol. 1987;138:3525–31.
26. Yeaman SJ, Fussey SPM, Danner DJ, James OFW, Mutimer DJ, Bassendine MF. Primary biliary cirrhosis: identification of two major M2 mitochondrial autoantigens. Lancet. 1988;1:1067–70.
27. Van de Water J, Fregeau D, Davis P *et al.* Autoantibodies of primary biliary cirrhosis recognise dihydrolipoamide acetyltransferase and inhibit enzyme function. J Immunol. 1988;141:2321–4.
28. Fussey SPM, Bassendine MF, James OFW, Yeaman SJ. Characterisation of the reactivity of autoantibodies in primary biliary cirrhosis. FEBS Lett. 1989;246:49–53.
29. Fussey SPM, Ali ST, Guest JR, James OFW, Bassendine MF, Yeaman SJ. Reactivity of primary biliary cirrhosis sera with *Escherichia coli* dihydrolipoamide acetyltransferase (E2p): characterisation of the main immunogenic region. Proc Natl Acad Sci USA. 1990;87: 3987–91.
30. Quinn J, Diamond AG, Palmer JM, Bassendine MF, James OFW, Yeaman SJ. Lipoylated and un-lipoylated domains of human PDC-E2 as autoantigens in primary biliary cirrhosis: significance of lipoate attachment. Hepatology. 1993;18:1384–91.
31. Snook JA, Chapman RW, Fleming K, Jewell DP. Anti-neutrophil nuclear antibody in ulcerative colitis, Crohn's disease and primary sclerosing cholangitis. Clin Exp Immunol. 1989;76:30–3.
32. Chapman RW, Cottone M, Selby WS, Shepherd HA, Sherlock S, Jewell DP. Serum autoantibodies, ulcerative colitis and primary sclerosing cholangitis. Gut. 1986;27:86–91.
33. Jones DEJ, Palmer JM, Yeaman SJ, Diamond AG, Bassendine MF. T-cell responses to the components of pyruvate dehydrogenase complex in primary biliary cirrhosis. Hepatology. 1994;19:791.
34. Palmer JM, Bassendine MF, James OFW, Yeaman SJ. Human pyruvate dehydrogenase complex as an autoantigen in primary biliary cirrhosis. Clin Sci. 1993;85:289–93.
35. Jones DEJ, Palmer JM, Yeaman SJ, Diamond AG, Bassendine MF. T-cell responses to human pyruvate dehydrogenase complex and its components in primary biliary cirrhosis. Gastroenterology. 1994;106:A912.
36. Van de Water J, Ansari AA, Surh CD *et al.* Evidence for the targeting by 2-oxo-

dehydrogenase enzymes in the T-cell response in primary biliary cirrhosis. J Immunol. 1991;146:89–94.
37. Kaufman DL, Clare-Saltzler M, Tian J *et al.* Spontaneous loss of T-cell tolerance to glutamic acid decarboxylase in murine insulin-dependent diabetes. Nature. 1993;366:69–72.
38. Tisch R, Xang XD, Singer SM, Liblau RS, Fugger L, McDevitt HO. Immune response to glutamic acid decarboxylase correlates with insulitis in non-obese diabetic mice. Nature. 1993;366:72–5.

22
Epidemiological and clinical features of primary biliary cirrhosis and primary sclerosing cholangitis

R. H. WIESNER

Epidemiology

Primary biliary cirrhosis occurs more frequently in females (90%) and has a median onset of 50 years of age (range 21–91 years). While primary biliary cirrhosis affects all races, it has predominantly been described in Caucasian populations. Whether this reflects better medical screening in this group of patients remains unknown. In the United Kingdom, up to 2% of cirrhotic deaths are related to primary biliary cirrhosis[3]. The incidence has been quite variable, ranging from 3.3 cases per million in Canada to 13.3 cases per million in Sweden[4,5]. Similarly, the prevalence in Canada is reported to be 22.4 cases per million, while in Sweden it has been reported to be 151 cases per million[4,5]. This variability in the incidence and prevalence remains poorly defined.

PRIMARY BILIARY CIRRHOSIS

Introduction

Primary biliary cirrhosis is a chronic cholestatic liver disease characterized by immunological destruction of interlobular and septal bile ducts leading to cholestasis, biliary cirrhosis, and frequently premature death from liver failure[1]. The aetiology of primary biliary cirrhosis remains unknown and, at this time, no totally effective therapy is available. Therapeutic intervention with liver transplantation has proved to be a life-saving procedure for those patients with end-stage disease[2].

Genetics

While primary biliary cirrhosis is known not to be inherited predominantly as an autosomal dominant or recessive trait, familial clustering has been reported in up to 2.4% of family members[6]. This includes occurrence in sisters, twins, mothers and daughters, as well as in identical twins. In addition, one study reported that first-degree healthy relatives with primary biliary cirrhosis had a prevalence of M2 antibody of 7.6%[7].

The results of histocompatibility testing have given controversial data. Early work suggested that there was no association of primary biliary cirrhosis with any HLA A, B or DR antigens[8]. In a predominantly Caucasian population in the United States, HLA DRw8 was found to be associated with primary biliary cirrhosis[9]. In another study, HLA DRw8 in association with C4 deficiency was found to be a risk factor for primary biliary cirrhosis[10]. Other studies have suggested that environmental factors may play an important role. In one study from Sheffield, primary biliary cirrhosis was associated with a particular water supply[11] and, in a more recent study, primary biliary cirrhosis is linked to a mycobacterial infection[12]. However, overall it is difficult to strongly implicate genetic or environmental factors, and our best estimate is that environmental factors, in combination with a genetically susceptible host, must both be present for primary biliary cirrhosis to develop.

Diagnosis

The diagnosis of primary biliary cirrhosis is based on a clinical picture of chronic cholestasis with an elevated serum alkaline phosphatase level being present for 6 months or more[1]. The antimitochondrial antibody and, in particular, the M2 antibody which is directed at the pyruvate dehydrogenase complex localized on the inner mitochondrial membrane, is quite diagnostic for primary biliary cirrhosis[13]. The presence of the M2 antibody is 98% sensitive and 96% specific for the diagnosis of primary biliary cirrhosis[13].

Liver biopsy is also important in confirming the diagnosis of primary biliary cirrhosis. The only hepatic lesion which is almost diagnostic of primary biliary cirrhosis is the florid duct lesion which is present in approximately 10–15% of liver biopsies performed in patients with early histological stage primary biliary cirrhosis[14] (Fig. 1). However, the presence of inflammatory bile duct destruction, portal fibrosis, ductopenia and biliary cirrhosis is usually quite confirmatory in the appropriate clinical setting. Cholangiography is important in differentiating primary biliary cirrhosis from primary sclerosing cholangitis, but often is not necessary in the clinical setting of a middle-aged female having a cholestatic biochemical profile and the presence of an M2 antibody[1].

Differential diagnosis

Primary biliary cirrhosis must be differentiated from a variety of other causes of chronic cholestasis, including drug-induced cholestasis, incomplete bile

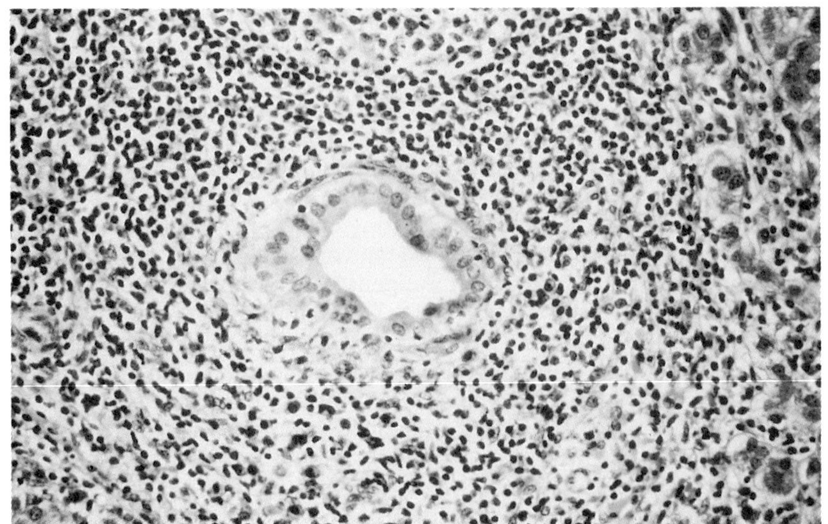

Fig. 1 The typical florid duct lesion characterized by epithelioid cells and epithelioid granulomas engulfing and destroying an interlobular bile duct

Table 1 Drugs associated with ductopenia

Chlorpromazine
Carbamazepine
Haloperidol
Erythromycin
Trimethoprim-sulphamethoxazole
Flucloxacillin
Itroconazole
Thiobendazole
Paraquat
Chlorpropamide
Spanish toxic oil syndrome

duct obstruction, primary sclerosing cholangitis, sarcoidosis and immune cholangiopathy. Drug-induced cholestasis is frequently excluded by taking a careful history to exclude the recent use of drugs known to cause chronic cholestasis. Drugs of particular interest known to be associated with ductopenia include chlorpromazine, thiobendazole, carbamazepine, erythromycin, haloperidol, and paraquat (a herbicidal agent) (Table 1)[15-19]. Primary sclerosing cholangitis is readily differentiated from primary biliary cirrhosis in that it occurs more often in males, it is frequently associated with chronic ulcerative colitis, and the M2 antibody is negative[20]. An endoscopic or transhepatic cholangiogram will show the classic intrahepatic and extrahepatic biliary stricturing which is the hallmark of primary sclerosing cholangitis. Incomplete bile duct obstruction can often be diagnosed on the basis of an ultrasound, which will often show dilated intrahepatic bile ducts. A cholangiogram will confirm the presence of incomplete biliary obstruction.

Table 2 Primary biliary cirrhosis compared to autoimmune cholangiopathy

	Primary biliary cirrhosis	*Autoimmune cholangiopathy*
Sex	Female	Female
Biochemical	Cholestatic	Cholestatic
AMA	Present	Absent
IgM	Elevated	± (normal)
Antinuclear antibody	Absent	Present
Smooth muscle antibody	Absent	Present
Portal infiltrates	Present	Present
Bile duct lesion	Present	Present
Response to steroids	Fair	Good

Modified from Sherlock S *et al.* Primary biliary cirrhosis: definition and epidemiological features. In: Meyer zum Buschenfelde KH, Hoofnagle J, Manns M, editors. Immunology and the liver. London, Kluwer; 1992:346.

Sarcoidosis can also cause difficulty in the differential diagnosis of primary biliary cirrhosis[21]. Clinically, sarcoidosis can present in an identical fashion to primary biliary cirrhosis, but the M2 antibody is negative and liver histology reveals multiple discrete hepatic granulomas as compared to the poorly formed granulomas commonly seen in primary biliary cirrhosis. Angiotensin-converting enzyme levels are elevated in both disease entities and, thus, are not able to differentiate between the two diseases. However, the Kveim–Siltzbach test is positive in sarcoidosis and negative in primary biliary cirrhosis and, therefore, is helpful in the differential diagnosis of these two clinical entities[21].

Finally, immune cholangiopathy is important to differentiate from primary biliary cirrhosis (Table 2)[22,23]. Both entities commonly occur in females but, here again, the M2 antibody is absent in patients with immune cholangiopathy. In addition, patients with immune cholangiopathy frequently have the presence of high-titre antinuclear antibodies and antismooth muscle antibodies, and frequently respond to corticosteroid therapy. Immune cholangiopathy most likely represents a variant of autoimmune chronic active hepatitis which predominantly affects bile ducts. Its response to corticosteroid therapy remains to be evaluated.

Associated diseases

Primary biliary cirrhosis is associated with a variety of other autoimmune diseases including the sicca syndrome, rheumatoid arthritis, thyroiditis, scleroderma, coeliac disease, pulmonary interstitial fibrosis and renal tubular acidosis[24]. In addition, portal adenopathy is frequently present. Female patients with primary biliary cirrhosis may have a higher incidence of breast cancer[25], while male primary biliary cirrhosis patients who develop cirrhosis appear to be at an increased risk for the development of hepatocellular cancer[26].

Clinical presentation

Primary biliary cirrhosis today most often presents without significant symptomatology in a patient in whom routine blood screening tests reveal an elevated serum alkaline phosphatase level[1]; indeed, 50% of patients diagnosed with primary biliary cirrhosis are asymptomatic. Clinical symptoms of primary biliary cirrhosis include the insidious onset of pruritus and fatigue, or the presentation of pruritus associated with pregnancy. Today, less than 20% of patients are jaundiced at the time of diagnosis and approximately 20% will have xanthelasma or xanthoma at the time of presentation. Initial presentation with a complication of portal hypertension such as variceal bleeding today occurs in less than 5% of patients.

Complications of primary biliary cirrhosis

In addition to the complications of portal hypertension, which include variceal bleeding, ascites and encephalopathy, patients with primary biliary cirrhosis frequently experience steatorrhoea associated with fat-soluble vitamin deficiency[27]. The aetiology of steatorrhoea is most often related to a decrease in the concentrations of bile acids in the duodenum, but infrequently steatorrhoea can be associated with concurrent chronic pancreatitis, coealiac sprue, or with the administration of medications such as cholestyramine or neomycin. When the bilirubin reaches $> 3\,mg/dl$ it is prudent to screen such patients for fat-soluble vitamin deficiencies, since vitamin A deficiency can lead to night-blindness, vitamin K deficiency can lead to coagulopathy, and vitamin D deficiency can be associated with osteomalacia or increased bone mineral loss. However, most often the metabolic bone disease associated with primary biliary cirrhosis is related to osteoporosis, for which the aetiology is thought to be associated with an imbalance between bone formation and bone reabsorption[28].

Natural history

In general, primary biliary cirrhosis follows a progressive course without spontaneous remissions. Figure 2 shows the natural history of primary biliary cirrhosis from a histopathologic viewpoint[29]. In general, primary biliary cirrhosis is associated with the progressive loss of interlobular and septal bile ducts, eventually leading to cholestasis, fibrosis and irreversible biliary cirrhosis. This model is based on one important but unproven hypothesis; that is, when the bile ducts are destroyed they do not regenerate. In contrast, hepatocytes have an almost infinite capacity to regenerate. In the above model there is a finite number of bile ducts within the liver, and as bile ducts are slowly destroyed their absolute number decreases, leading to ductopenia. As this occurs, the disease progresses histologically from stage 1 (characterized by portal inflammation) to stage 4 (characterized by thick strands of fibrosis linking portal tracts and central veins). This progression is accompanied by signs and symptoms of cholestasis, and correlates with the development of

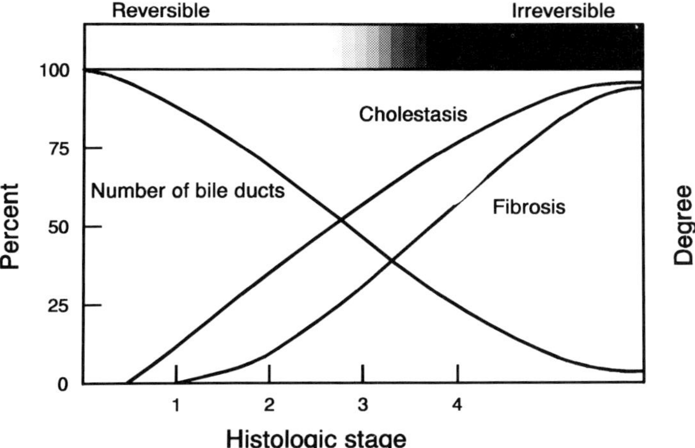

Fig. 2 Histopathological evolution of primary biliary cirrhosis from reversible immunological bile duct stage, which potentially should be responsive to medical therapy to an irreversible fibrotic/cirrhotic stage resistant to medical intervention. Reprinted with permission from Wiesner RH. Primary biliary cirrhosis: an assessment of current medical therapies. In: Krawitt EL, Wiesner RH, editors. Autoimmune liver diseases. New York: Raven Press; 1991:175–89

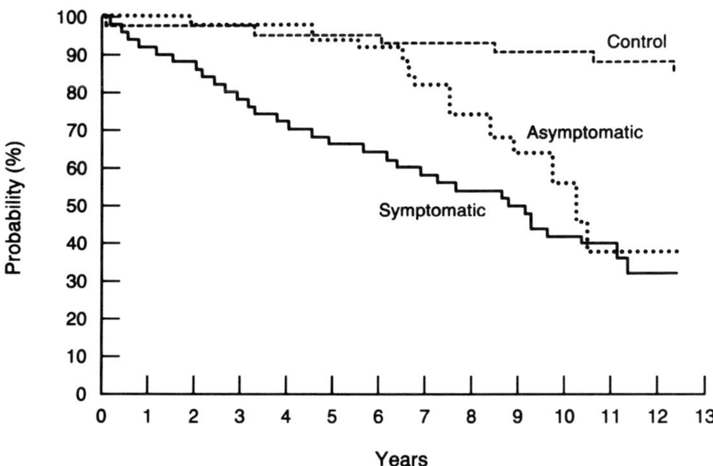

Fig. 3 Kaplan Meier survival stimates of patients with asymptomatic and symptomatic primary biliary cirrhosis compared to an age-, sex-, and race-matched control

jaundice and diminished hepatic synthetic function.

Asymptomatic primary biliary cirrhosis patients clearly survive longer than symptomatic patients, but not as long as healthy age- and sex-matched controls[30] (Fig. 3). The median survival for asymptomatic patients in a prospective study was approximately 10 years. In this study, 32/44 asymptomatic primary biliary cirrhosis patients followed for 4–6 years developed a progressive rise in serum bilirubin levels and a progressive decrease in serum albumin levels. During this follow-up, 84% of patients developed symptoms related to their liver disease and experienced a four-fold increase in mortality compared to the general population[30]. Other studies have documented that symptomatic primary biliary cirrhosis patients with stage 3 or 4 histological disease have a median survival of 7–9 years[31,32] (Fig. 3).

Statistical models have been devised to predict the probability of survival for individual patients with primary biliary cirrhosis, and these models appear to be important with regard to application to liver transplantation. The Mayo model relies on non-invasive variables such as serum bilirubin, albumin, prothrombin time, the presence of oedema, and a patient's age, details of which can be readily obtained at any clinic[33]. These models are not only important for the selection and timing of liver transplantation, but may also serve as important indicators of disease progression in the evaluation of new therapeutic modalities.

PRIMARY SCLEROSING CHOLANGITIS

Primary sclerosing cholangitis is a chronic syndrome characterized by chronic cholestasis caused by diffuse inflammation and fibrosis that involves the entire biliary tree[34,35]. The pathological process obliterates intrahepatic and extrahepatic bile ducts, ultimately leading to biliary cirrhosis, portal hypertension and hepatic failure[36]. The aetiology of primary sclerosing cholangitis remains unknown; however, its close association with inflammatory bowel disease, most commonly chronic ulcerative colitis, has remained quite intriguing[37]. Similar to primary biliary cirrhosis, at this time there is no totally effective therapy available, and therapeutic intervention with liver transplantation has proven to be effective for those patients with end-stage disease[38].

Epidemiology

The prevalence of primary sclerosing cholangitis in the United States is unknown at this time. However, because of the frequent association (75%) of primary sclerosing cholangitis with chronic ulcerative colitis, we can estimate the prevalence of primary sclerosing cholangitis on the basis of studies which have shown a 2.4–7.5% prevalence of primary sclerosing cholangitis in patients with chronic ulcerative colitis[39,40]. Because the prevalence of chronic ulcerative colitis ranges from 40 to 225 cases per 100 000 population, the prevalence of primary sclerosing cholangitis in the United States can be estimated to be 2–7 cases per 100 000 population[41-43]. This estimate has recently been supported by the results of an epidemiological study from Sweden which reported the prevalence of chronic ulcerative colitis and primary sclerosing cholangitis to be 171 cases per 100 000 population and 6.3 cases per 100 000 population, respectively[44]. These results probably underestimate the true prevalence of primary sclerosing cholangitis, since primary sclerosing cholangitis can occur in patients with normal serum levels of alkaline phosphatase and 20–30% of patients with primary sclerosing cholangitis do not have associated inflammatory bowel disease. Thus, primary sclerosing cholangitis appears to be more common than previously suspected, and may have a prevalence which is similar to that reported for primary biliary cirrhosis. In the United States, primary sclerosing cholangitis is the third most common indication for liver transplantation in adults[45].

Genetics

Like primary biliary cirrhosis, primary sclerosing cholangitis is known not to be inherited, predominantly as an autosomal dominant or recessive trait. But familial clustering has been reported, with up to 175 of family members having either associated chronic ulcerative colitis or primary sclerosing cholangitis[46–48]. In recent years it has become evident that genetic factors play an important role in primary sclerosing cholangitis. Findings to support this statement include the fact that several HLA haplotypes have been found to be associated with primary sclerosing cholangitis, including HLA B8, DR2, DR3, and DRw52a[49].

Several investigations have found a strong association of primary sclerosing cholangitis with the HLA haplotype B8, DR3[50,51], both of which are known to be associated with other autoimmune diseases, such as autoimmune chronic active hepatitis, type I diabetes mellitus, myasthenia gravis, thyroiditis and coeliac disease. Still others have found that the HLA haplotype DR2, in addition to B8 and DR3, is an independent factor which appears to influence the initiation of primary sclerosing cholangitis[52]. An initial report of HLA DRw52a occurring in 100% of Caucasian North American primary sclerosing cholangitis patients has not been confirmed in a group of Swedish patients using a more specific assay[53–55]. Farrant *et al.* analysed the frequency of DR B3*0101 allele, which encodes for DRw52a, and this was indeed found to be the most strongly associated allele present in 55% of primary sclerosing cholangitis but also present in 22% of controls[56]. Finally, some studies have suggested that primary sclerosing cholangitis patients with HLA DR4 have a more progressive disease[57], while other investigators have indicated that those patients with DRw52a have a more progressive disease[56]. It is obvious that further studies are needed to better define the relationship between HLA haplotype and genetic predisposition to primary sclerosing cholangitis, as well as the relationship between HLA haplotypes and prognosis.

Diagnosis

Criteria used to diagnose primary sclerosing cholanigits have evolved with time. Originally, the diagnosis of primary sclerosing cholangitis was established only at surgery by palpating the fibrotic common bile duct and by biopsy of the common bile duct to exclude bile duct cancer[58]. Later, operative cholangiography revealed beading and irregularity of the

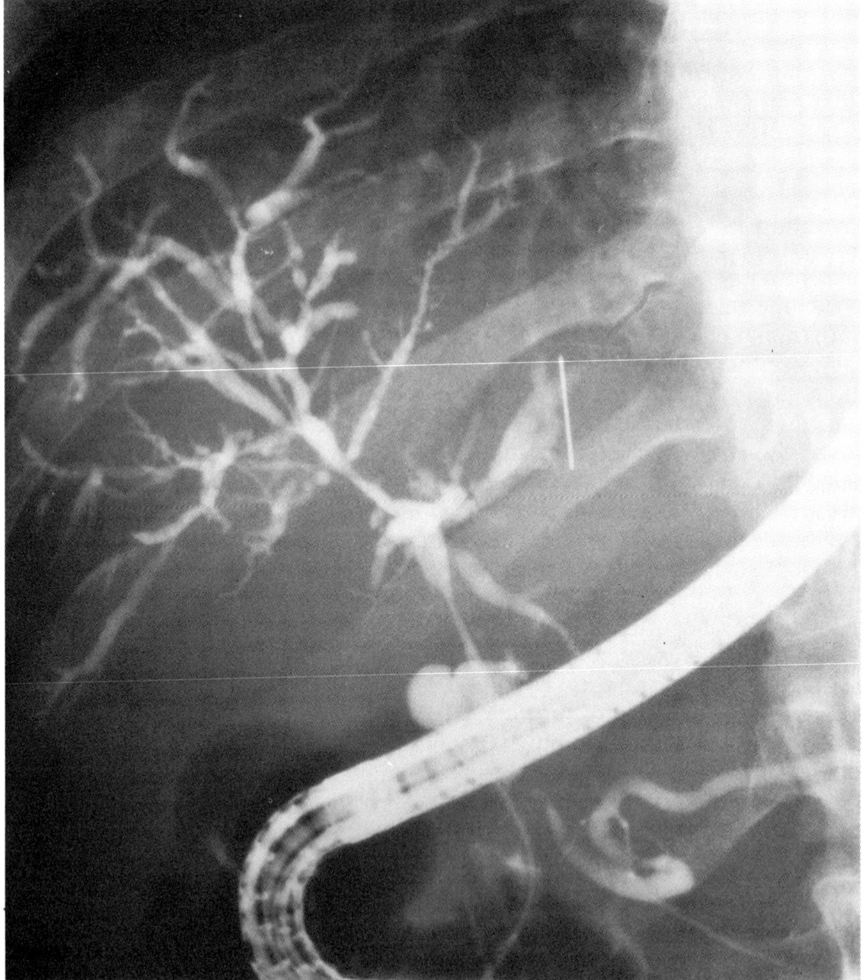

Fig. 4 A typical cholangiogram from a patient with primary sclerosing cholangitis showing irregular narrowing and beading of both the extrahepatic and intrahepatic biliary tree along with areas of telangiectasia

extrahepatic and intrahepatic bile ducts which, today, represent the characteristic radiological features that are diagnostic of primary sclerosing cholangitis in the appropriate clinical setting (Fig. 4). The recognition of the relationship between primary sclerosing cholangitis and inflammatory bowel disease provided an additional diagnostic clue that often allowed clinicians to make an earlier diagnosis of primary sclerosing cholangitis in patients with inflammatory bowel disease who had chronic abnormal biochemical liver tests.

In the past, primary sclerosing cholangitis was diagnosed most often in advanced histological stages when the patient was extremely ill and markedly jaundiced. More recently, non-surgical diagnostic tests, such as the transhepatic cholangiogram and the endoscopic retrograde cholangiogram, coupled with increased awareness of primary sclerosing cholangitis and its association with chronic ulcerative colitis, have led to an earlier diagnosis[59]. Indeed, primary sclerosing cholangitis is a cholangiographic diagnosis provided that other causes of secondary sclerosing cholangitis are excluded. The causes of secondary sclerosing cholangitis are listed below.

The onset of primary sclerosing cholangitis is most often insidious and usually occurs in middle-aged men[34]. The mean age at the time of diagnosis of primary sclerosing cholangitis is 40 years, and two-thirds of patients are male[34]. Most patients have had symptoms for 1–2 years before the diagnosis is actually made. The gradual onset of progressive fatigue and pruritus followed by jaundice is the most frequent symptom-complex leading to the diagnosis. Clinical cholangitis marked by recurrent fever, right upper quadrant pain, and jaundice is uncommon except in patients who have had previous reconstructive biliary surgery, or in those patients who have developed a dominant stricture of the extrahepatic bile duct[60]. A liver biopsy can be helpful in confirming the diagnosis, but rarely are there specific findings. Hepatic histological abnormalities are found on liver biopsy in virtually all patients with primary sclerosing cholangitis. Early histological changes include enlargement of the portal tracts characterized by oedema, portal fibrosis and proliferation of interlobular bile ducts. Other changes include periductal inflammation and fibrosis, duct obliteration and loss of interlobular bile ducts (ductopenia). The most specific finding is the obliterative duct lesion, which is seen in < 10% of liver biopsies obtained from primary sclerosing cholangitis patients[36] (Fig. 5). The end-stages of primary sclerosing cholangitis are marked by histological findings which include loss of interlobular and septal bile ducts, portal fibrosis and biliary cirrhosis (with or without the presence of cholestasis).

Differential diagnosis

The differential diagnosis of primary sclerosing cholangitis for the most part consists of excluding secondary causes of sclerosing cholangitis[60,61]. This includes biliary calculi with bacterial cholangitis, previous biliary tract surgery other than simple cholecystectomy, congenital abnormalities of the biliary tract, cholangiopathy associated with acquired immune deficiency syndrome, ischaemic stricturing, bile duct neoplasm, exposure to bile duct toxins (such as floxuridine), and drug hepatotoxicity which leads to ductopenia as noted under the section on primary biliary cirrhosis. In the typical clinical setting a middle-aged male having long-standing chronic ulcerative colitis presents with an elevated serum alkaline phosphatase level. A cholangiogram shows beading and irregularity of the intrahepatic and extrahepatic bile ducts and, in this setting, the diagnosis of primary sclerosing cholangitis is easily made. It must be pointed out that while the cholangiographic findings of primary sclerosing cholangitis are quite typical,

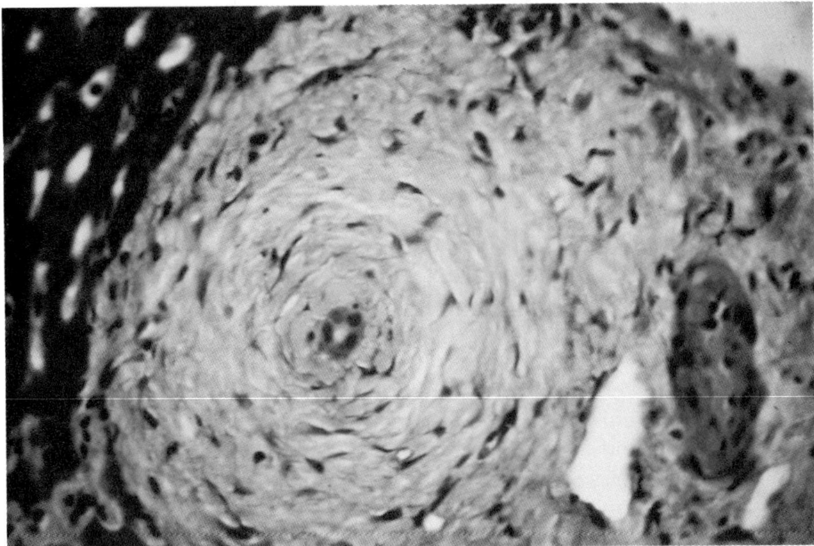

Fig. 5 A liver biopsy specimen from a patient with primary sclerosing cholangitis showing the fibro-obliterative bile duct lesion characterized by concentric fibrosis which is obliterating the interlobular bile duct

they are not specific, and are found in a variety of other secondary causes of sclerosing cholangitis.

In contrast to primary biliary cirrhosis where the presence of antimitochondrial antibody is quite pathognomonic of the disease, the presence of traditional autoantibodies is infrequent in primary sclerosing cholangitis[61]. Testing for antimitochondrial antibodies is almost always negative or, if found, they are present in low titres. Other autoantibodies, such as antinuclear antibodies and antismooth muscle antibodies, are found infrequently; generally they are present in less than one-third of primary sclerosing cholangitis patients. On the contrary, the presence of anticolon antibodies and neutrophil cytoplasmic antibodies has been documented in the majority of primary sclerosing cholangitis patients[62]. These antibodies, however, are seen in a number of other autoimmune disorders, including in patients with chronic ulcerative colitis who do not have primary sclerosing cholangitis, and thus are not specific. The relationship to the pathogenesis remains poorly defined in that the presence and the titres of these autoantibodies do not correlate with the presence or severity of primary sclerosing cholangitis.

Associated diseases

Primary sclerosing cholangitis, like primary biliary cirrhosis, is associated with a variety of other autoimmune diseases. These include inflammatory bowel disease, coeliac disease, retroperitoneal fibrosis, rheumatoid arthritis, thyroiditis and a host of other diseases thought to be of autoimmune origin[60].

Of importance is that primary sclerosing cholangitis patients appear to be predisposed to the development of cholangiocarcinoma[60]. In patients with primary sclerosing cholangitis, 10–15% appear to develop cholangiocarcinoma during the course of the disease. The highest incidence appears to occur in those patients with long-standing chronic ulcerative colitis and cirrhotic stage primary sclerosing cholangitis. Indeed, we consider primary sclerosing cholangitis to be a premalignant condition of the biliary tree just as chronic ulcerative colitis is considered a premalignant condition of the colon. Because primary sclerosing cholangitis patients often have long-standing relatively quiescent colitis, they are at risk for developing both cholangiocarcinoma and colon cancer. Unfortunately, it has been difficult to diagnose bile duct cancer early in primary sclerosing cholangitis patients since fine-needle aspiration, brush cytology, and exfoliative bile cytology have been rather insensitive in detecting cholangiocarcinoma in the presence of primary sclerosing cholangitis. The difficulty in making the diagnosis of cholangiocarcinoma in primary sclerosing cholangitis is supported by the recent report from the University of Pittsburgh in which 10.6% of patients with primary sclerosing cholangitis undergoing liver transplantation were found to have an unsuspected cholangiocarcinoma[45]. Recent reports have suggested that the measurement of serum concentrations of the glycoprotein CA 19-9 may be promising for the detection of cholangiocarcinoma[63]. Further prospective study to evaluate the usefulness of CA 19-9 as a screening test for cholangiocarcinoma in the primary sclerosing cholangitis patient is at present under way. Preliminary data suggest that this test is helpful in confirming the diagnosis of cholangiocarcinoma, but whether it is going to be sensitive to detect early cholangiocarcinoma remains questionable.

Natural history

On the basis of a number of recent prospective studies there is growing evidence that primary sclerosing cholangitis is typically a progressive disease. The largest of these studies, from the Mayo Clinic, reported on 174 patients with primary sclerosing cholangitis who had a mean follow-up of 6 years[34]. The median survival from the time of diagnosis of primary sclerosing cholangitis in all patients was 11.9 years, and both symptomatic and asymptomatic patients had a decreased survival rate compared with that of a US population matched for age, sex and race (Fig. 6). Histological stage was also prognostic of overall survival (Fig. 7). These findings have been confirmed by a number of other centres which have reported median survival times from diagnosis of primary sclerosing cholangitis to be between 9 and 11 years[35].

A subgroup of patients with primary sclerosing cholangitis without symptoms at the time of diagnosis has also been evaluated[64]. At the Mayo Clinic, 45 patients with primary sclerosing cholangitis without symptoms had a mean follow-up of 6.25 years. During this follow-up period, 76% had progression of disease on the basis of clinical and pathological findings and 31% had liver failure resulting in death and/or need for liver transplantation.

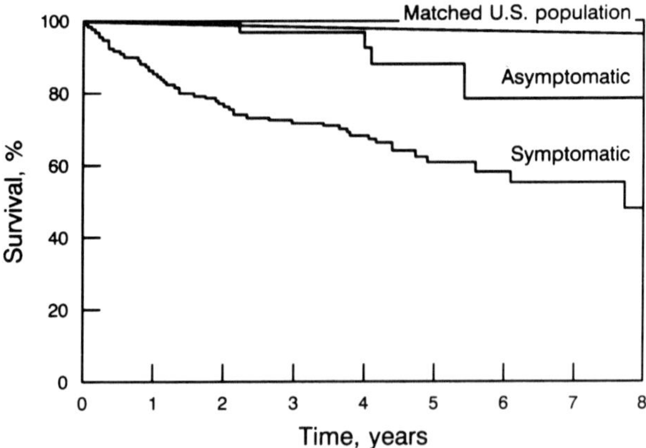

Fig. 6 Kaplan Meier estimated survival in primary sclerosing cholangitis patients who are asymptomatic and symptomatic compared to a control population matched for age, sex, and race

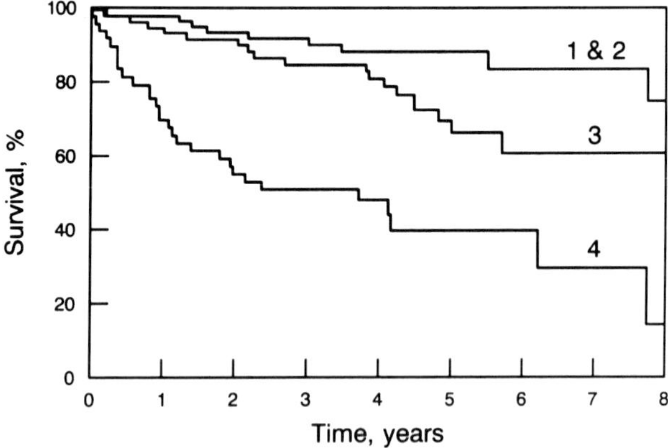

Fig. 7 Kaplan Meier estimated survival in primary sclerosing patients based on initial histological stage

However, other institutions have found primary sclerosing cholangitis to be a more benign disease. Helzberg *et al.*, from Yale, reported a 75% 9-year survival, and studies from Norway estimated the mean survival of patients with primary sclerosing cholangitis to be 17 years from the time of diagnosis[65,66]. Reasons for these differences have recently been put into perspective[67]. First, primary sclerosing cholangitis progresses silently for a number of years and can be detected only by prospective follow-up of liver function tests and hepatic histologies – observations which were not performed in a number of key studies. Second, early detection of the disease would be associated with a longer survival time, which seems to be the case in the Norwegian studies, in which patients with inflammatory bowel disease who had minimal abnormalities in liver function tests were aggressively evaluated with cholangiography. Third, the starting point for survival analysis is important in determining overall survival time. Comparing one group of patients in whom follow-up began at the time of cholangiographic diagnosis of primary sclerosing cholangitis with a second group of patients in whom the diagnosis of primary sclerosing cholangitis was back-dated to the time of first onset of symptoms or first biochemical abnormalities would obviously lead to differences in overall survival time. Overall, we belive the weight of evidence indicates that primary sclerosing cholanigits is indeed a progressive disease in most cases, and that therapeutic intervention should be in the early stages of the disease, since primary sclerosing cholangitis, like primary biliary cirrhosis, is a disease in which ductopenia develops which leads to cholestasis, fibrosis and eventually cirrhosis.

As in primary biliary cirrhosis, survival models have been formulated for primary sclerosing cholangitis to predict survival on the basis of clinical, biochemical and histological features of the disease. The use of sophisticated statistical approaches, most notably the Cox multivariate regression analysis, has enabled us to develop a prognostic model based on four independent variables, which include age, serum bilirubin, the presence or absence of splenomegaly, and histological stage on liver biopsy[68]. Using these models one can estimate survival for the individual primary sclerosing cholangitis patient at any point in the disease course. One can also use the prognostic risk score to evaluate the effect of timing on liver transplantation in this disease entity. Additional studies are at present under way to further refine these models and evaluate their utility in monitoring the effect of experimental therapy on disease progression.

References

1. Sherlock S, Dooley JC. Primary biliary cirrhosis. In: Diseases of the liver and biliary system, 9th edn. Oxford: Blackwell Scientific Publications; 1993;236–48.
2. Markus BH, Dickson ER, Grambsch PM *et al.* Efficacy of liver transplantation in patients with primary biliary cirrhosis. N Engl J Med. 1989;320:1709–13.
3. Hamlyn AN, Sherlock S. The epidemiology of primary biliary cirrhosis: a survey of mortality in England and Wales. Gut. 1974;15:473–9.
4. Witt-Sullivan H, Heathcote J, Cauch K *et al.* The demography of primary biliary cirrhosis in Ontario, Canada. Hepatology. 1990;12:98–105.
5. Danielsson A, Boqvist L, Uddenfeldt P. Epidemiology of primary biliary cirrhosis in a defined rural population in the northern part of Sweden. Hepatology. 1990;11:458–64.
6. Myszor M, James OFW. The epidemiology of primary biliary cirrhosis in north-east England: an increasingly common disease. Q J Med. 1990;75:377–85.
7. Triger DR. Epidemiology: is there an environmental contribution? Presented at the International Association for Study of the Liver, Brighton, UK, 1992.
8. Bassendine MF, Dewar PJ, James OFW. HLA-DR antigens in primary biliary cirrhosis: lack of association. Gut. 1985;26:625–8.
9. Gores GJ, Moore SB, Fisher LD, Powell FC, Dickson ER. Primary biliary cirrhosis: association with class II major histocompatibility complex antigens. Hepatology. 1987;7:889–92.
10. Manns MP, Bremm A, Schneider PM *et al.* HLA DRw8 and complement C4 deficiency as risk factors in primary biliary cirrhosis. Gastroenterology. 1991;101:1367–73.
11. Triger DR. Primary biliary cirrhosis: an epidemiological study. Br Med J. 1980;281:772–5.
12. Vilagut L, Vila J, Vinas O *et al.* Mycobacterium gordonae in primary biliary cirrhosis: possible etiology for the disease. J Hepatol. 1993;18(Suppl. 1):59.

13. Van de Water J, Cooper A, Surh CD *et al.* Detection of autoantibodies to recombinant mitochondrial proteins in patients with primary biliary cirrhosis. N Engl J Med. 1989;320:1377–80.
14. Ludwig J, Dickson ER, McDonald GSA. Staging of chronic nonsuppurative destructive cholangitis (syndrome of primary biliary cirrhosis). Virchow Arch [A]. 1978;379:103–12.
15. Degott C, Feldmann G, Larrey D *et al.* Drug-induced prolonged cholestasis in adults: a histological semiquantitative study demonstrating progressive ductopenia. Hepatology. 1992;15:244–51.
16. Forbes GM, Jeffrey GP, Shilkin KB, Reed WD. Carbamazepine hepatotoxicity: another cause of the vanishing bile duct syndrome. Gastroenterology. 1992;102:1385–8.
17. Manivel JC, Bloomer JR, Snover DC. Progressive bile duct injury after thiabendazole administration. Gastroenterology. 1987;93:245–9.
18. Walker CO, Combes B. Biliary cirrhosis induced by chlorpromazine. Gastroenterology. 1966;51:631–40.
19. Dincsoy HP, Saelinger DA. Haloperidol-induced chronic cholestatic liver disease. Gastroenterology. 1982;83:694–700.
20. Chapman RWG, Margorgh BA, Rhodes JM *et al.* Primary sclerosing cholangitis: a review of its clinical features, cholangiography, and hepatic histology. Gut. 1980;21:870–7.
21. Keeffe EB. Sarcoidosis and primary biliary cirrhosis. Literature review and illustrative cases. Am J Med. 1987;83:977–80.
22. Ben-Ari Z, Dhillon AP, Sherlock S. Autoimmune cholangiopathy? Part of the spectrum of autoimmune chronic active hepatitis. Hepatology. 1993;18:10–15.
23. Michieletti P, Wanless IR, Katz A *et al.* Antimitochondrial antibody negative primary biliary cirrhosis: a distinct syndrome of autoimmune cholangitis. Gut. 1994;35:260–5.
24. Culp KS, Fleming CR, Duffy J, Baldus WP, Dickson ER. Autoimmune associations in primary biliary cirrhosis. Mayo Clin Proc. 1982;57:365–70.
25. Goudie BM, Burt AD, Boyle P *et al.* Breast cancer in women with primary biliary cirrhosis. Br Med J. 1985;291:1597–8.
26. Collier JD, Mitchison H, Kelly P, Bassendine MF, James OFW. Increased risk of developing hepatocellular carcinoma in male patients with primary biliary cirrhosis. Hepatology. 1994;19:521.
27. Lanspa SJ, Chan AT, Bell JS III, Go VL, Dickson ER, DiMagno EP. Pathogenesis of steatorrhea in primary biliary cirrhosis. Hepatology. 1985;5:837–42.
28. Hodgson SF, Dickson ER, Wahner HW, Johnson KA, Mann KG, Riggs BL. Bone loss and reduced osteoblastic function in primary biliary cirrhosis. Ann Intern Med. 1985;103:855–60.
29. Wiesner RH. Primary biliary cirrhosis: an assessment of current medical therapies. In: Krawitt EL, Wiesner RH, editors. Autoimmune liver diseases. New York: Raven Press; 1991:175–89.
30. Balasubramaniam K, Grambsch PM, Wiesner RH, Lindor KD, Dickson ER. Diminished survival in asymptomatic primary biliary cirrhosis: a prospective study. Gastroenterology. 1990;98:1567–71.
31. Roll J, Boyer JL, Barry D, Klatskin G. The prognostic importance of clinical and histological features in asymptomatic and symptomatic primary biliary cirrhosis. N Engl J Med. 1983;308:1–7.
32. Mitchison HI, Lucey MR, Kelly PJ, Neuberger JM, Williams R, Jam OF. Symptom development and prognosis in primary biliary cirrhosis: a study of two centers. Gastroenterology. 1990;99:778–84.
33. Dickson ER, Grambsch PM, Fleming TR, Fisher LD, Langworthy A. Prognosis in primary biliary cirrhosis: model for decision making. Hepatology. 1989;10:1–7.
34. Wiesner RH, Grambsch PM, Dickson ER *et al.* Primary sclerosing cholangitis: natural history, prognostic factors, and survival analysis. Hepatology. 1989;10:430–7.
35. Farrant JM, Hayllar KM, Wilkinson ML *et al.* The natural history and prognostic variables in primary sclerosing cholangitis. Gastroenterology. 1991;100:1710–17.
36. Ludwig J, LaRusso NF, Wiesner RH. The syndrome of primary sclerosing cholangitis. Prog Liv Dis. 1990;9:555–66.
37. Wiesner RH. Etiopathogenesis of primary sclerosing cholangitis. In: Gentilini P, Arias IM, McIntyre N, Rodes J, editors. Cholestasis. International Congress Series 1059. Amsterdam, Elsevier; 1994:153–60.

38. Wiesner RH. Advances in therapy for primary sclerosing cholangitis. Eur J Gastroenterol Hepatol. 1992;4:276–83.
39. Schrumpf E, Fausa O, Elgjo K, Kolmannskog F. Hepatobiliary complications of inflammatory bowel disease. Semin Liver Dis. 1988;8:201–9.
40. Shepherd HA, Selby WS, Chapman RWG et al. Ulcerative colitis and persistent liver dysfunction. Q J Med. 1983;52:503–13.
41. Bonneview O, Riis P, Anthonisen P. An epidemiologic study of ulcerative colitis in Copenhagen County. Scand J Gastroenterol. 1968;3:432–8.
42. Mendeloff AI. The epidemiology of idiopathic inflammatory bowel disease. In: Kirnser JB, Shorter RG, editors. Inflammatory bowel disease, 2nd edn. Philadelphia, Lea & Febiger; 1980:5–19.
43. Stonnington CM, Phillips SF, Melton LJ III, Zinsmeister AR. Chronic ulcerative colitis: incidence and prevalence in a community. Gut. 1987;28:402–9.
44. Rolny P, Ryden B-O, Tysk C, Wallerstedt S. Prevalence of primary sclerosing cholangitis in patients with ulcerative colitis. Gastroenterology. 1991;100:1319–23.
45. Marsh JW Jr, Shunzaburo I, Makowka L et al. Orthotopic liver transplantation for primary sclerosing cholangitis. Ann Surg. 1988;207:21–5.
46. Quigley EMM, LaRusso NF, Ludwig J, MacSween RNM, Birnie GG, Watkinson G. Familial occurrence of primary sclerosing cholangitis and ulcerative colitis. Gastroenterology. 1983;85:1160–5.
47. Jorge AD, Esley C, Ahumada J. Family incidence of primary sclerosing cholangitis associated with immunologic diseases. Endoscopy. 1987;19:114–17.
48. Quigley EMM, Beaver SJ, Wiesner RH, Larusso NF. Family occurrence of inflammatory bowel disease in primary sclerosing cholangitis. Gastroenterology. 1987;92:1585 (abstr.).
49. Chapman RW. The immunogenetics of primary sclerosing cholangitis. In: Meyer zum Buschenfelde K-H, Hoofnagle J, Manns M, editors. Immunology of the liver. Boston/London: Kluwer; 1993:318–23.
50. Chapman R, Vargiese Z, Gaul R et al. Association of primary sclerosing cholangitis with HLA-B8. Gut. 1983;24:38–41.
51. Schrumpf E, Fansa O, Forre O et al. HLA antigens and immunoregulatory T cells in ulcerative colitis associated with hepatobiliary disease. Scand J Gastroenterol. 1982;17:187–91.
52. Donaldson PT, Farran JM, Wilkinson ML et al. Dual association of HLA DR2 and DR3 with primary sclerosing cholangitis. Hepatology. 1991;13:129–33.
53. Prochazka EJ, Terasaki PI, MinSik Park DVM et al. Association of primary sclerosing cholangitis with HLA-DRw52a. N Engl J Med. 1990;322:1842–4.
54. Munoz S, Westerberg S, Martin P et al. HLA-DRw52a: lack of universal association with primary sclerosing cholangitis. Gastroenterology. 1991;100:A778(abstr.).
55. Zetterquist H, Broome V, Einarsson K, Olerup O. HLA class II genes in primary sclerosing cholangitis and chronic inflammatory bowel disease: no HLA-DRw52a association in Swedish patients with sclerosing cholangitis. Gut. 1992;33:942–6.
56. Farrant JM, Doherty DG, Donaldson PT et al. Amino acid substitutions at position 38 of the DR B polypeptide confer susceptibility to and protection from primary sclerosing cholangitis. Hepatology. 1992;16:390–5.
57. Mehal WZ, Lo YM, Wordsworth P et al. HLA DR4 is a marker for rapid disease progression in primary sclerosing cholangitis. Gastroenterology. 1994;106:100–7.
58. Wiesner RH, LaRusso NF. Clinicopathic features of the syndrome of primary sclerosing cholangitis. Gastroenterology. 1980;79:200–6.
59. Elias E, Summerfield JA, Dick R, Sherlock S. Endoscopic retrograde cholangiopancreatograph in the diagnosis of jaundice with ulcerative colitis. Gastroenterology. 1974;67:907–11.
60. Wiesner RH, Porayko MK, LaRusso NF, Ludwig J. Primary sclerosing cholangitis. In: Schiff L, Schiff ER, editors. Diseases of the liver, 7th edn. Philadelphia: Lippincott; 1993:411–26.
61. Wiesner RH, LaRusso NF, Ludwig J, Dickson ER. Comparison of clinicopathologic features of primary sclerosing cholangitis and primary biliary cirrhosis. Gastroenterology. 1985;88:108–14.
62. Duerr RH, Targan SR, Landers CJ et al. Neutrophil cytoplasmic antibodies: a line between

primary sclerosing cholangitis and ulcerative colitis. Gastroenterology. 1991;100:1385–91.
63. Nichols JC, Gores FJ, LaRusso NF, Wiesner RH, Nagorney DM, Ritts RE, Jr. Diagnostic role of serum CA 19-9 for cholangiocarcinoma in patients with primary sclerosing cholangitis. Mayo Clin Proc. 1993;68:874–9.
64. Porayko MK, Wiesner RH, LaRusso NF *et al.* Patients with asymptomatic primary sclerosing cholangitis frequently have a progressive disease. Gastroenterology. 1990;98: 1594–602.
65. Helzberg JH, Petersen JM, Boyer JL. Improved survival with primary sclerosing cholangitis: a review of clinicopathologic features and comparison of symptomatic and asymptomatic patients. Gastroenterology. 1987;92:1869–75.
66. Aadland E, Schrumpf E, Fausa O *et al.* Primary sclerosing cholangitis: a long-term follow-up study. Scand J Gastroenterol. 1987;22:655–64.
67. Porayko MK, LaRusso NF, Wiesner RH. Is primary sclerosing cholangitis a progressive disease? Semin Liv Dis. 1991;11:18–25.
68. Dickson ER, Murtaugh PA, Wiesner RH *et al.* Primary sclerosing cholangitis: refinement and validation of survival models. Gastroenterology. 1992;103:1893–901.

23
Mechanisms of action of ursodeoxycholic acid in cholestasis

R. POUPON and R. E. POUPON

INTRODUCTION

Chronic cholestatic diseases form a homogeneous group of diseases with several points in common. Most of them result from the destruction of intrahepatic bile ducts, or from a developmental defect. Most chronic cholestatic conditions can progress towards cirrhosis. We postulated that some liver lesions and the progression towards cirrhosis could at least in part be mediated by endogenous bile acid accumulation in blood, liver and peripheral tissues.

In cholestatic conditions, bile acid circulation and metabolism are altered, hepatic clearance is diminished, and blood and tissue concentrations are increased; the formation of deoxycholic and lithocholic acids is decreased. Cholic and chenodeoxycholic acids become the main circulating bile species. Urinary excretion of bile acids, which is negligible in physiological conditions, increases as certain atypical bile acids emerge (hydroxylated bile acids, and 3 hydroxy-Δ-5-cholanoic acid). The proportion of sulphated and glucuronidated bile acids is strongly increased.

Contrary to endogenous human bile acids, especially chenodeoxycholic acid, ursodoxycholic acid (UDCA) and its two metabolites, tauro- and glyco-UDCA, have a very low detergency and are not toxic *in vitro* or in man. In particular, UDCA has no toxicity up to concentrations of 500 μmol/l in several *in vitro* models. Humans detoxify and excrete lithocholate, however, which does not accumulate in the enterohepatic circulation. In primary biliary cirrhosis (PBC), UDCA administration has a beneficial effect on the long-term course of the disease.

Although we do not know precisely how chenodeoxycholic and cholic acid accumulation damages the liver, it is now possible to sketch a simplified mechanism of action of UDCA in cholestasis. UDCA (a) decreases the accumulation of cholic and chenodeoxycholic acid, (b) inhibits their intestinal reuptake, and (c) increases their canalicular excretion.

SERUM BILE ACIDS IN CHOLESTASIS: EFFECT OF UDCA THERAPY

Continuous administration of UDCA induces marked changes in plasma bile acid composition and distribution in PBC[1–5]. In our randomized study[6], we found that, irrespective of the histological stage of the disease, UDCA became the major circulating bile acid. The levels and proportions of cholic acid and, to a lesser extent, chenodeoxycholic acid, decreased markedly. The observation that UDCA lowered cholic acid levels more than chenodeoxycholic acid levels could be explained by the fact that chenodeoxycholic acid absorption is less dependent on ileal absorption, as it can be absorbed throughout the small intestine by non-ionic passive diffusion. In addition, UDCA is partly converted into chenodeoxycholic acid during chenodeoxycholic acid feeding[7]. Levels of atypical bile acids, such as 3-monohydroxy-Δ-5-cholanoic acid, also fall significantly. In contrast, levels of total secondary bile acids are not modified. These changes are independent of the histological stage of PBC. However, certain differences in absolute concentrations observed before UDCA administration persist during treatment. For example, in advanced stages, bile acid concentrations before and during UDCA administration were higher than in early stages. Changes in urinary bile acid excretion have also been described: levels of 1- and 6-hydroxylated endogenous bile acids are reduced and these species replaced by hydroxylated derivatives of UDCA[3,8]. Thus, during UDCA administration, the liver and peripheral tissues are exposed to a lower level of endogenous bile acids and to an increased concentration of UDCA and its hydroxylated metabolites.

INHIBITION OF INTESTINAL BILE ACID ABSORPTION BY UDCA

Active ileal absorption is the main mechanism controlling the bile acid pool in health and cholestasis. Experimental studies have shown a natural inhibition of this active intestinal transport between pairs of bile acids *in vitro* and *in vivo*[9].

In contrast to chenodeoxycholic acid, UDCA does not suppress bile acid synthesis in man[10] and it increases the rate of cholic acid and chenodeoxycholic acid catabolism[11–14]. This has been also observed in patients with PBC[13,14]. To test the hypothesis that UDCA might promote intestinal excretion of primary bile acids by inhibiting active ileal transport of endogenous bile acid conjugates, we and others[15,16] used [75Se]HCAT, a structural analogue of taurocholate that is not deconjugated by bacteria and that is highly sensitive and specific in the investigation of active ileal absorption of bile acids. During UDCA therapy the fractional catabolic rate and the percentage retention of [75Se]HCAT fell significantly, while no significant change occurred in subjects receiving the placebo. Similar findings have been observed in cholestatic patients, regardless of the aetiology (unpublished results). Finally, similar effects have also been obtained in patients with ileostomies, who served as a model to investigate the effects of UDCA and chenodeoxycholic acid on ileal excretion of primary bile acids[17].

Several arguments, however, suggest that decreased intestinal absorption is not the only explanation for the hepatoprotective effect of UDCA in cholestatic liver diseases. First, cholestyramine, which also reduces bile acid concentrations by impairing their intestinal absorption, does not appear to have a frank beneficial effect in terms of biochemical parameters in chronic cholestatic conditions[18,19]. Second, in experimental models (the isolated and *in-situ* perfused rat liver), intravenous infusion of UDCA protects against chenodeoxycholic acid (and lithocholate) induced liver injury[20–23]. These findings indicate that UDCA has a direct effect on liver cells.

EFFECTS OF UDCA ON HEPATOBILIARY TRANSPORT PATHWAYS

On the basis of the above-mentioned studiees it has been suggested that UDCA has a cytoprotective effect on liver cells, which appears to be specific for bile acid-induced injury. Indeed, UDCA does not protect against acetaminophen, CCl_4, α-naphthyl-isothiocyanate, or ischaemic reperfusion injury[24–26].

The vectorial transport of bile acids across hepatocytes is dependent on the polarized distribution of transporters located on the basolateral and canalicular membranes. The maximal uptake capacity greatly exceeds the maximum hepatic excretory capacity, indicating that excretion across the canalicular membrane is rate-limiting for overall hepatic bile acid transport. Detailed reviews of this uptake process have recently been published[27,28]. The uptake of bile acids across basolateral membranes requires the intervention of one or more transport systems. Following uptake, intracellular transport involves specific binding proteins and a transcytotic vesicular pathway. Canalicular secretion occurs via one of several transport proteins, and probably through a vesicular mechanism. In physiological (non-cholestatic) conditions, periportal hepatocytes and, thus, the periportal canaliculus are mainly responsible for extraction of bile acids from the blood and their excretion in the bile. In cholestatic conditions due to the destruction of a certain proportion of interlobular bile ducts, recruitment of medio- and peri-lobular hepatocytes probably permits bile acids to bypass cholestatic portal and periportal areas.

The capacity of the liver to take up bile acids varies between species and bile acids. In general, maximal transport and intrinsic clearance are inversely proportional to the degree of bile acid hydrophobicity. Thus, tauro-UDCA has the highest intrinsic clearance, at least in the rat[29].

Several lines of evidence suggest that UDCA protects liver cells through an increase in the intrinsic ability of hepatocytes to secrete bile acids into bile. When taurocholate is simultaneously infused with UDCA to rats, not only is the cholestasis due to excess taurocholate prevented, but canalicular excretion of both taurocholate and total bile acids increases[20]. The same observations have been reported using UDCA plus chenodeoxycholate or deoxycholate[21,23] or lithocholate[22]. *In vitro*, the cytoprotection provided by tauro-UDCA was related to its ability to reduce the intrahepatocytic taurochenodeoxycholate content[30]. Again, *in vitro*, tauro-UDCA increased the efflux of chenodeoxycholate from preloaded hepatocytes[30]. In the isolated perfused rat liver, tauro-UDCA increased the clearance V_{max}/K_m, i.e. intrinsic hepatic clearance of taurocholate[31,32].

The mechanism(s) by which UDCA, or its conjugates, augment the uptake of other bile acids has rarely been studied. It has been proposed that this effect could be mediated by an increase in hepatocyte volume. In the intact liver, taurocholate excretion into bile is stimulated following hypotonic amino acid (or insulin) induced cell swelling[33,34]; excretory V_{max} doubles when the intracellular space increases by 10–15%; Tauro-UDCA (10–50 μmol/l) induces hepatocyte swelling. Stimulation of taurocholate excretion by tauro-UDCA strongly depends on the extent of tauro-UDCA-induced swelling rather than the tauro-UDCA concentration. The stimulatory effect of cell swelling on taurocholate excretion into bile is abolished in the presence of colchicine, suggesting a microtubule-dependent mechanism. From these findings it has been proposed that the swelling-induced stimulation of taurocholate excretion into bile is due to a microtubule-dependent insertion of bile acid transporters into the canalicular membrane[34]. Recent evidence has also been provided that the targeting of transporters to the canaliculus could be mediated through a sustained increase in cytosolic calcium induced by tauro-UDCA[35]. Bile acid flux throughout the canaliculus towards periportal zones and the interlobular canal could be facilitated by the contractions induced by tauro-UDCA[36].

Hepatobiliary transport of organic anions, such as bilirubin and BSP, can be facilitated by most bile salts, including UDCA. UDCA increases the maximal biliary secretion of bilirubin in the rat[37], showing that its effect is not restricted to hepatobiliary bile acid transport pathways.

OTHER POSSIBLE MECHANISMS

Immune modulation

Our controlled trial unexpectedly showed that some of the immunological markers of PBC improved during UDCA therapy, suggesting that bile acids and/or UDCA interfere with immune regulation. This led us to explore the effect of cholestasis and bile acids on the immune system. HLA molecules, specifically class I species, are the main targets of the cytotoxic reaction. Abnormal expression of class I molecules on hepatocytes is a salient feature of PBC and primary sclerosing cholangitis. We[38] and others[39] have found that long-term administration of UDCA reduces both cholestasis and the abnormal expression of HLA class I molecules on hepatocytes. It has also been reported that such a reduction can occur on biliary cells. Experimental data indicate that this effect is mediated by a decrease in serum and tissue bile acid accumulation. Whatever the mechanism, the reduction in hepatocyte or biliary cell MHC class I antigen expression induced by UDCA could block periportal and lobular cell necrosis by suppressing the cytotoxic T cell target; this would provide a rational explanation for the improvement in bile duct paucity and periportal necrosis observed in patients on UDCA.

Stabilization of hepatocellular membranes

There is some evidence that UDCA conjugates can stabilize plasma membranes directly against disruption by more toxic bile salts. UDCA has anti-cytolytic properties in erythrocytes and model membranes (with a cholesterol–lecithin molar ratio ≥ 0.5) exposed to high bile acid concentrations[40,41]. However, the clinical relevance of these findings is unclear, since most studies have been performed with very high concentrations of bile acids.

Hypercholeresis

Unconjugated UDCA can induce bicarbonate-rich hypercholeresis in rats, and it has been postulated that this property might be related to its therapeutic effect[42]. Biliary levels of unconjugated UDCA do not markedly increase during UDCA administration to patients with PBC[43] or cystic fibrosis[44]. As the hypercholeresis induced by UDCA administration to rats was linearly related to the recovery of unconjugated UDCA in the bile, it seems unlikely that the choleresis induced by cholehepatic circulation of unconjugated UDCA plays a role in its action in cholestatic patients.

CONCLUSION

Until the 1980s the role of bile acids in the initiation of liver injury in man was only suspected on the basis of the toxicity of whole bile and bile salts, and studies showing elevations in serum and tissue levels of bile salts in liver diseases. The beneficial effects of UDCA in PBC have provided the first firm evidence that bile acids may in some way be related to liver injury in man.

There are many questions regarding the hepatoprotective effect of UDCA that should be addressed in the near future. In particular, we do not know how chronic cholestasis induces liver fibrosis and if UDCA can prevent or counteract this process. Most cholestatic diseases have an immune pathophysiological basis: we must learn much more about the impact of cholestasis and bile acids on the immune system, particularly on endogenous or exogenous peptide presentation in cells exposed to high concentrations of bile components. We have seen that the trafficking of transporters in hepatocytes may be affected by bile acids; efforts must be made to learn more about this important issue. Finally, structural analogues of UDCA, or combinations of drugs should be studied, in order to determine if better therapeutic efficacy could be obtained.

References

1. Chrétien Y, Poupon R, Gherardt MF *et al*. Bile acid glycine and taurine conjugates in serum of patients with primary biliary cirrhosis: effect of ursodeoxycholic treatment. Gut. 1989;30:1110–15.

2. Poupon RE, Chrétien Y, Poupon R, Paumgartner G. Serum bile acids in primary biliary cirrhosis: effect of ursodeoxycholic acid therapy. Hepatology. 1993;17:599–604.

3. Stiehl A, Rudolph G, Raedsch R *et al.* Ursodeoxycholic acid-induced changes of plasma and urinary bile acids in patients with primary biliary cirrhosis. Hepatology. 1990;3:492–7.

4. Crosignani A, Podda M, Bertoloni E, Battezzati PM, Zuin M, Setchell KDR. Failure of ursodeoxycholic acid to prevent a cholestatic episode in a patient with benign recurrent intrahepatic cholestasis: a study of bile acid metabolism. Hepatology. 1991;13:1076–83.

5. Batta AK, Salen G, Arora R *et al.* Effect of ursodeoxycholic acid on bile acid metabolism in primary biliary cirrhosis. Hepatology. 1989;10:414–19.

6. Poupon RE, Balkau B, Eschwège E, Poupon R and the UDCA–PBC Study Group. A multicenter, controlled trial of ursodiol for the treatment of primary biliary cirrhosis. N Engl J Med. 1991;324:1548–54.

7. Federowski T, Salen G, Collaliolo A, Tint G, Mosbach E, Hall J. Metabolism of ursodeoxycholic acid in man. Gastroenterology. 1977;73:1131–7.

8. Batta AK, Arora R, Salen G, Tint GS, Eskreis D, Katz S. Characterization of serum and urinary bile acids in patients with primary biliary cirrhosis by gas liquid chromatography mass spectrometry. Effect of ursodeoxycholic acid treatment. J Lipid Res. 1989;12:1953–62.

9. Wilson F. Intestinal transport of bile acids. Am J Physiol. 1981;241:G83–92.

10. Tint G, Salen G, Shefer S. Effect of ursodeoxycholic acid on cholesterol and bile acid metabolism. Gastroenterology. 1986;91:1007–18.

11. Hardison W, Grundy S. Ursodeoxycholate and its taurine conjugate on bile acid synthesis and cholesterol absorption. Gastroenterology. 1984;87:130–5.

12. Nilssell K, Angelin B, Einarsson K. Comparative effect of ursodeoxycholic acid and chenodeoxycholic acid on bile acid kinetics and biliary lipid secretion in humans: evidence for different modes of action on bile acid synthesis. Gastroenterology. 1983;85:1248–56.

13. Roda E, Mazzella F, Bazzoli N *et al.* Effect of ursodeoxycholic acid administration on biliary lipid secretion in primary biliary cirrhosis. Dig Dis Sci. 1989;34(Suppl):52S–8S.

14. Roda E, Mazzella G, Bazzoli F *et al.* Primary bile acids kinetics in primary biliary cirrhosis before and after UDCA administration. In: Paumgartner G, Stiehl A, Barbara L, Roda E, editors. Strategies for the treatment of hepatobiliary diseases. Dordrecht: Kluwer; 1990:91–2.

15. Marteau P, Chazouillères O, Myara A, Jian R, Rambaud JC, Poupon R. Effect of chronic administration of ursodeoxycholic acid on the ileal absorption of endogenous bile acids in man. Hepatology. 1990;12:1206–8.

16. Eusufzai S, Ericsson S, Cederlund T, Einarsson K, Angelin B. Effect of ursodeoxycholic acid treatment on ileal absorption of bile acids in man as determined by the SeHCAT test. Gut. 1991;32:1044–8.

17. Stiehl A, Raedsch R, Rudolph G. Acute effects of ursodeoxycholic and chenodeoxycholic acid on the small intestinal absorption of bile acids. Gastroenterology. 1990;98:424–8.

18. Schaffner F, Klion F, Latuff A. The long term use of cholestyramine in the treatment of primary biliary cirrhosis. Gastroenterology. 1965;48:293–8.

19. Datta D, Sherlock S. Cholestyramine for long term relief of the pruritus complicating intrahepatic cholestasis. Gastroenterology. 1966;50:323–32.

20. Kitani K, Kanai S. Tauroursodeoxycholate prevents taurocholate induced cholestasis. Life Sci. 1982;30:515–23.

21. Heuman DM, Mills AS, McCall J, Hylemon PB, Pandak WM, Vlahcevic ZR. Conjugates of ursodeoxycholate protect against cholestasis and hepatocellular necrosis caused by more hydrophobic bile salts. *In vivo* studies in the rat. Gastroenterology. 1991;1:203–11.

22. Schölmerich J, Baumgartner U, Miyai K, Gerok W. Tauroursodeoxycholate prevents taurolithocholate-induced cholestasis and toxicity in rat liver. J Hepatol. 1990;10:280–3.

23. Schmucker D, Ohta M, Kanai S, Sato Y, Kitani K. Hepatic injury induced by bile salts: correlation between biochemical and morphological events. Hepatology. 1990;12:1216–21.

24. Chazouillères O, Ballet F, Legendre C *et al.* Effect of bile acids on ischemia-reperfusion liver injury. J Hepatol. 1991;13:318–22.

25. Ando M, Yasunaga M, Shirasawa H, Okita K. Therapeutic effect of ursodeoxycholate (UDCA) for alpha-naphthyl-isothiocyanate (ANIT) induced intrahepatic cholestasis. Gastroenterology. 1991;100:392(abstr.).

26. Michael S, Simko V, Oberstein E. Ursodeoxycholic (UDCA) in in vitro rat liver slices exposed to hepatotoxic CCl_4 or acetominophen (ACP). Gastroenterology. 1991;100:774a(abstr.).
27. Nathanson M, Boyer J. Mechanisms and regulation of bile secretion. Hepatology. 1991;14:551–6.
28. Suchy F. Hepatocellular transport of bile acids. Semin Liver Dis. 1993;13:235–47.
29. Poupon R, Chrétien Y, Parquet M, Rey C, Ballet F, Infante R. Hepatic transport of bile acids in the isolated perfused rat liver: structure-kinetics relationship. Biochem Pharmacol. 1988;37:209–12.
30. Ohiwa T, Katagiri K, Hoshino M, Hayakawa T, Nakai T. Tauroursodeoxycholate and tauro-beta-muricholate exert cytoprotection by reducing intrahepatocyte taurocholate content. Hepatology. 1993;17:470–6.
31. Deroubaix X, Coche T, Depiereux E, Feytmans E. Saturation of hepatic transport of taurocholate in rats in vivo. Am J Physiol. 1991;260:G189–96.
32. Häussinger D, Hallbrucker C, Saha N, Lang F, Gerok W. Cell volume and bile acid excretion. Biochem J. 1992;288:681–9.
33. Hallbrucker C, Lang F, Gerok W, Haüssinger D. Cell swelling increases bile flow and taurocholate excretion into bile in isolated perfused rat liver. Biochem J. 1992;281:593–5.
34. Häussinger D, Saha N, Hallbrucker C, Lang F, Gerok W. Involvement of microtubules in the swelling-induced stimulation of transcellular taurocholate transport in perfused rat liver. Biochem J. 1993;291:355–60.
35. Boyer J, McGrath J, Ng O. Microtubule dependent targeting of transporters to apical membrane determines the canalicular excretion of bile acids in hepatocyte couplets. Hepatology. 1993;18:107(abstr.).
36. Oda M, Yokomori H, Ishii K et al. Ursodeoxycholic acid enhances bile canalicular contractions. Hepatology. 1990;12:999(abstr.).
37. Galan AI, Jimenez R, Munoz ME, Gonzales J. Effect of ursodeoxycholate on maximal biliary secretion of bilirubin in the rat. Biochem Pharmacol. 1990;39:1175–80.
38. Calmus Y, Gane P, Rouger P, Poupon R. Hepatic expression of class I and class II major histocompatibility complex molecules in primary biliary cirrhosis: effect of ursodeoxycholic acid. Hepatology. 1990;11:12–15.
39. Beuers U, Spengler U, Kruis W et al. Ursodeoxycholic acid for treatment of primary sclerosing cholangitis: A placebo-controlled trial. Hepatology. 1992;16:707–14.
40. Heuman DM. Hepatoprotective properties of ursodeoxycholic acid. Gastroenterology. 1993;104:6:1865–70.
41. Güldütuna S, Immer G, Imohof BS, You T, Leuschner U. Molecular aspects of membrane stabilization by ursodeoxycholate. Gastroenterology. 1993;104:1736–44.
42. Dumont M, Erlinger S, Uchman S. Hypercholeresis induced by ursodeoxycholic acid and 7-ketolithocholic acid in the rat: possible role of bicarbonate transport. Gastroenterology. 1980;79:82–9.
43. Crosignani A, Podda M, Battezzati PM et al. Changes in bile acid composition in patients with primary biliary cirrhosis induced by ursodeoxycholic acid administration. Hepatology. 1991;14:1000–7.
44. Nakagawa M, Colombo C, Setchell KDR. Comprehensive study of the biliary bile acid composition of patients with cystic fibrosis and associated liver disease before and after UDCA administration. Hepatology. 1990;2:322–34.

24
Cytoprotection by ursodeoxycholic acid

U. LEUSCHNER, S. GÜLDÜTUNA, S. BHATTI, P. SIPOS, T. YOU and
G. ZIMMER

INTRODUCTION

The term 'cytoprotection' is usually applied to substances which protect
organs, isolated cells, membranes, cell organelles or certain cell enzymes
against the effect of other toxic substances. Cytoprotection is usually
investigated by means of *in-vitro* experiments, and it often remains unresolved
whether such effects are reproducible or relevant *in vivo*. The cytoprotective
effect of a substance may become apparent only when one or more metabolic
steps have taken place changing the structure of the molecule. Thus the
definition of cytoprotection is rather imprecise.

Bile acids are amphiphilic molecules which can have more hydrophobic,
apolar or more polar, hydrophilic properties. This attribute enables bile
acids to act as detergents. Cytotoxicity and cytoprotection are connected to
these detergent properties and the balance of hydrophobicity/hydrophilicity[1–3].
The least toxic bile acid is ursodeoxycholic acid (UDCA), cholic acid (CA)
is slightly more toxic, followed by chenodeoxycholic acid (CDCA), then
deoxycholic acid (DCA) and lithocholic acid (LCA), which is the most
toxic[1,2]. Sulphation reduces hepatotoxicity markedly, conjugation with
taurine and glycine to a smaller extent.

HEPATOCYTE DAMAGE BY BILE SALTS: ELECTRON MICROSCOPY

The first evidence that certain bile acids might injure hepatocytes was
provided some 30 years ago. Intravenous administration of sodium tauro-
LCA (TLCA) to hamsters for 4 h led to a dilatation of the bile capillaries,
a shortening or destruction of the microfilaments of the ectoplasm, and the
formation of vacuoles at the basolateral surface of the hepatocyte[4,5]. After
20 h proliferation of smooth endoplasmic reticulum (SER) had occurred,

whereas the mitochondria remained more or less unchanged. Similar results were found in other species following oral administration of CDCA or other unconjugated bile acids[6-13].

The dose- and time-related progression of cell damage was demonstrated by the following experiments: CDCA was administered to rats via an endopharyngeal tube in increasing doses from 20 to 1000 mg/kg a day for 5–60 days. The first alterations observed at lower doses and shorter treatment times were numerous indentations in the basolateral (sinusoidal) cell membrane and cytoplasmic vacuoles. The bile capillaries were dilated and the number of microvilli was reduced. At a dose of 100 mg/kg a day the smooth endoplasmic reticulum began to proliferate within a few days, and from a dose of 250 mg upwards fusion of vesicles from the sinusoidal membranes with the vesicles of the SER and the Golgi apparatus occurred. At a dose of 500 mg/kg a day the rough endoplasmic reticulum (RER) became markedly dilated. Lysosmes, cytoplasm and the cell nucleus were unchanged and the mitochondria were only slightly altered. At 1000 mg/kg a day several animals died[10,14]. On the other hand, intravenous administration of 100 mg/kg bodyweight of sulphated LCA and TLCA only induced mild alterations in hepatocyte structure[8]. Conjugates or sulphate esters of toxic bile acids are less harmful. UDCA and its conjugates did not damage hepatocytes, even in very high doses and during long-term administration[11-15].

MEMBRANE DAMAGE BY BILE SALTS

This sequence of the appearance of ultrastructural alterations indicates that the changes in the outer cell membranes may be due to a direct toxic effect of bile acids, e.g. when toxic bile acids encounter the sinusoidal membrane for the first time after diffusion through the space of Disse. Subsequently, they are rapidly transported through the hepatocyte, concentrated around the bile capillary, and finally excreted into the bile. At this point they could then induce the described changes in the area of the bile capillaries (microfilaments). It is only when toxic bile acids accumulate within the hepatocytes that changes in the SER, RER and Golgi apparatus become visible.

These hints for a direct membrane-damaging effect of bile salts are supported by publications reporting that, during liver perfusion, bile acids interact with the canalicular hepatocyte membrane and enhance the secretion of membrane-bound phospholipids and enzymes into the bile[16-18]. For instance, TCDCA stimulated the secretion of 5′-nucleotidase and alkaline phosphatase (AP) into the bile more than did TCA[18]. The 5′-nucleotidase is located almost exclusively in the canalicular portion of the hepatocyte membrane[19], together with high concentrations of AP[20,21]. However, it is not only membrane proteins that are excreted into the bile; the membrane also becomes porous to intracellular substances. For example this is shown by an increased excretion of the cytoplasmic enzyme lactate dehydrogenase (LDH)[19]. Under physiological conditions it is unlikely that the macromolecular LDH is secreted into the bile[22,23] and that this occurs only when the membrane becomes 'leaky'.

A further indication of a direct membrane effect of bile acids is provided by the observation that bile acids induce the synthesis of 5'-nucleotidase and AP at the canalicular membrane[24,25]. Investigations with red blood cells also support a direct interaction. When human erythrocytes were incubated in a TCDCA or TDCA solution for 15 min it resulted in maximal haemolysis[26], and in erythrocyte membranes toxic bile salts led to a change in membrane polarity[27]. Since erythrocytes do not possess cell organelles the membrane damage could not have been caused by bile acid-induced metabolites, and must be the result of a direct membrane effect.

NEW ASPECTS ON DIRECT BILE SALT–MEMBRANE INTERACTIONS

Although most of the results quoted here indicate a direct membrane-damaging effect of hydrophobic bile salts, cellular alterations induced in liver perfusion studies or hepatocyte cultures could also have been caused by metabolites produced in the cells themselves; i.e. the alterations could be an indirect effect. However, two observations suggest that there are in fact direct membrane effects:

1. Similar membrane alterations to those seen in hepatocytes are observed in isolated erythrocytes which do not possess cell organelles (see above).
2. UDCA is able to prevent the destruction of the pericanalicular microfilaments by toxic bile acids, but not the dilatation of the bile capillary.

Since basolateral and canalicular membranes seem to play an important role in the development of hepatocyte injury, we investigated whether apolar and polar bile acids have a direct influence on isolated liver cell membranes.

Basolateral hepatocyte membranes were isolated from rat livers according to the method of Meier *et al.*[28], and changes in membrane structure were investigated using electron paramagnetic resonance spectroscopy (EPR) with two different spin labels. The 16-DSA (doxyl stearic acid) label provides information on changes occurring in the deep, apolar parts of the membranes, and the 5-DSA label reports from the superficial layers. In the 16-DSA label the reporter group – a nitroxide stable radical – is attached to a stearic acid molecule at C_{16} (apolar); in the 5-DSA label the reporter group is fixed to C_5 (more polar). The reporter groups provide information on the polarity and molecular motion in their environments by absorbing and remitting magnetic energy. The spin labels are incorporated into the plasma membrane lipid bilayers parallel to the phospholipid fatty acid chains, with the carboxyl group oriented towards the polar head groups of the phospholipid molecules[29,30].

Incubation of 1 mg of labelled membranes with 1 μmol CDCA for 90 min significantly increased membrane fluidity compared to membranes incubated in buffer; that is, the membranes become porous and water was able to intrude into the membrane structure. However, when membranes were preincubated with 0.25 or 0.5 μmol UDCA and subsequently incubated with 1 μmol CDCA, UDCA prevented the damaging effect of CDCA. Membrane injury by CDCA was also demonstrated by the increase of phospholipids in the supernatant, caused by solubilization of phospholipids from the membranes. When the membranes were preincubated with UDCA, the release of phospholipids from the membranes by CDCA was prevented[31].

In order to discover at exactly which position within the basolateral membrane UDCA exerts its stabilizing effect, we investigated the individual membrane layers by using different spin labels. When spin-labelled membranes were incubated with CDCA, alterations were found in the signal from the 16-DSA label, i.e. within the deeper membrane layers. UDCA prevented the alterations in the signal, indicating that it stabilized the deep, apolar domain, whereas TUDCA and GUDCA had no effect. Experiments with the 5-DSA label showed that CDCA had a smaller effect on the superficial membrane layers, whereas TUDCA and GUDCA increased the order parameter in this more polar superficial domain. UDCA had no effect at all in this region.

Therefore UDCA seems to be incorporated into the deeper membrane layers, at the same site where CDCA exerts its damaging effect. The steroid nucleus of UDCA is possibly located at a similar position in the membrane to that of cholesterol, which suggests that UDCA might be able to act in a similar manner as do cholesterol molecules when it stabilizes plasma membranes.

If UDCA fulfils a similar role to cholesterol within the phospholipid membrane, then UDCA should not be effective in stabilizing phospholipid-poor, protein-rich membranes. Furthermore, if the hypothesis is correct that UDCA can substitute for cholesterol in a phospholipid-rich membrane, then investigations with large unilamellar vesicles (LUV) with different cholesterol content should support this hypothesis.

We therefore investigated the effect of UDCA on isolated mitochondria and phospholipid vesicles which had been treated with CDCA. When isolated hepatocyte mitochondria were preincubated with 1 mmol/l UDCA for 5–60 min, followed by incubation with 1 mmol/l CDCA, the glutamate dehydrogenase (GLDH) release from the mitochondrial matrix was reduced only when the preincubation time was less than 20 min. More than 20 min preincubation with UDCA no longer significantly diminished the GLDH release compared to incubation with CDCA alone. Therefore UDCA does not appear to remain attached to, or to be incorporated into, the membranes. The lack of stabilization of protein-rich mitochondrial membranes by UDCA has also been corroborated by EPR investigations using a 4-maleimido TEMPO spin label (protein label) and by electron microscopic investigations[32].

Large unilamellar vesicles (LUV)[33] consisting of egg-yolk lecithin with different cholesterol concentrations provided a standardized membrane model on which to test the stabilizing effect of UDCA. The vesicles were loaded with carboxy-fluorescein (CF) and subsequently incubated with different concentrations of CDCA. The CF efflux and phospholipid release were measured. Low concentrations of CDCA led to CF efflux from the vesicles depending on the cholesterol content of the membranes. CF efflux was higher at lower cholesterol content. CF was released before any change in vesicle size had occurred as measured by laser-light scattering. Above the critical micellar concentration of CDCA, LUV were solubilized and phospholipid and cholesterol concentrations in the supernatant increased[33].

LUV with different cholesterol contents were then incubated with UDCA and the phospholipid concentration in the supernatant was determined after centrifugation at 100 000 **g** (gravimetrical stress). The effect of UDC concerning LUV stabilization was greatest in vesicles without cholesterol and lowest in cholesterol-rich vesicles[34].

In conclusion, UDCA does not appear to be incorporated into protein-rich membranes, whereas in phospholipid membranes UDCA may possess a similar stabilizing effect to that of cholesterol. Low concentrations of toxic bile salts induce transient hole formation (leakiness) in membranes and vesicles; in high concentrations membrane solubilization occurs.

These results are consistent with the current views on the cytotoxic and cytoprotective effects of bile salts. In electron microscopic investigations on hepatocyte morphology[11,13-15], in studies on albumin and enzyme release into bile[17,18], and also in investigations on hepatocyte cultures[26,35], hydrophobic bile salts have been shown to be toxic, whereas UDCA is non-toxic and may even counteract the toxic effect of hydrophobic bile salts.

HYPOTHESES ON BILE ACID TOXICITY AND CYTOPROTECTION

Hydrophobic bile acids probably exert their cytotoxic effect by intruding into the lipid bilayer of membranes[36]. Increasing bile salt concentrations result in the self-aggregation of bile salt molecules and alterations in the orientation of lipids and bile salt molecules[37]. Thus at concentrations below those necessary for the micellar solubilization of phospholipids[37], transient membrane holes are formed[33,37], allowing inulin or carboxyfluorescein to escape from the vesicles, and the release of enzymes from intact cells, e.g. LDH[26,35].

EPR investigations have shown that toxic bile salts increase membrane fluidity and allow water to intrude into the membranes[38,39]. It is conceivable that this 'softening' process enables the formation of the inclusion vacuoles at the sinusoidal cell membrane seen in electron microscopic studies[5-7]. Such vacuoles have also been described after carbon tetrachloride and allyl alcohol intoxication, or during hypoxia, and are an indication of membrane damage[40,41]. The inclusion vacuoles bud off from the basolateral cell membrane and contain the contents of the space of Disse.

Alterations at the basolateral hepatocyte membrane can be induced by low bile acid concentrations, whereas changes at the canalicular membranes seem to require rather higher concentrations. Since bile acids are found physiologically in much higher concentrations at the canalicular hepatocyte pole, the canalicular membranes need to be more resistant than the basolateral membranes, and this is reflected in their higher cholesterol content[31]. Thus inclusion vacuoles are rarely observed at the canalicular membrane, and the polarity of isolated canalicular membranes does not increase upon incubation with CDCA[31]. The dilatation of bile capillaries results from the destruction of microfilaments[42], rather than damage to the canalicular membrane itself.

There are several possible explanations for the hepatoprotective effect of UDCA:

1. UDCA reduces the toxicity of hydrophobic bile acids in the extracellular compartment, as shown in experiments with hydrophilic and hydrophobic bile salts in buffer[31]. UDCA forms mixed micelles with CDCA and DCA, thus increasing the hydrophilicity of the bile salt solution.
2. UDCA may interact with mixed CDCA or DCA phospholipid micelles which have formed in the outer leaflet of phospholipid-rich membranes[36,37]. The micelles thus become less hydrophobic and cannot solubilize membrane lipids.
3. UDCA may be incorporated into the apolar domain of membranes and thus prevent the access of toxic apolar bile acids[31], stabilizing the membrane structure in a similar manner to phosphatidylserine, phosphatidylethanolamine or cholesterol[31,34,37].
4. UDCA could help to preserve membrane function, e.g. by reducing the expression of HLA class I antigens[43,44].
5. The effect of UDCA could result from a simultaneous influence on membrane structure and function.
6. UDCA could prevent the destruction of ectoplasmic microfilaments at the canalicular membrane; however, it does not counteract the dilatation of bile capillaries[45].

In summary, at least six possible direct cytoprotective mechanisms can be hypothesized for UDCA, based on the effects observed with cell membranes or in adjacent compartments (space of Disse, ectoplasm). In addition, indirect metabolic aspects of cytoprotection may exist. The influence of UDCA on calcium homeostasis and the interactions of UDCA, toxic bile salts, and oxygen-free radicals have not been discussed here; however, these are fascinating topics for future investigation.

References

1. Attili AF, Angelico M, Cantafora A, Alvaro D, Capocaccia L. Bile acid-induced liver toxicity: relation to the hydrophobic balance of bile acids. Med Hypoth. 1986;19:57–69.
2. Armstrong MJ, Carey MC. The hydrophobic–hydrophilic balance of bile salts. Inverse correlation between reverse-phase high performance liquid chromatographic mobilities and micellar cholesterol-solubilizing capacities. J Lipid Res. 1982;23:70–80.
3. Nakayama F, Miyazaki K, Koga A. Effect of chenodeoxycholic and ursodeoxycholic acids on isolated human hepatocytes. Gastroenterology. 1980;78:1228 (abstr.).
4. Schaffner F, Javitt NB. Morphologic changes in hamster liver during intrahepatic cholestasis induced by taurolithocholate. Lab Invest. 1966;15:1783–92.
5. Priestly BG, Côté G, Plaa GL. Biochemical and morphological parameters of taurolithocholate-induced cholestasis. Can J Physiol Pharmacol. 1971;49:1078–91.
6. Miyai K, Price VM, Fisher MM. Bile acid metabolism in mammals. Ultrastructural studies on the intrahepatic cholestasis induced by lithocholic and chenodeoxycholic acids in the rat. Lab Invest. 1971;24:292–302.
7. Fisher MM, Magnusson R, Phillips MJ, Miyai K. Bile acid metabolism in mammals. IV.

Sex differences in chenodeoxycholic acid metabolism in the rat. Lab Invest. 1972;27: 254–62.

8. Leuschner U, Czygan P, Stiehl A. Licht- und elektronenmikroskopische Untersuchungen zur Toxizität von sulfatierter und nichtsulfatierter Lithocholsäure. Verh Dtsch Ges Inn Med. 1975;81:1311–13.

9. Leuschner U. Leberschäden bei Chenosäurebehandlung: Tierexperimentelle Ergebnisse und Befunde bei Patienten mit Chenosäure-Therapie. Verh Bd Z Gastroenterol. 1976;9:60–4.

10. Leuschner U, Schneider M, Loos R, Kurtz W. Morphologic investigations on the toxicity of orally applied CDCA in the liver, gastrointestinal tract, kidney and adrenal gland of the rat. Res Exp Med. 1977;171:41–55.

11. Leuschner U, Schneider M, Korte L. The influence of chenodeoxycholic acid and ursodeoxycholic acid on the hepatic structure of the rat. Z Gastroenterol. 1979;17:244–55.

12. Miyai K, Javitt NB, Gochman N, Jones HM, Baker D. Hepatotoxicity of bile acids in rabbits. Ursodeoxycholic acid is less toxic than chenodeoxycholic acid. Lab Invest. 1982;46:428–37.

13. Miyazaki K, Nakayama F, Koga A. Effect of chenodeoxycholic and ursodeoxycholic acids on isolated adult human hepatocytes. Dig Dis Sci. 1984;29:1123–30.

14. Leuschner U. Liver tissue injury due to chenodeoxycholic acid: metabolic pathways and toxicity. In: Paumgartner G, Stiehl A, Gerok W, editors. Biological effects of bile acids. Lancaster: MTP; 1979:191–203.

15. Fedorowski T, Salen G, Zaki G, Shefer S, Mosbach EH. Comparative effects of ursodeoxycholic acid and chenodeoxycholic acid in the rhesus monkey. Gastroenterology. 1978;74: 75 81.

16. Barnwell SG, Godfrey PP, Lowe PJ, Coleman R. Biliary protein output by isolated perfused rat livers. Effects of bile salts. Biochem J. 1983;210:549–57.

17. Barnwell SG, Lowe PJ, Coleman R. Effect of taurochenodeoxycholate or tauroursodeoxycholate upon biliary outputs of phospholipids and plasma membrane enzymes, and the extent of cell damage, in isolated perfused rat livers. Biochem J. 1983;216:107–11.

18. Kitani K, Ohta M, Kanai S. Tauroursodeoxycholate prevents biliary protein excretion induced by other bile salts in the rat. Am J Physiol. 1985;248:G407–17.

19. Stolzenbach F. Lactate dehydrogenase. Methods Enzymol. 1966;9:278–88.

20. Blitzer BL, Boyer JL. Cytochemical localization of Na^+,K^+-ATPase in rat hepatocytes. J Clin Invest. 1978;62:1104–8.

21. Holdsworth G, Coleman R. Enzyme profiles of mammalian bile. Biochim Biophys Acta. 1975;389:47–50.

22. Godfrey PP, Warner MJ, Coleman R. Enzymes and proteins in bile. Variations in output in rat cannula bile during and after depletion of bile-salt pool. Biochem J. 1981;196:11–16.

23. Mullock BM, Dobrota M, Hinton RH. Sources of the proteins of rat bile. Biochim Biophys Acta. 1978;543:497–507.

24. Hatoff DE, Hardison WGM. Induced synthesis of alkaline phosphatase by bile acids in rat liver cell culture. Gastroenterology. 1979;77:1062–7.

25. Hatoff DE, Hardison WGM. Bile acids modify alkaline phosphatase induction and bile secretion pressure after bile duct obstruction in the rat. Gastroenterology. 1981;80:666–72.

26. Heuman DM, Pandak WM, Hylemon PB, Vlahcevic ZR. Conjugates of ursodeoxycholate protect against cytotoxicity of more hydrophobic bile salts: in vitro studies in rat hepatocytes and human erythrocytes. Hepatology. 1991;14:920–6.

27. Leuschner U, Fischer H, Kurtz W et al. Ursodeoxycholic acid in primary biliary cirrhosis: Results of a controlled double-blind trial. Gastroenterology. 1989;97:1268–74.

28. Meier PJ, Sztul ES, Reuben A, Boyer JL. Structural and functional polarity of canalicular and basolateral plasma membrane vesicles isolated in high yield from rat liver. J Cell Biol. 1984;98:991–1000.

29. Smith ICP, Butler KW. Oriented lipid systems as model membranes. In: Berliner LJ, editor. Spin labeling, theory and applications. New York: Academic Press; 1976:411–48.

30. Gaffney BJ, Lin CD. Spin-label measurements of membrane-bound enzymes. In: Martonosi A, editor. The enzymes of biological membranes, vol. 1. New York: Wiley, 1976:71–90.

31. Güldütuna S, Zimmer G, Imhof M, Bhatti S, You T, Leuschner U. Molecular aspects of membrane stabilization by ursodeoxycholate. Gastroenterology. 1993;104:1736–44.

32. Bhatti S, Elze A, Güldütuna S, Zimmer G, You T, Leuschner U. Calcium enhances

mitochondrial damage induced by chenodeoxycholate (CDC) in vitro, whereas ursodeoxycholate (UDC) reduces glutamate dehydrogenase (GLDH) release but does not preserve mitochondrial ultrastructure. Gastroenterology. 1994;106:A867.

33. Güldütuna S, Weiß A, Deisinger B *et al.* The effect of chenodeoxycholate (CDC) on large unilamellar vesicles (LUV) with variable cholesterol concentration. Gastroenterology. 1994; 106:A902.

34. Güldütuna S, Weiß A, Deisinger B *et al.* Ursodeoxycholate (UDC) mimics the membrane stabilizing effect of cholesterol on large unilamellar vesicles (LUV). Gastroenterology. 1994; 106:A902.

35. Galle PR, Theilmann L, Raedsch R, Otto G, Stiehl A. Ursodeoxycholate reduces hepatotoxicity of bile salts in primary human hepatocytes. Hepatology. 1990;12:486–91.

36. Schubert R, Beyer K, Wolburg H, Schmidt K-H. Structural changes in membranes of large unilamellar vesicles after binding of sodium cholate. Biochemistry. 1986;25:5263–9.

37. Schubert R, Schmidt K-H. Structural changes in vesicle membranes and mixed micelles of various lipid compositions after binding of different bile salts. Biochemistry. 1988;27: 8787–94.

38. Keith AD, Sharnhoff M, Cohn GE. A summary and evaluation of spin labeling used as probes for biological membrane structures. Biochim Biophys Acta. 1973;300:379–419.

39. Griffith OH, Jost PC. Lipid spin labels in biological membranes. In: Berliner LJ, editor. Spin labeling theory and applications. New York: Academic Press; 1976:453–523.

40. Hübner G. The pathic reactions of the liver tissue. An electron microscopic study. Stuttgart: Fischer; 1968.

41. Altmann HW. Allgemeine morphologische Pathologie des Cytoplasmas. Die Pathobiosen. Handb Allg Path II/I Berlin, Göttingen, Heidelberg: Springer, 1955.

42. Phillips MJ, Oda M, Mak E, Fisher MM, Jeejeebhoy KN. Microfilament dysfunction as a possible cause of intrahepatic cholestasis. Gastroenterology. 1975;69:48–58.

43. Calmus Y, Gane P, Rouger P, Poupon R. Hepatic expression of class I and class II major histocompatibility complex molecules in primary biliary cirrhosis. Effect of ursodeoxycholic acid. Hepatology. 1990;11:12–15.

44. Leuschner U, Güldütuna S, Dienes HP *et al.* Bile acids during treatment of primary biliary cirrhosis. Ursodeoxycholic acid improves membrane stability and influences histological immune reactions in liver tissue. In: Paumgartner G, Stiehl A, Gerok W, editors. Bile acids as therapeutic agents. Dordrecht/Boston/London: Kluwer; 1991:297–99.

45. Thibault N, Maurice M, Maratrat M, Cordier A, Feldmann G, Ballet F. Effect of touroursodeoxycholate on actin filament alteration induced by cholestatic agents. A study in isolated rat hepatocyte couplets. J Hepatol. 1993;19:367–76.

25
Methionine enkephalin and aminopeptidase-M activity in blood in children with cholestasis before and after treatment with ursodeoxycholic acid

R. M. JANAS, J. TRETTER, K. WARNAWIN, J. PAWLOWSKA, J. RUJNER and J. SOCHA

INTRODUCTION

Enkephalins, endogenous opioid pentapeptides, are markedly elevated in blood in patients with cholestatic liver diseases, but not in patients with other disorders[1-4]. Adults with acute parenchymal diseases were shown to exhibit an approximately six-fold increase of plasma methionine enkephalin[1]. Similarly, plasma leucine enkephalin was highly elevated in patients with acute liver diseases as well as in patients with chronic liver disorders[3]. The enkephalin increase was seemingly proportional to the degree of liver damage. The pathophysiological significance of these observations remains unclear. It has been speculated that the enkephalins accumulated in blood penetrate the blood–brain barrier[5], and contribute to the pathogenesis of pruritus of cholestasis[6] or hepatic encephalopathy[1]. Preliminary results from experiments showing that administration of nalmefene or naloxone, opiate receptor antagonists, ameliorated pruritus of cholestasis[2,7] and, in some patients, precipitated a severe opioid withdrawal reaction on starting the drug[2], seem to support this thesis. Like exogenous opiates the opioid peptides are potent vasodilators; therefore, their potential involvement in ascites formation has also been speculated upon[4].

The origin of circulating enkephalins is unclear. The adrenal glands[8], sympathetic nerves[9] and gastrointestinal endocrine cells[10] have been shown to contain opioid peptides. Although increased enkephalin secretion has not been excluded, the accumulation of enkephalins in cholestasis was postulated to be a result of their diminished inactivation by the liver[1] or, alternatively, by serum proteinases. Our study was undertaken in order to determine if enkephalins accumulate in blood of children with cholestasis of different aetiology. There are no literature data available on this question. We also tested the hypothesis of whether impairment of the hepatic or blood plasma enkephalin degrading proteinases may be responsible for the accumulation of enkephalins in blood. Additionally, we studied the effect of ursodeoxycholic acid treatment on both the accumulation and degradation of enkephalins in the patients.

MATERIALS AND METHODS

Patients

The protocol of this study was accepted by the Hospital Ethics Committee.

Group 1: Fifteen boys and girls, aged 3 months–14.5 years, mean 7.5 months, with arteriohepatic dysplasia (Alagille syndrome).

Group 2: Nine boys and girls, aged 3 months–12 years, mean 5 years, with progressive intrahepatic familial cholestasis (Byler's disease).

Group 3: Nineteen boys and girls aged 2 months–3 years, mean 1.5 year, with extrahepatic biliary duct atresia.

Control group: Eight healthy boys and girls aged 3–12 years, mean 6 years.

Disease controls: Boys and girls aged 2–8 years, mean 4 years, with hyperthyroidism ($n = 3$), hypothyroidism ($n = 4$) or renal failure ($n = 4$).

Treatment with ursodeoxycholic acid

The patients from groups 1–3 ($n = 21$) were treated with ursodeoxycholic acid as Ursofalk® at a dose of 15 mg/kg per day for 4–5 weeks.

Liver biopsy specimens

Liver specimens were obtained for diagnostic examination, and it was possible to use part of each specimen in this study.

Group 1: Nine intraoperative biopsy specimens from children (aged approximately 3 months) with extrahepatic biliary duct atresia.

Group 2: Seven percutaneous blind needle biopsy specimens from children aged 1.5–14 years, mean 6 years, with chronic active hepatitis due to HBV infection.

Liver extracts

Liver biopsy specimens (10–40 mg each) were intensively washed with an excess of ice-cold saline in order to remove blood, and homogenized in 1:9 (weight/volume) 25 mmol/l tris-HCl, pH 7.5, containing 0.15 mol/l NaCl. The homogenates were centrifuged at 3000 **g** for 15 min at 4°C. The resulting extracts were harvested and assayed for enkephalin degrading activity.

Radioimmunoassay

Radioimmunoassay of the methionine enkephalin in blood plasma, or in some experiments in blood serum, was performed using [^{125}I]methionine enkephalin and C-terminally directed, specific methionine enkephalin antibody from Incstar (Stillwater, Minnesota, USA). Enkephalins were separated from the plasma proteins with C18 Sep-Pak columns (Incstar), according to the procedure detailed by Thornton et al.[4].

Assay of enkephalin-degrading activity

The incubation mixture consisted of $160\,\mu l$ of $25\,mmol/l$ Tris-HCl, pH 7.5, $20\,\mu l$ prediluted (10–50 times) serum or liver extract was incubated with 50–$100\,pmol/l$ [^{125}I]methionine enkephalin (Incstar, specific activity approximately $500\,Ci/mmol$) at $37°C$. The reaction was terminated by boiling or acidification with $1\,mol/l$ hydrochloric acid.

Degradation of the label was quantified with aluminium silicate binding assay, as described by Janas et al.[11]. Intact [^{125}I]methionine enkephalin was almost completely adsorbed by the aluminium silicate: $91 \pm 4\%$, mean $\pm$ SEM, $n > 20$. Reverse-phase high-performance liquid chromatography analysis showed that the aluminium silicate-bound radioactivity represented the intact [^{125}I]methionine enkephalin. As a result of the hydrolytic activity of serum or liver extract proteinases, radioactive products that were not adsorbed by the silicate ($4 \pm 3\%$, mean $\pm$ SEM, $n > 20$), appeared in the reaction medium. The main radioactive product was identified as [^{125}I]tyrosine: 85–90% of the total radioactivity of the products, whereas unidentified 3–4 amino acid fragments of [^{125}I]methionine enkephalin constituted 10–15% (data not shown).

Inhibition and substrate specificity of enkephalin-degrading activity

Degradation of a fixed amount of [^{125}I]methionine enkephalin (final concentration $100\,pmol/l$) was quantified in the presence of increasing concentrations of protease inhibitors, puromycin or bestatin, or unlabelled methionine enkephalin (all from Sigma, St Louis, Missouri, USA). The concentration of an inhibitor causing half-maximal inhibition of the label degradation (ED_{50}) was calculated from the inhibitory curve. The Michaelis constant (K_m) was determined from Lineweaver–Burk plots assuming equal affinity of the enzyme to labelled and unlabelled methionine enkephalin according to the method described by Movsas et al.[12].

Incubation of isolated erythrocytes with bile acids

Human erythrocytes were isolated from heparinized blood with Ficoll-Hypaque (Pharmacia Fine Chemicals AB, Uppsala, Sweden) and suspended in saline:haematocrit 20%. Aliquots (0.5 ml) of the erythrocyte suspension were incubated at $37°C$ for 60 min in the presence of increasing concentrations (0–$1500\,\mu mol/l$) of taurodeoxycholic acid, cholic acid or both (from Sigma). After incubation, erythrocytes were removed by centrifugation, and the post-incubation media used for determination of enkephalin-degrading activity by aluminium silicate binding assay.

Table 1 Enkephalin-degrading activity and methionine enkephalin concentration in blood of healthy children and children with thyroid or renal disorders (disease controls) expressed as means $\pm$ SD

	Healthy controls	Disease controls
Enkephalin-degrading activity (pg ml^{-1} min^{-1})	290 $\pm$ 24 ($n = 8$)	234 $\pm$ 44 ($n = 11$)
Methionine enkephalin (pg/ml)	50 $\pm$ 35 ($n = 8$)	60 $\pm$ 15 ($n = 10$)

Table 2 Enkephalin-degrading activity, methionine enkephalin, alkaline phosphatase, total bilirubin, and alanine aminotransferase in blood of children with Alagille syndrome before and after the treatment with ursodeoxycholic acid, expressed as means $\pm$ SD

	Before treatment	After treamtent
Enkephalin-degrading activity (pg ml^{-1} min^{-1})	1416 $\pm$ 640 ($n = 15$)	1810 $\pm$ 920 ($n = 9$)
Methionine enkephalin (pg/ml)	150 $\pm$ 49 ($n = 12$)	152 $\pm$ 70 ($n = 9$)
Alkaline phosphatase (U/l)	1202 $\pm$ 485 ($n = 14$)	1142 $\pm$ 523 ($n = 9$)
Total bilirubin (mg/dl)	4.2 $\pm$ 1.8 ($n = 15$)	4.3 $\pm$ 2.0 ($n = 8$)
Alanine aminotransferase (U/l)	130 $\pm$ 62 ($n = 12$)	136 $\pm$ 49 ($n = 8$)

Other assays

Alkaline phosphatase, total bilirubin and alanine aminotransferase in plasma were determined by commercially available laboratory tests.

Statistical analysis

Values are expressed as means $\pm$ SD unless otherwise stated. The Mann–Whitney U-test was used to determine the significance of differences between means; $p < 0.05$ was considered significant.

RESULTS

The plasma concentrations of methionine enkephalin and serum enkephalin-degrading activity in healthy children and children with thyroid disorders or renal failure (disease controls) are shown in Table 1. The mean values of methionine enkephalin: 50 $\pm$ 35 pg/ml and 60 $\pm$ 15 pg/ml (means $\pm$ SD), respectively, were not statistically different ($p > 0.05$). Similarly, the differences in enkephalin-degrading activity: 290 $\pm$ 24 pg ml^{-1} min^{-1} and 234 $\pm$ 44 pg ml^{-1} min^{-1} (means $\pm$ SD), respectively, were not significantly different ($p > 0.05$).

In children with Alagille syndrome (Table 2), the plasma methionine enkephalin concentrations: 150 $\pm$ 49 pg/ml (mean $\pm$ SD) were significantly elevated as compared to the control group ($p < 0.05$). Serum enkephalin-degrading activity: 1416 $\pm$ 640 pg ml^{-1} min^{-1} (mean $\pm$ SD) were also significantly elevated ($p < 0.001$). Alkaline phosphatase: 1202 $\pm$ 485 U/l, total bilirubin: 4.2 $\pm$ 1.8 mg/dl, and alanine aminotransferase: 130 $\pm$ 62 U/l (means $\pm$ SD) were increased in comparison to normal values. Treatment with ursodeoxycholic acid for a period of 4–5 weeks did not affect ($p > 0.05$) any of these parameters (Table 2).

Table 3 Enkephalin-degrading activity, methionine enkephalin, alkaline phosphatase, total bilirubin and alanine aminotransferase in the blood of children with Byler's disease before and after treatment with ursodeoxycholic acid expressed as means $\pm$ SD

	Before treatment	*After treatment*
Enkephalin-degrading activity (pg ml^{-1} min^{-1})	494 ± 35 ($n = 9$)	446 ± 60 ($n = 8$)
Methionine enkephalin (pg/ml)	180 ± 98 ($n = 9$)	185 ± 80 ($n = 7$)
Alkaline phosphatase (U/l)	997 ± 280 ($n = 8$)	1090 ± 290 ($n = 7$)
Total bilirubin (mg/dl)	7.3 ± 4.5 ($n = 8$)	5.5 ± 3.4 ($n = 8$)
Alanine aminotransferase (U/l)	65 ± 18 ($n = 9$)	49 ± 9 ($n = 6$)

Table 4 Enkephalin-degrading activity, methionine enkephalin, alkaline phosphatase, total bilirubin and alanine aminotransferase in the blood of children with extrahepatic biliary duct atresia before and after treatment with ursodeoxycholic acid, expressed as means $\pm$ SD

	Before treatment	*After treatment*
Enkephalin-degrading activity (pg ml^{-1} min^{-1})	1232 ± 485 ($n = 17$)	1164 ± 520 ($n = 13$)
Methionine enkephalin (pg/ml)	170 ± 78 ($n = 15$)	148 ± 39 ($n = 10$)
Alkaline phosphatase (U/l)	1576 ± 852 ($n = 18$)	1732 ± 625 ($n = 13$)
Total bilirubin (mg/dl)	10.5 ± 4.2 ($n = 17$)	3.0 ± 4.8 ($n = 14$)
Alanine aminotransferase (U/l)	151 ± 73 ($n = 15$)	186 ± 92 ($n = 12$)

The statistical significance of elevation of the methionine enkephalin: 180 ± 98 pg/ml (mean $\pm$ SD) in children with Byler's disease (Table 3) was at the same level as in children with Alagille syndrome ($p < 0.05$). Enkephalin-degrading activity: 494 ± 35 pg ml^{-1} min^{-1} (mean $\pm$ SD) was about double the value found for the healthy children ($p < 0.05$). Alkaline phosphatase: 997 ± 280 U/l, total bilirubin: 7.3 ± 4.5 mg/dl, and alanine aminotransferase: 65 ± 18 U/l (means $\pm$ SD) were elevated in these patients as compared to normal values. Treatment with ursodeoxycholic acid for a period of 4–5 weeks did not significantly affect ($p > 0.05$) any of these parameters (Table 3).

The plasma methionine enkephalin concentration: 170 ± 78 pg/ml (mean $\pm$ SD) in children with extrahepatic biliary duct atresia (Table 4) was significantly elevated as compared to healthy controls ($p < 0.05$). The elevation of enkephalin-degrading activity: 1232 ± 485 pg ml^{-1} min^{-1} (mean $\pm$ SD) was also statistically significant ($p < 0.001$) as compared to healthy controls. Alkaline phosphatase: 1576 ± 852 U/l, total bilirubin: 10.5 ± 4.2 mg/dl, and alanine aminotransferase: 151 ± 73 U/l (means $\pm$ SD) were elevated as compared to normal values. Treatment with ursodeoxycholic acid for a period of 4–5 weeks did not affect ($p > 0.05$) any of the above parameters (Table 4).

Enkephalin-degrading activity in the extracts of the liver specimens (Fig. 1) from patients with extrahepatic biliary duct atresia: 42 ± 18 pg mg^{-1} min^{-1}, or chronic active hepatitis due to HBV infection: 36 ± 14 pg mg^{-1} min^{-1} (means $\pm$ SD) were not statistically different ($p > 0.05$).

Endogenous methionine enkephalin was stable in the EDTA plasma samples; however, in the corresponding serum samples it was slowly degraded

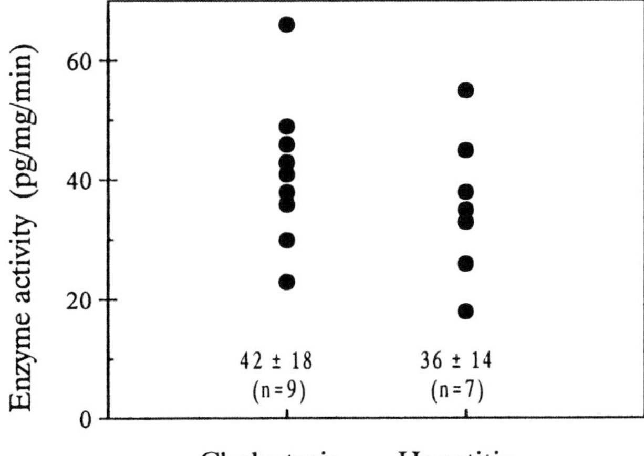

Fig. 1 Enkephalin-degrading activity in liver biopsy specimens from patients with cholestasis due to extrahepatic biliary duct atresia and from patients with chronic active hepatitis due to HBV infection. Liver biopsy specimens were homogenized and centrifuged as detailed in Materials and methods. [^{125}I]Methionine enkephalin-degrading activity of each liver extract was quantified with the aluminium silicate-binding assay. Each point is an averaged value from two determinations for each liver extract. Data are also expressed as means ± SD

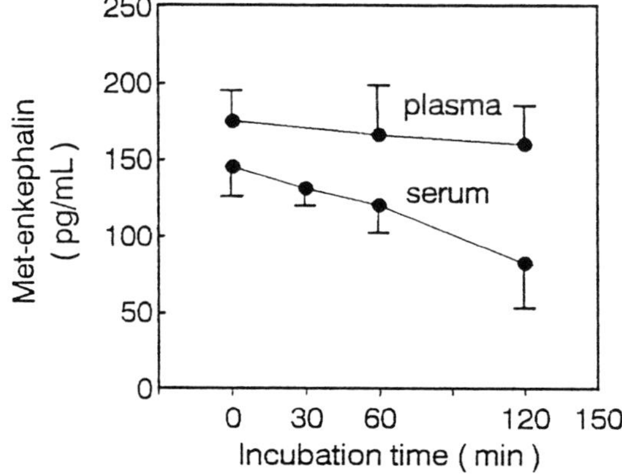

Fig. 2 Degradation of endogenous methionine enkephalin in blood plasma and serum samples. Blood was obtained from the same four patients with Byler's disease. EDTA was used as the anticoagulant to obtain plasma. The samples were incubated at 37°C for the specified periods and radioimmunoassayed in duplicate for the methionine enkephalin concentration as detailed in Materials and methods. Values are expressed as means ± SEM

when incubated at 37°C (Fig. 2). After 120 min the mean level of the methionine enkephalin immunoreactivity in the serum samples decreased by about 50%.

Inhibition characteristics and substrate specificity data of the enkephalin-degrading activity in the extracts from the liver biopsy specimens from patients with extrahepatic biliary duct atresia or chronic active hepatitis,

Table 5 Characteristics of enkephalin-degrading activity in serum samples and liver extracts

| | Inhibitors ($\mu mol/l$) | | Michaelis constant towards methionine enkephalin ($\mu mol/l$) |
	Bestatin ED_{50}	Puromycin ED_{50}	
Blood serum			
Cholestasis	1.8 ± 0.2	21 ± 4	282 ± 33
Control	1.8 ± 0.3	20 ± 1	270 ± 98
Liver extracts			
Atresia	2.4 ± 0.1	38 ± 7	286 ± 70
Hepatitis	1.8 ± 0.2	49 ± 11	233 ± 32

Serum samples were obtained from the patients with Alagille syndrome ($n = 2$), Byler's disease ($n = 2$) or extrahepatic biliary duct atresia ($n = 3$), and from the healthy children (controls, $n = 6$). The liver extracts were prepared from biopsy specimens from the patients with extrahepatic biliary duct atresia ($n = 5$) or chronic active hepatitis ($n = 4$). The samples were analysed separately, and the results are expressed as means $\pm$ SEM

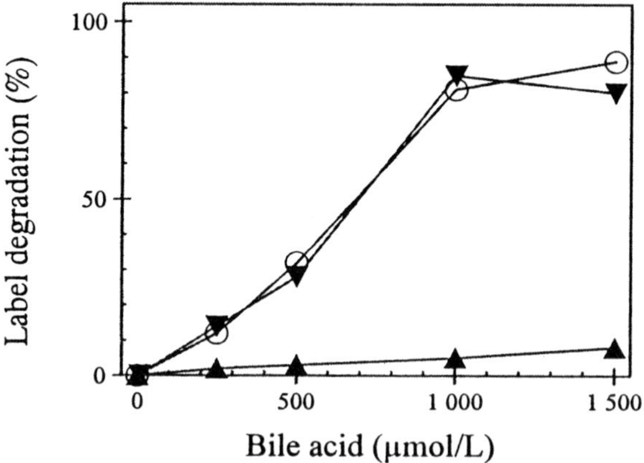

Fig. 3 Influence of bile acids on erythrocyte haemolysis resulting in the appearance of enkephalin-degrading activity in the incubation media. Isolated human erythrocytes ($100\,\mu l$ of the packed cells in four volumes of saline) were incubated in the presence of increasing concentrations of ($\bigcirc$) taurodeoxycholic acid, ($\blacktriangle$) cholic acid or both ($\blacktriangledown$), for $60\,min$ at $37°C$. After centrifugation the $[^{125}I]$methionine enkephalin-degrading activity in $20\,\mu l$ aliquots of the post-incubation media was quantified with the aluminium silicate-binding assay. Data are expressed as means from two representative experiments

and in the serum samples from healthy children and children with Byler's disease, are summarized in Table 5. Bestatin inhibited enkephalin-degrading activity at a half-maximal concentration of about $2\,\mu mol/l$, whereas puromycin was 10–20 times less effective. The mean values of the Michaelis constant, calculated towards unlabelled methionine enkephalin, were about $250\,\mu mol/l$.

The effect of taurodeoxycholic and cholic acids on erythrocyte haemolysis and the resulting appearance of the enkephalin-degrading activity in the incubation media are shown in Fig. 3. Isolated erythrocytes did not degrade labelled methionine enkephalin (data not shown). There was no enkephalin-degrading activity in the media where the isolated erythrocytes were incubated alone for 60 min at 37°C. Addition of taurodeoxycholic acid at concentrations of 250–500 μmol/l caused notable haemolysis and appearance of enkephalin-degrading activity in the incubation media. That was not the case if cholic acid was used. Moreover, cholic acid did not diminish erythrocyte haemolysis caused by taurodeoxycholic acid (Fig. 3).

DISCUSSION

Children with cholestasis due to arteriohepatic dysplasia (Alagille syndrome), progressive intrahepatic familial cholestasis (Byler's disease) or extrahepatic biliary duct atresia exhibited a 3–4-fold increase of plasma methionine enkephalin concentration as compared to the healthy children and children with non-hepatic disorders. The increase was of similar magnitude as that reported for adult patients with acute or chronic liver diseases[1–4]. In our patients the serum enkephalin-degrading activity was highly elevated. The highest elevation (5–6-fold) was found in children with Alagille syndrome or extrahepatic biliary duct atresia, whereas children with Byler's disease exhibited an approximately 2-fold increase. Treatment with ursodeoxycholic acid at a dose of 15 mg/kg a day for a period of 4–5 weeks did not lower either plasma methionine enkephalin immunoreactivity or enkephalin-degrading activity in these children. Moreover, other parameters of liver disease – alkaline phosphatase, total bilirubin and alanine aminotransferase – also remained unaffected. The hepatoprotective effects of long-lasting urso-deoxycholic acid therapy, resulting in improvement of the markers of cholestasis, have been summarized in a recent review[13]. It therefore seems possible that administration of ursodeoxycholic acid in our patients for a longer period of time could result in decreasing plasma methionine enkephalin concentrations or serum enkephalin-degrading activity, or both. Such a study is in progress at our hospital.

When considering the possible origin of methionine enkephalin accumulating in blood, we assumed that either the serum enkephalin-degrading activity had been impaired or, as others have suggested[1], that the hepatic enkephalin-degrading potential had been affected. Our results, however, point rather to increased enkephalin degradation in the blood in our patients. Moreover, our data suggest that hepatic enkephalin degradation in patients with extrahepatic biliary duct atresia was not impaired, at least in comparison with the patients with chronic active hepatitis due to HBV infection, in whom we did not find cholestasis or cirrhosis. Recently, Antoniello et al.[14] reported that insulin and glucagon degradation were not affected by hepatic cirrhosis. Enkephalin uptake and degradation by isolated hepatocytes have been reported[15,16]. Therefore, it seems possible that, in cholestasis, an excess of bile acids may inhibit hepatic uptake, transport or degradation of enkephalins, whereas the hepatic enkephalin-degrading potential may remain unchanged. The results from the LaRusso laboratory showing the inhibitory effect of bile acids on the uptake and processing of cholecystokinin octapeptide and other small hydrophobic peptides by isolated perfused rat liver[17], and isolated rat hepatocytes[18] can be viewed as supporting this hypothesis. The increase of serum enkephalin-degrading activity that we have found in our patients with cholestasis may be considered to be a homeostatic response to the increased level of enkephalin and, possibly, of other opioid peptides. Circulating enkephalins are protected from degradation through interaction with enkephalin-binding substances in plasma[19]. However, a fraction of free enkephalins would still be susceptible to the degrading enzymes. Indeed, our data indicate that endogenous methionine enkephalin was stable in those plasma samples in which the degrading enzymes were inactivated by EDTA. In parallel serum samples, methionine immunoreactivity decreased during incubation at 37°C, although the disappearance rate was incomparably lower than that for the exogenous (free) enkephalin[20]. Also, the data from this experiment suggest that, in cholestasis, methionine enkephalin is secreted into the blood in a form protected from degradation.

The o igin and potential pathophysiological role of enkephalin-degrading activity in blood of patients with cholestasis is unclear. It may be of hepatic origin, similar to alanine aminotransferase or alkaline phosphatase. However, our data with isolated erythrocytes suggest that these cells contain an abundance of enkephalin-degrading activity that could be released by addition of taurodeoxycholic acid. This observation seems to be worthy of further studies. Our inhibitory and substrate specificity data (Table 5) suggest that aminopeptidase-M[21] is a major enkephalin-degrading enzyme both in blood serum and liver extracts. Moreover, the serum concentration of this enzyme in cholestasis seems to be elevated. However, taking into account recent reports[22,23], the potential involvement of yet other proteinases in enkephalin degradation should be considered.

In summary, we have shown that methionine enkephalin concentrations and enkephalin-degrading activity are significantly elevated in the blood of children with cholestasis of different aetiology. The hepatic enkephalin-degrading potential was not altered in patients with cholestasis. The clinical and pathophysiological significance of these observations is not yet clear, and seems to be worthy of further studies.

References

1. Thornton JR, Losowsky MS. Methionine enkephalin is increased in plasma in acute liver disease and is present in bile and urine. J Hepatol. 1989;8:53–9.
2. Thornton JR, Losowsky MS. Opioid peptides and primary biliary cirrhosis. Br Med J. 1988;297:1501–4.
3. Thornton JR, Losowsky MS. Plasma leucine enkephalin is increased in liver disease. Gut. 1989;30:1392–5.
4. Thornton JR, Dean H, Losowsky MS. Is ascites caused by impaired hepatic inactivation of blood-borne endogenous opioid peptides? Gut. 1988;29:1167–72.
5. Banks WA, Kastin AJ. Peptide transport systems for opiates across the blood-brain barrier. Am J Physiol. 1990;259:E1–10.
6. Jones EA, Bergasa NV. The pruritus of cholestasis: from bile acids to opiate antagonists. Hepatology. 1990;5:884–7.
7. Bergasa NV, Talbot TL, Alling DW et al. A controlled trial of naloxone infusions for the pruritus of cholestasis. Gastroenterology. 1992;102:544–9.
8. Chaminade M, Foutz AS, Rossier J. Co-release of enkephalins and precursors with

catecholamines by the perfused cat adrenal in situ. Life Sci. 1983;33:21–4.

9. Schultzberg M, Hokfelt T, Lundberg JM, Terenius L, Elfvin LG, Elde R. Enkephalin-like immunoreactivity in nerve terminals in sympathetic ganglia and adrenal medulla and in adrenal medullary gland cells. Acta Physiol Scand. 1978;103:475–7.

10. Polak JM, Bloom SR, Sullivan SN, Facer P, Pearse AGE. Enkephalin-like immunoreactivity in the human gastrointestinal tract. Lancet. 1977;1:972–4.

11. Janas RM, Marks DL, LaRusso NF. An aluminium silicate binding assay for quantitation of degradation of cholecystokinin octapeptide and other short peptides. Analyt Biochem. 1992;206:6–12.

12. Movsas B, Mannor GE, Yallow RS. Degradation of the 34-amino acid gastrin by rat tissue homogenates. Life Sci. 1985;36:89–95.

13. Heuman DM. Hepatoprotective properties of ursodeoxycholic acid. Gastroenterology. 1993;104:1865–9.

14. Antoniello S, Larocca S, Cavalcanti E, Auletta M, Salvatore F, Cacciatore L. Insulin and glucagon degradation in liver are not affected by hepatic cirrhosis. Clin Chim Acta. 1989;183:343–50.

15. Hothi SH, Randall DP, Titheradge MA. [Leu]enkephalin stimulates carbohydrate metabolism in isolated hepatocytes and kidney tubule fragments by interaction with angiotensin II receptors. Biochem J. 1989;257:705–10.

16. Leach RP, Allan EH, Titheradge MA. The stimulation of glycogenolysis in isolated hepatocytes by opioid peptides. Biochem J. 1985;227:191–7.

17. Gores GJ, Miller LJ, LaRusso NF. Hepatic processing of cholecystokinin peptides. II. Cellular metabolism, transport, and biliary excretion. Am J Physiol. 1986;250:G350–6.

18. Gores GJ, Kost LJ, Miller LJ, LaRusso NF. Processing of cholecystokinin by isolated hepatocytes. Am J Physiol. 1989;257:G242–8.

19. Possenti R, DeMarco V, Cherubini O, Roda LG. Enkephalin-binding systems in human plasma. Neurochem Res. 1983;8:423–32.

20. Shibanoki S, Weinberger SB, Ishikawa K, Martinez JL, Jr. Further characterization of the in vitro hydrolysis of [Leu]- and [Met]enkephalin in rat plasma. HPLC–ECD measurement of substrate and metabolite concentrations. Regul Peptides. 1991;32:267–78.

21. Benter IF, Hirsh EM, Tuchman AJ, Word PE. N-terminal degradation of low molecular weight opioid peptides in human cerebrospinal fluid. Biochem Pharmacol. 1990;40:465–72.

22. Janas RM, Marks DL, LaRusso NF. Purification and partial characterization of a heat-resistant, cytosolic neuropeptidase from rat liver. Biochem Biophys Res Commun. 1994;198:574–81.

23. Swain MG, Vergalla J, Jones EA. Plasma endopeptidase 24.11 (enkephalinase) activity is markedly increased in cholestatic liver diseases. Hepatology. 1993;18:556–8.

26
Treatment with ursodeoxycholic acid, as monotherapy and in combination with other agents, in primary biliary cirrhosis

H. R. VAN BUUREN, F. H. J. WOLFHAGEN and S. W. SCHALM

INTRODUCTION

Numerous studies have now confirmed the original observations of Leuschner and co-workers[1] that, in patients with primary biliary cirrhosis (PBC), ursodeoxycholic acid (UDCA) improves the results of several laboratory liver function tests, especially alkaline phosphatase, γ-glutamyl transferase and alanine and aspartate aminotransferases[2-12]. UDCA also lowers[6,10] or stabilizes serum bilirubin[5-8]. Whether UDCA also improves symptoms and liver histology, and modifies the natural history and the ultimate prognosis of the disease, can only be judged from the results of placebo controlled trials. At least 11[2-12] such trials have now been reported, either in abstract form or as full articles (Table 1).

Table 1 UDCA in primary biliary cirrhosis: controlled trials

Reference	Year	No. of patients	Follow-up (months)	Type of report
2	1989	20	9	Article
3	1990	45	6	Article
4	1990	16	18	Abstract
5	1991	50	29	Article
6	1991	146	24	Article
7	1992	178	48	Abstract
8	1992	222	24	Abstract
9	1993	153	48	Abstract
10	1993	88	6	Article
11	1993	12	6	Article
12	1994	46	24	Article

EFFECT OF UDCA ON SYMPTOMS

The effect of UDCA on the most common symptoms in PBC (fatigue and pruritus) has not been assessed or reported by all investigators. In nine of the randomized controlled trials the effect of UDCA on pruritus was reported. A positive effect was reported in only three[5,6,11]. In two of these studies interpretation of the reported beneficial effect is problematic, either due to the limited information provided[5] or due to the design of the study (crossover study in 12 patients with two consecutive 3-month treatment periods)[11]. The clinical importance of the reported statistically significant difference in patients experiencing pruritus in the other study seems limited[6]. In only one[5] of the five studies reporting on the effect of UDCA on fatigue[4-7,12] was a favourable effect of UDCA established.

In conclusion, controlled investigations have failed to demonstrate a clear beneficial effect of UDCA on symptoms.

EFFECT OF UDCA ON LIVER HISTOLOGY

There are six reports[2,4-7,12], two of them in abstract form[4,7] which provide results of controlled evaluations of liver histology during UDCA treatment.

Leuschner et al.[2] noted improved hepatic morphology in six, and deterioration in two out of 10 patients treated with UDCA during 9 months; among eight placebo patients one improved and four clearly deteriorated. A composite histology score improved by a mean of 18% in the UDCA group and decreased with a mean of 18% in the placebo patients. However, statistical evaluation failed to show significant differences. In Poupon's study[6] paired histological evaluation in 95 patients after 2 years treatment with UDCA was performed. Compared with the placebo group there was a significant improvement in a number of histological characteristics in the patients receiving UDCA, including bile-duct paucity, ductular proliferation, poly- and mononuclear cell infiltration, piecemeal necrosis, parenchymal necrosis, lobular inflammation and cholestasis. There was no difference in the degree of fibrosis. Changes in histological stage were not specifically mentioned. According to a composite histology score, 28/50 (56%) UDCA and 13/45 (29%) placebo patients improved; 10/50 (20%) UDCA and 22/45 (49%) placebo patients worsened ($p < 0.002$).

O'Brien et al.[4], in a study of 16 patients, were the only group to report a significant effect of UDCA on the histological stage of the disease. They also noted a significant difference in favour of the UDCA group when they compared portal infiltrates, cholestasis, bile duct proliferation, bile duct loss and periportal fibrosis. Piecemeal necrosis was not significantly changed. Hadziyannis et al.[5] and Lindor et al.[7] reported absence of a favourable effect of UDCA on histological progression in their studies including 235 patients. In the study of Turner et al.[12] seven UDCA- and 15 placebo-treated patients who were non-cirrhotic at entry were compared for the development of histological cirrhosis over the 2 study years. One of seven (14%) of the UDCA patients who completed 2 years' treatment and were biopsied was documented as having developed cirrhosis, compared to eight of 14 (57%) placebo patients. These differences were not significant. The authors concluded that there was a trend for delay in *de-novo* cirrhosis in the UDCA-treated group, but that the numbers were too small for meaningful statistical comparison.

In conclusion, there is limited documentation of a beneficial effect of UDCA on liver histology in PBC. At present there is no convincing evidence that UDCA influences fibrogenesis or halts histological progression. Unfortunately, it is unlikely that such major effect on hepatic histology will ever be established more conclusively, since most investigators, in particular those conducting large trials[6,8], have chosen to interrupt placebo treatment after 2 years of controlled evaluation, and subsequent open treatment of all patients with UDCA.

EFFECT OF UDCA ON CLINICAL PROGRESSION

Considering the number of patients studied, and the length of follow-up, the effect of UDCA on the eventual outcome of the disease could be assessed in six controlled studies[5-9,12].

In Poupon *et al.*'s 2-year controlled trial[6] no deaths were reported, but the treatment failure rate in both treatment groups was significantly different. Failure was defined as a doubling of bilirubin to more than 70 μmol/l or an increase to more than 200 μmol/l (UDCA group three patients, placebo seven patients), development of ascites (UDCA one, placebo three), oesophageal variceal bleeding (UDCA one, placebo two) or side-effects (both groups one patient). After an additional period of 2 years, in which all patients received UDCA, the failure rate in the original UDCA and placebo groups was 12% and 26% respectively, which was significantly different. During this additional 2-year period two patients in the UDCA group required liver transplantation compared with 12 in the original placebo group, a difference which was statistically significant. Survival was comparable: five and seven patients had died, from all causes, in the original UDCA and placebo groups respectively. Lindor *et al.*[7] found that treatment failure (defined as death, liver transplantation, histological progression, development of oesophageal varices, ascites or encephalopathy, doubling of serum bilirubin, progression of pruritus and fatigue, drug toxicity or withdrawal) was delayed in the patient group receiving UDCA ($p < 0.0003$). Of the individual components of the treatment failure score, only the doubling of bilirubin was significantly different between the two groups (three versus 15 patients). Seven patients on UDCA died or required transplantation compared to 12 in the placebo group, a non-significant difference. Although UDCA had a significantly favourable effect on serum bilirubin, an interim analysis at 3 years of the Greek trial[5] indicated that UDCA was not associated with a significant change in the natural course of the disease: four of 25 UDCA-treated and five of 25 placebo-treated patients had either died or required liver transplantation. Five patients in the UDCA group and four in the placebo group had developed ascites, variceal bleeding or encephalopathy.

In the large Canadian multi-centre study[8], after 2 years of treatment, 5/111 (4.5%) and 9/111 (8.1%) patients treated with UDCA and placebo respectively had died; 7/111 (6.3%) patients treated with UDCA versus 10/111 (9%) placebo patients had required transplantation. These differences were not significant. The percentage rise in serum bilirubin was significantly less in the UDCA group. In the study of Combes et al.[9] there was no difference in frequencies or time to development of treatment failures between both UDCA and control groups. More details from this study await publication. Turner et al.[12] concluded from their study that there appeared not to be a significant difference between UDCA and placebo treatment on the rate of developing liver failure requiring transplantation or resulting in death from a liver-related cause. These authors also found a significant, albeit modest, change in serum bilirubin between the placebo and UDCA-treated patients favouring the latter.

These results clearly indicate that during long-term administration of UDCA serum bilirubin levels tend to stabilize, with fewer patients showing a marked increase or a doubling. Nevertheless, despite this apparent beneficial effect on a major prognostic variable of the disease, the currently available data indicate that UDCA is unlikely to be associated with a major beneficial effect on the ultimate course of the disease. This finding would also imply that serum bilirubin in PBC patients receiving bile acid therapy is no longer the major indicator of disease progression[13,14] and that prognostic scores, like the Mayo model[15], may need adaptation for predicting prognosis. Mortality was not significantly different between UDCA and placebo study groups, although there was a trend for lower mortality in UDCA-treated patients in some studies. Only in the French study[6] was a significant difference in liver transplantation requirement found. This finding is remarkable considering the slowly progressive character of the disease and the relative short treatment period of 2 years.

A beneficial effect of UDCA on the ultimate course of the disease might be limited to subgroups of patients, e.g. patients with histological stage I or II disease. Hopefully the results of some of the larger ongoing trials[7-9], and of meta-analyses using the individual data of the larger controlled trials, will show whether such subgroups can be identified.

UDCA AND REMISSIONS OF THE DISEASE

One way to assess the efficacy of UDCA in PBC is to study its potential to modify the natural course of the disease; another approach may be to study its potential to induce complete remissions of the disease[16,17]. Disease remission is a well-established therapeutic concept in haematological diseases, such as leukaemia or malignant lymphomas, and in autoimmune disorders including chronic autoimmune hepatitis. For PBC, criteria for disease remission have been proposed by Beukers and Schalm[17]. These include disappearance of PBC-related complaints, especially pruritus and fatigue, and the capability to perform normal daily activities (symptomatic remission); normal values for bilirubin, AST and IgM, and serum alkaline phosphatase not exceeding 1.5 times the upper limit of normal (biochemical remission) and inflammatory infiltrate absent or restricted to the portal tracts without bile duct destruction and absence of granulomas (histological remission). A complete remission is defined as a symptomatic, biochemical and histological remission. The potential of UDCA to induce complete remissions in PBC, using these criteria, has been studied by the Dutch Multicentre PBC Study Group in 110 patients with non-advanced disease (Child–Pugh class A patients) in an open study lasting 1 year[18]. Twelve patients attained a biochemical remission and seven a biochemical and symptomatic remission. In six of these seven patients a liver biopsy could be performed after 1 year. The criteria for histological remission were fulfilled in three of these six patients. Thus, a complete remission was achieved in 3% (confidence interval 1–9%) of PBC patients with compensated disease during 1 year of UDCA treatment.

TOLERANCE AND ADVERSE EFFECTS OF UDCA IN PBC

UDCA is a drug free from serious adverse effects. Diarrhoea or pruritus may occur. These side-effects are usually transient or respond to lowering the dose. A review of the results of the 11 controlled trials[2–12], in which 478 patients were treated with UDCA and 471 with placebo, confirms the excellent tolerance of UDCA in PBC. The dose of UDCA varied from 8.7 to 15 mg/kg. Adverse effects of UDCA were reported in 15 of the 478 (3.1%) patients treated with UDCA: six patients had a worsening of pruritus, five (transient) diarrhoea, one constipation, two a skin rash and one mental depression. Treatment was discontinued in eight (1.6%) of these patients. Eight (1.6%) of the 471 patients treated with placebo experienced adverse effects: worsening of pruritus in four, constipation in one, depression in one and gastric ulcer in one. Placebo treatment was interrupted in five of these patients (1%). In patients with advanced disease (cirrhosis with Child–Pugh class B or C disease) UDCA treatment may be associated with an increase in bilirubin and clinical deterioration[19]. There is as yet no evidence that such patients benefit from UDCA treatment, and in general liver transplantation should be the primary consideration in these advanced cases. In patients with advanced disease in whom UDCA treatment is considered, careful monitoring and a low initial dose of UDCA seem advisable.

UDCA IN PBC: CONCLUSIONS

UDCA is a well-tolerated and safe drug for treating PBC. UDCA improves biochemical parameters of the liver disease in nearly all patients with non-advanced disease. There is no conclusive evidence that UDCA ameliorates symptoms. UDCA may improve several elements of liver histology, but a beneficial effect on liver fibrosis or on progression towards more advanced histological stages of the disease has not been documented. The finding in one study that significantly less patients treated with UDCA for 4 years required liver transplantation than a comparable group who received UDCA for 2 years, awaits confirmation by other groups. No significant effect on mortality has been reported. UDCA slows the progression of PBC when doubling of serum bilirubin is used as a criterion. It is doubtful whether this effect on bilirubin corresponds with a truly beneficial effect on the course of the disease. In the large majority of patients treatment with UDCA does not seem capable of inducing disease remissions.

Considering the overall benefit–risk ratio, UDCA is currently the most attractive first-line treatment option in PBC. It is evident, however, that the drug is only partially effective, and that there is still a genuine need for more effective medical therapy.

UDCA IN COMBINATION WITH OTHER AGENTS IN PBC

A number of individual drugs – including azathioprine, prednisone, cyclosporin, methotrexate and UDCA – have shown some efficacy in the treatment of PBC, but major effects on histology or the ultimate course of the disease have not been shown. Therefore, it has been suggested[17,20] that there should be a rethink of treatment strategies in PBC and a focus on the evaluation of combinations of drugs which have shown some efficacy in the past to achieve complete remissions (Fig. 1). A number of investigators have now explored the efficacy of combined treatment of UDCA with other potentially effective drugs (Table 2).

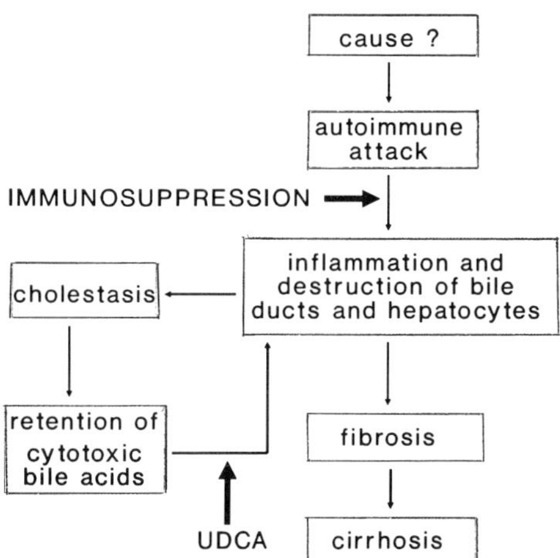

Fig. 1 Hypothesis on the pathophysiology of primary biliary cirrhosis and sites of action of UDCA and immunosuppressive therapy. The model illustrates the potential synergistic effect of combined immunosuppressive and bile acid treatment

UDCA IN COMBINATION WITH COLCHICINE

Raedsch et al. performed a randomized controlled study in 22 patients with PBC with a follow-up of 12 months[21,22]. The patients were randomized to UDCA plus 1 mg colchicine/day or UDCA plus placebo. All patients were pretreated with UDCA alone for 12 months. No significant differences were found between the groups regarding aminotransferases, bilirubin, cholinesterase, albumin and cholesterol. There was no additional effect of colchicine on symptoms such as pruritus. Histological evaluation showed no differences between the groups; there was no evidence for an effect on fibrosis in the colchicine-treated patients[22].

Podda et al. performed a similar trial in 88 patients[23]. The results of this trial have not yet been published. A preliminary analysis showed no evidence for an additional effect of colchicine (oral communication).

In a study performed by Shibata et al. 12 patients received a combination of 600 mg UDCA and 1 mg colchicine daily for more than 2 years[24]. Analysis showed no clear additional effect of colchicine on liver biochemical parameters.

At present colchicine does not seem to improve the results that can be obtained with UDCA treatment alone.

Table 2 Studies evaluating UDCA in combination with other agents in PBC

Agents	Reference	Year	Type of study	No. of patients	Follow-up (months)
UDCA + colchicine	21,22	1992	RCT	22	12
	23	1992	RCT	88	–*
	24	1992	Open	12	24
UDCA + methotrexate	25	1992	Open	14	17
	26	1993	Open	8	6
UDCA + prednisone/ azathioprine	Dutch multicentre study	1994	RCT	41	–*

RCT = randomized controlled trial
*Ongoing trials

UDCA IN COMBINATION WITH METHOTREXATE

Kaplan[25] reported on 14 PBC patients who were treated with either UDCA ($n = 9$) or methotrexate ($n = 5$) and then received additional treatment with methotrexate or UDCA. UDCA alone improved itching in three of the four patients, but had no effect on fatigue in three patients with this symptom. The addition of methotrexate improved fatigue in all three patients. Methotrexate alone improved itching and fatigue in all five patients. UDCA had no additional effect on symptoms. UDCA and methotrexate had an additive effect on serum alkaline phosphatase and bilirubin. UDCA lowered ALT in both groups, whereas methotrexate administered first increased ALT levels. The order in which the drugs were given had no effect on the ultimate levels of alkaline phosphatase and bilirubin. No toxicity of methotrexate was reported.

Buscher and colleagues[26] studied the effect of methotrexate 15 mg weekly added to UDCA 10–15 mg/kg daily in eight patients. Within 2–4 weeks of the combined treatment seven patients complained of increased fatigue and one of transient abdominal discomfort. Serum transaminases markedly increased during the first months of treatment and thereafter gradually improved. Alkaline phosphatase clearly decreased in six of the eight patients. Bilirubin, elevated in two patients, decreased slightly, while albumin and cholinesterase did not change. Within 8 weeks pre-existing pruritus disappeared in seven patients, and fatigue in three of the seven patients with this symptom.

These preliminary results suggest that combination therapy of UDCA and methotrexate may be more effective than UDCA given alone. Obviously, the results of controlled studies in more patients have to be awaited before more definitive conclusions can be drawn.

UDCA AND PREDNISONE/AZATHIOPRINE

The effect of combined treatment with UDCA and prednisone in seven symptomatic PBC patients was retrospectively evaluated by Wolfhagen *et al.*[23]. After starting the combined treatment five of the seven patients became asymptomatic. Serum alkaline phosphatase and AST decreased in all patients. AST became normal in four patients and alkaline phosphatase in two. Bilirubin, only slightly elevated in one patient, remained stable during a median follow-up of 1.5 years. Figure 2 shows the additional effect of prednisone on liver biochemical tests in one of these patients. The combined treatment was reported to be well tolerated by all patients.

In 1992, stimulated by these observations and by the results of previous studies showing a beneficial effect of prednisone on complaints, liver biochemical liver tests and clinical progression[13] and a significant effect of azathioprine on survival[27], a randomized double-blind controlled trial evaluating combined UDCA and low-dose prednisone/azathioprine treatment was initiated by the Dutch Multicentre PBC study group.

Inclusion criteria of this ongoing study are absence of disease remission after at least 1 year treatment with UDCA and compensated (Child–Pugh class A) liver disease. Patients are randomly assigned to groups receiving either UDCA 8–10 mg/kg per day plus one capsule containing prednisone 10 mg/day and azathioprine 50 mg/day or UDCA plus one capsule containing placebo for 1 year. A subgroup of patients is also randomly assigned to treatment with either etidronate/calcium or calcium alone. The main aim of the study is to determine whether the combined treatment can increase the number of patients with disease remission. At present 41 patients have entered this trial. An interim analysis of the first 18 patients who completed the study showed that alkaline phosphatase, AST and IgM decreased significantly in the combined-treatment group compared with the placebo group. Changes in bilirubin, at entry abnormal in six patients, and albumin

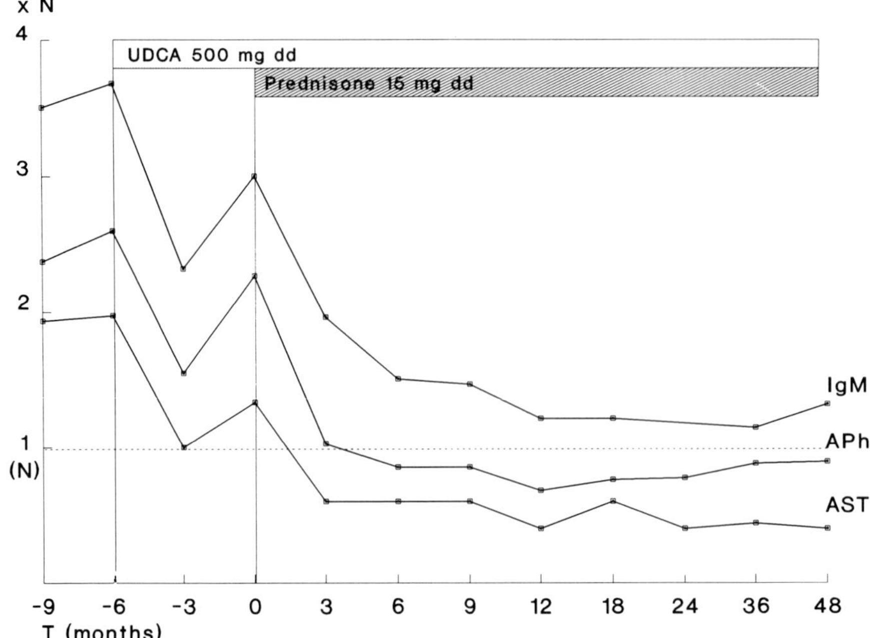

Fig. 2 Effect of prednisone added to UDCA on alkaline phosphatase (APh), AST and IgM, expressed as multiples of the upper limit of normal (N), during 4 years of combined treatment. There was normalization of AST and APh, and disappearance of fatigue, within 3 months of combined treatment

were not significant. There was no evidence for an accelerated bone loss in the prednisone-treated patients. Data on symptoms and liver histology, and thus on the number of patients with complete remissions, are currently not available.

These preliminary results seem encouraging, and at least suggest that low dose immunosuppressive treatment enhances the effect of UDCA alone. The trial will be continued until at least 60 patients have been included.

References

1. David R, Kurtz W, Strohm WD, Leuschner U. Die Wirkung von Ursodeoxycholsäure bei chronischen Leberkrankheiten. Eine Pilotstudie. Z Gastroenterol. 1985;23:420(abstr.).
2. Leuschner U, Fischer H, Kurtz W *et al.* Ursodeoxycholic acid in primary biliary cirrhosis: results of a controlled double-blind trial. Gastroenterology. 1989;97:1268–74.
3. Oka H, Toda G, Ikeda Y *et al.* A multi-center double-blind controlled trial of ursodeoxycholic acid for primary biliary cirrhosis. Gastroenterol Jpn. 1990;25:774–80.
4. O'Brien CB, Senior JR, Sternlieb JM *et al.* Ursodiol treatment of primary biliary cirrhosis. Gastroenterology. 1989;98:A617(abstr.).
5. Hadziyannis SJ, Hadziyannis ES, Lianidou E, Makris A. Long-term treatment of primary biliary cirrhosis with ursodeoxycholic acid: the third year of a controlled trial. In: Paumgartner G, Stiehl A, Gerok W, editors. Bile acids as therapeutic agents. Dordrecht: Kluwer; 1991:287–96.

6. Poupon RE, Balkau B, Eschwège E, Poupon R and the UDCA-PBC study group. A multicenter, controlled trial of ursodiol for the treatment of primary biliary cirrhosis. N Engl J Med. 1991;324:1548–54.

7. Lindor KD, Baldus WP, Jorgensen RA, Ludwig J, Murtaugh PA, Dickson ER. Ursodeoxycholic acid (UDCA) is beneficial therapy for patients with primary biliary cirrhosis. Hepatology. 1992;16:91A(abstr.).

8. Heathcote EJL, Cauch K, Walker V, Bailey RJ. The Canadian multi-centre double-blind randomized controlled trial of ursodeoxycholic acid in primary biliary cirrhosis. Hepatology. 1992;16:91A(abstr.).

9. Combes B, Carithers RL, Maddrey WC *et al.* A randomized, double-blind, placebo-controlled trial of ursodeoxycholic acid (UDCA) in primary biliary cirrhosis. Hepatology. 1993;18:175A(abstr.).

10. Battezzati PM, Podda M, Cianchi FB *et al.* Ursodeoxycholic acid for symptomatic primary biliary cirrhosis. Preliminary analysis of a double-blind multicenter trial. J Hepatol. 1993;17:332–8.

11. Hwang SJ, Chan CY, Lee SD, Wu JC, Tsay SH, Lo KJ. Ursodeoxycholic acid in the treatment of primary biliary cirrhosis: a short-term, randomized double-blind controlled, cross-over study with long-term follow up. J Gastroenterol Hepatol. 1993;8:217–23.

12. Turner IB, Myszor M, Mitchison HC *et al.* A two year trial examining the effectiveness of ursodeoxycholic acid in primary biliary cirrhosis. J Gastroenterol Hepatol. 1994;9:162–8.

13. Mitchison HC, Palmer JM, Bassendine MF *et al.* A controlled trial of prednisolone treatment in primary biliary cirrhosis. Three-year results. J Hepatol. 1992;15:336–44.

14. Reichen J. Pharmacologic treatment of cholestasis. Semin Liver Dis. 1993;13:302–15.

15. Dickson ER, Gramsbsch PM, Fleming TR *et al.* Prognosis in primary biliary cirrhosis: model for decision making. Hepatology. 1989;10:1–7.

16. Wiesner RH, Grambsch PM, Lindor KD, Ludwig J, Dickson ER. Clinical and statistical analyses of new and evolving therapies for primary biliary cirrhosis. Hepatology. 1988;8:668–76.

17. Beukers R, Schalm SW. Immunosuppressive therapy for primary biliary cirrhosis. J Hepatol. 1992;14:1–6.

18. Wolfhagen FHJ, van Buuren HR, van Berge Henegouwen GP and the Dutch Multicenter PBC study group. Can ursodeoxycholic acid induce complete remissions in primary biliary cirrhosis? J Hepatol. 1993;18:S43(abstr.).

19. Keppelhout JC, Mulder CJJ, van Berge Henegouwen GP, de Vries RA, Brandt K-H. Ursodeoxycholic acid treatment in primary biliary cirrhosis with the emphasis on late stage disease. Neth J Med. 1992;41:11–16.

20. Kaplan MM. New strategies needed for treatment of primary biliary cirrhosis. Gastroenterology. 1993;104:651–3.

21. Raedsch R, Stiehl A, Walker S, Scherrmann JM, Kommerell B. Kombinierte Ursodeoxycholsäure plus Colchizin-Behandlung bei primär biliärer Zirrhose: Ergebnisse einer Placebo-kontrollierten Doppelblindstudie. Z Gastroenterol. 1992;30:55–7.

22. Raedsch R, Stiel A, Rudi J *et al.* Combined urso plus colchicine treatment in primary biliary cirrhosis: efficacy, pharmacology and urso-colchicine interactions. Proceedings of the XII international Falk bile acid meeting, Basel, 1992:48–9.

23. Podda M and the Italian multicenter group for the study of UDCA in PBC. Long-term effects of the administration of ursodeoxycholic acid (UDCA) alone or with colchicine in patients with primary biliary cirrhosis (PBC). A double-blind multicenter study. Proceedings of the XII international Falk bile acid meeting, Basel, 1992:50–1.

24. Shibata J, Fujiyama S, Honda Y, Sato T. Combination therapy with ursodeoxycholic acid and colchicine for primary biliary cirrhosis. J Gastroenterol Hepatol. 1992;7:277–82.

25. Kaplan MM. The therapeutic effects of ursodiol and methotrexate are additive and well tolerated in primary biliary cirrhosis. Hepatology. 1992;16:92A(abstr.).

26. Buscher H-P, Zietzschmann Y, Gerok W. Positive responses to methotrexate and ursodeoxycholic acid in patients with primary biliary cirrhosis responding insufficiently to ursodeoxycholic acid alone. J Hepatol. 1993;18:9–14.

27. Christensen E, Neuberger J, Crowe J *et al.* Beneficial effect of azathioprine and prediction of prognosis in primary biliary cirrhosis. Gastroenterology. 1985;89:1084–91.

28. Wolfhagen FHJ, van Buuren HR, Schalm SW. Combined treatment with ursodeoxycholic acid and prednisone in primary biliary cirrhosis. Neth J Med. 1994;44:84–90.

27
Methotrexate alone or in combination with ursodeoxycholic acid as possible treatment in primary biliary cirrhosis

W. VAN STEENBERGEN, R. SCIOT, P. VAN EYKEN, V. DESMET and J. FEVERY

INTRODUCTION

Primary biliary cirrhosis (PBC) is a chronic, progressive cholestatic disorder, characterized by the destruction of small intrahepatic bile ducts, and ultimately leading to the development of cirrhosis, portal hypertension and liver failure. Although the exact aetiology of this disease remains unknown, two processes appear to cause the hepatic damage. The first is a profound but incompletely understood abnormality of immune regulation, with an attack by activated cytotoxic T-lymphocytes on the biliary epithelium, leading to the chronic non-suppurative destruction of the small bile ducts[1,2]. The second is related to the intracellular accumulation of potentially toxic endogenous bile acids, leading to a chemical damage of hepatocytes in areas of the liver where bile drainage is impeded by obliteration of bile ducts[2,3]. At present there is no proven, generally accepted treatment for primary biliary cirrhosis. Therapeutic interventions have been aimed at both pathogenic mechanisms. Immunomodulating and anti-inflammatory agents such as corticosteroids, azathioprine, d-penicillamine, chlorambucil, colchicine and cyclosporin have been used in order to suppress the immunologically mediated destruction of bile duct epithelial cells. Most of these drugs show some efficacy with regard to symptoms, liver tests and histology, but are also characterized by major side-effects which make their long-term use hazardous[1,2,4,5]. Based on its positive effects in two patients with primary sclerosing cholangitis[6], a low-dose oral pulse treatment with methotrexate (MTX) has been evaluated in patients with non-cirrhotic PBC. In preliminary uncontrolled observations, marked improvements in symptoms, biochemical tests of liver function and histology have been reported[2,7–9].

Ursodeoxycholic acid (UDCA), a hydrophilic and less toxic bile acid which is given to replace the detergent endogenous bile acids, leads to biochemical improvement[3,10-14]. Improvement in histology and slowing of the progression of PBC is mainly reported by the group of Poupon[10,15], but not by others[11,12,16]. Some patients treated with UDCA even progress to a complicated cirrhosis despite improvements in clinical symptoms and biochemical liver test results[17].

In view of the apparent limited efficacy of these individual drug regimens, combination therapy of UDCA with immunomodulating agents seems indicated as a more effective treatment for PBC[1,5,18]. Preliminary results indicative of an additive effect of MTX and UDCA in lowering serum alkaline phosphatase and bilirubin levels have been reported by Kaplan[19].

The present study reports on the clinical, biochemical and histological evolution of patients with PBC who are treated with MTX, either used alone or in combination with UDCA.

PATIENTS AND METHODS

Open study

In the open study, 13 patients with PBC (10 women and three men with a mean age of 58 years) were studied. Before treatment, histological stages I, II, III and IV according to Ludwig *et al.*'s classification[20], were present in two, four, six and one patient, respectively. All patients were treated with a weekly low-dose oral pulse treatment of MTX (15 mg/week, taken as 5 mg every 12 h three times each week)[7] during a period of 1 year. Statistical analysis of differences in liver tests measured at entry and at 1, 3, 6, 9 and 12 months was done with analysis of variance for repeated measurements. In nine of these 13 patients, liver biopsy specimens were evaluated before and after 1 year of treatment. A histological scoring system was used, based on the presence of fibrosis, inflammation, necrosis and cholestasis.

Controlled study

In a further study, 14 patients who were admitted between August 1991 and April 1992 were randomly assigned to receive either no treatment ($n = 6$) or a combination of MTX 15 mg/week with UDCA 500 mg daily given at bedtime ($n = 8$). Details of these patients are given in Table 1. Exclusion criteria were the presence of cirrhosis, excessive alcohol consumption, serological or histological evidence for chronic viral hepatitis B or C, serological evidence for a previous hepatitis B infection[21], mental depression, pregnancy and evidence of a chronic infection. One of the actively treated patients had a typical histological picture of a vanishing bile duct disease, but proved to be negative for antimitochondrial antibodies (AMF). Radiologically, there was no evidence for primary sclerosing cholangitis. This patient had high titres of antinuclear antibodies with a homogeneous immunofluorescence pattern, no smooth muscle antibodies, normal serum

Table 1 Clinical, biochemical and immunological features in six untreated and eight MTX/UDCA-treated patients with non-cirrhotic PBC at entry to the study

Parameters	Untreated (n = 6)	MTX/UDCA (n = 8)
Female/male	4/2	8/0
Mean age ($\pm$ SD) (years)	56 $\pm$ 7	47 $\pm$ 8
Histological stage		
I	n = 2	n = 2
II	n = 2	n = 2
III	n = 2	n = 4
Pruritus (score)		
1	n = 3 (50%)	n = 1 (12.5%)
2	n = 3 (50%)	n = 6 (75.0%)
3	n = 0	n = 1 (12.5%)
Fatigue (score)		
1	n = 3 (50%)	n = 2 (25.0%)
2	n = 2 (33%)	n = 2 (25.0%)
3	n = 1 (17%)	n = 3 (37.5%)
4	n = 0	n = 1 (12.5%)
Blood sedimentation rate (mm)	24.0 $\pm$ 10.7	45.5 $\pm$ 30.3
Haemoglobin (g/100 ml)	13.8 $\pm$ 0.8	13.8 $\pm$ 0.9
WBC ($\times 10^9$/l)	6.5 $\pm$ 1.8	6.9 $\pm$ 1.7
Platelets ($\times 10^9$/l)	216 $\pm$ 48	247 $\pm$ 56
Prothrombin time (INR)	1 $\pm$ 0	1 $\pm$ 0
Albumin (g/100 ml)	4.2 $\pm$ 0.3	4.3 $\pm$ 0.4
γ-Globulins (g/100 ml)	1.4 $\pm$ 0.3	1.6 $\pm$ 0.6
Immunoglobulin M (mg/100 ml)	525 $\pm$ 259	605 $\pm$ 310
Creatinine (mg/100 ml)	0.8 $\pm$ 0.2	0.8 $\pm$ 0.1
Alkaline phosphatase ($\times$ N)*	2.4 $\pm$ 1.2	5.0 $\pm$ 2.7
GOT ($\times$ N)*	1.3 $\pm$ 0.3	2.1 $\pm$ 0.9
GPT ($\times$ N)*	1.6 $\pm$ 0.8	2.5 $\pm$ 1.2
GGT ($\times$ N)*	11.2 $\pm$ 5.0	17.0 $\pm$ 10.4
Bilirubin (mg/100 ml)	0.6 $\pm$ 0.3	0.9 $\pm$ 0.7
Cholesterol (mg/100 ml)	245 $\pm$ 46	294 $\pm$ 95
Mayo risk score	4.2 $\pm$ 0.4	3.9 $\pm$ 0.5
Antinuclear antibodies positive	n = 3 (50%)	n = 6 (75.0%)
Smooth muscle antibodies positive	n = 0	n = 1 (12.5%)
Antimitochondrial antibodies positive	n = 6 (100%)	n = 7 (87.5%)
Antimitochondrial antibody profiles†		
A–B	n = 3 (50%)	n = 3 (43%)
C–D	n = 3 (50%)	n = 4 (57%)

*Enzyme activities were standardized by dividing the measured values by the upper reference value of the laboratory, so that values are expressed as multiples of the upper limit of normal values ($\times$ N).

†Antimitochondrial antibody profiles according to Klein and Berg[25] two-sample Wilcoxon test.

IgG and increased IgM levels, and could best be defined as having the AMF-negative 'autoimmune cholangitis' variant of PBC[22,23]. The median time period between the first observation of abnormal liver tests and inclusion in the study was 4.5 years (range 1.3–15 years) and 1.1 year (range 0.1–13 years) for the untreated and for the MTX/UDCA-treated patients, respectively.

One patient (MTX/UDCA no. 5), who had a histological stage II at entry, did not tolerate UDCA because of increasing pruritus. She took only MTX during the whole study period. In patient no. 7, MTX had to be discontinued after 6 months of treatment because of an interstitial pneumonitis. MTX/UDCA patient no. 1 showed poor drug compliance. MTX was interrupted after 6 months for at least 11 months because of suspicion of a fungal infection around a dental implant.

In all patients, clinical symptoms – especially pruritus and fatigue – and the following laboratory tests were evaluated at entry (time 0) and at 1, 3, 6, 12, 18 and 24 months of follow-up: blood sedimentation rate, red and white blood cell count, platelet count, prothrombin time, serum albumin, γ-globulins, urea, creatinine, alkaline phosphatase, bilirubin, glutamic oxaloacetic (GOT) and glutamic pyruvic (GPT) transaminases, γ-glutamyl-transpeptidase (γ-GT), cholesterol, and an examination of urine for the presence of proteinuria and red blood cells. Total and individual serum bile acids were analysed by gas chromatography[24] at entry and at 1, 3, 6, 12 and 24 months.

Serum IgM and the presence of antimitochondrial antibodies, antinuclear antibodies and smooth muscle antibodies were evaluated at entry and at 24 months. Antimitochondrial antibody subtyping was performed at entry and at 24 months in Professor P. Berg's laboratory according to published methods[25]. The severity of itching and fatigue was evaluated at each visit and scored on a scale of 1–4, as previously described[26]. The Mayo risk score was calculated at entry and at 24 months[27].

Liver biopsy specimens were obtained at entry and at 24 months, except for two patients, one in the untreated and one in the combination therapy group, who refused to have a second liver biopsy after 2 years of follow-up. All biopsies were reassessed by two pathologists (R.S. and P.V.E.) and scored quantitatively, essentially as described by Poupon et al.[10]. The following histological features were each scored on a scale of 0–3: fibrosis, portal inflammation, piecemeal necrosis, ductular proliferation, parenchymal inflammation, parenchymal necrosis, bilirubinostasis, cholate stasis and cholestatic liver cell rosettes. These values were used to calculate a liver histology score for each liver biopsy specimen: the lowest possible score was 0 and the highest 27. The degree of bile duct paucity was calculated as the number of interlobular bile ducts divided by the number of portal tracts. The histological stage was determined according to the Ludwig classification[20].

Clinical, biochemical and histological variables were compared between the two groups with the Wilcoxon rank-sum test. For each patient, and for each parameter analysed, the difference between the last and initial value was computed, and comparisons were then made between the two treatment groups by the two-sample Wilcoxon test.

A two-tailed p-value below 0.05 was considered to indicate a significant difference. A comparison of the evolution of the biochemical parameters was also performed with multivariate ANOVA.

RESULTS

Open study

After 1 year of treatment with MTX in the uncontrolled study a significant decrease was found for alkaline phosphatase (871–618 U/l; $p = 0.04$), for IgM (585–326 mg/100 ml; $p = 0.04$), and for γ-globulins (1.49–1.04 g/100 ml; $p = 0.002$). No significant differences in histological parameters before and after treatment were found. Side-effects of the treatment consisted of a severe MTX pneumonitis that occurred in one patient and responded well to treatment with corticosteroids.

Controlled study

The evolution of pruritus and of fatigue was not significantly better in the MTX/UDCA-treated group than in the untreated group. Six of the actively treated patients initially presented with a pruritus score of 2 and had a score of 1 (thus a complete absence of pruritus) after 24 months of treatment. A similar improvement in pruritus, however, was also noticed in three patients in the untreated group.

After 24 months the levels of alkaline phosphatase, SGPT, and γ-GT were significantly reduced in the MTX/UDCA-treated group as compared to the untreated group. Alkaline phosphatase decreased to 43% of its initial value in the treated group and became normal in four of the eight treated cases. A statistical decrease in alkaline phosphatase was only observed from entry to month 1 and from month 1 to month 3 of the study. After 3 months no further decline in alkaline phosphatase could be observed. In one patient (MTX/UDCA no. 7), alkaline phosphatase fell dramatically from 9.7 to 1.9 times the upper limit of normal at month 6 of treatment. At that time, MTX had to be discontinued because of an interstitial pneumonitis. Although the UDCA component of the treatment was continued, alkaline phosphatase rose up again to 6 times the upper limit of normal. In five MTX/UDCA-treated patients, transaminases rose transiently after 3 months of treatment. IgM levels declined markedly in four of the eight MTX/UDCA-treated patients. However, after 2 years of treatment, the IgM concentration was not significantly reduced in the treated group as compared to the untreated group.

Compliance to the UDCA therapy was assessed by measuring the amount of serum UDCA relative to the total level of bile acids in serum after an overnight fast. The mean percentages of UDCA in the untreated and in the treated groups were 3% and 1%, respectively, at entry, and 1% and 49%, respectively, at 24 months.

There was no significant improvement in the MTX/UDCA-treated group relative to the untreated group for any of the individual histological parameters studied. At entry the mean total histological scores were 7.6 ± 3.9 and 10.3 ± 3.9 in the untreated and in the treated group, respectively; after 24 months the corresponding scores were 8.4 ± 6.3 and 10.8 ± 5.0.

One patient developed an interstitial pneumonitis after 6 months of treatment with MTX. She responded well to discontinuation of the immuno-modulating agent and to a temporary treatment with corticosteroids. Thrombocytopenia below $100\,000/mm^3$ occurred in two patients after 18 months of treatment with MTX, and in one untreated patient who had evolved into cirrhosis and hypersplenism. A drop in white blood cell count to $3700/mm^3$ occurred in one of the treated cases at 24 months.

DISCUSSION

Despite the use of various immunosuppressive and anti-inflammatory agents, and of the hepatoprotective UDCA, there is still no convincing and significant breakthrough in the treatment of PBC. Recently, attention has been focused on the use of MTX. A clinical and biochemical improvement with 25–60% significant decreases in alkaline phosphatase and with decreases in serum transaminases, γ-GT, γ-globulins, IgM, and titres of antimitochondrial antibodies have been reported in our own uncontrolled observations and in those of others[7–9,28]. Liver histology has been reported to be improved in five out of nine patients with pre-cirrhotic PBC, who have been treated with MTX for 12–34 months[7]. In our own open study on 13 patients who were all treated for 12 months, we could not demonstrate a significant improvement in histological features. A 40–60% decrease in alkaline phosphatase and significant improvements in other liver tests, IgM, and antimitochondrial antibody titres have been observed during treatment with UDCA[10–14]. Significant improvements in histological parameters have been described by some[10,13,14], but not by others[12,16].

We decided to combine the immunomodulating and anti-inflammatory properties of MTX[29–32] with the potentially beneficial effects of UDCA, in an attempt to obtain more satisfactory results than those described with both drugs used alone. The treatment schedule and the study protocol were restricted to patients with the more early histological stages I, II and III of the disease. Patients with cirrhosis have irreversible disease and do not seem to respond to MTX[33].

In controlled conditions we could not demonstrate a significant clinical or histological improvement in the MTX/UDCA-treated patients relative to the untreated cases. Improvements in liver tests mainly consisted of a 60% decrease in alkaline phosphatase, which is comparable to the decreases observed after treatment with MTX[7,8,28] or with UDCA alone[10,13]. Further-more, alkaline phosphatase is not considered a parameter of prognostic significance in patients with PBC[34,35]. Hence, the fact that MTX and UDCA decreased the serum alkaline phosphatase levels is of limited significance.

Failure to show an effect of the present combination therapy on the clinical and histological evolution in patients with non-cirrhotic PBC may point to a real absence of a significant effect of this drug regimen, or might be influenced by the limited number of patients included, which limits the power of this study. On the basis of our experience, however, the empirical use of MTX cannot be recommended for patients with PBC.

Another point of concern is the inherent hepatotoxicity that can be associated with MTX therapy[36-38]. Others have questioned this[39]. According to published guidelines, previous or active alcoholism, renal insufficiency and a combination of obesity and diabetes mellitus should be considered as contraindications for therapy with MTX[40]. The occurrence of interstitial pneumonitis led to discontinuation therapy in two of our 21 patients treated with MTX. Approximately 3–5% of patients with rheumatoid arthritis develop interstitial pneumonitis on MTX[41]. In conclusion, this study shows no significant benefit of a combination therapy with MTX and UDCA, except for a decrease in alkaline phosphatase, SGPT, and γ-GT. This therapy, therefore, cannot yet be recommended as empirical therapy for patients with non-cirrhotic PBC.

References

1. Sherlock S. Primary biliary cirrhosis and vanishing bile ducts. In: McIntyre N, Benhamou J-P, Bircher J, Rizetto M, Rodes J, editors. Oxford textbook of clinical hepatology. Oxford: Oxford University Press; 1991:743–50.
2. Kaplan MM. Primary biliary cirrhosis. In: Schiff L, Schiff ER, editors. Diseases of the liver. Philadelphia: Lippincott, 1993:377–410.
3. Poupon R, Chrétien Y, Poupon RE, Ballet F, Calmus Y, Darnis F. Is ursodeoxycholic acid an effective treatment for primary biliary cirrhosis? Lancet. 1987;1:834–6.
4. Wiesner RH, Grambsch PM, Lindor KD, Ludwig J, Dickson ER. Clinical and statistical analyses of new and evolving therapies for primary biliary cirrhosis. Hepatology. 1988;8: 668–76.
5. Kaplan MM. New strategies needed for treatment of primary biliary cirrhosis. Gastroenterology. 1993;104:651–3.
6. Kaplan MM, Arora S, Pincus SH. Primary sclerosing cholangitis and low-dose oral pulse methotrexate therapy. Clinical and histologic response. Ann Intern Med. 1987;106:231–5.
7. Kaplan MM, Knox TA. Treatment of primary biliary cirrhosis with low-dose weekly methotrexate. Gastroenterology. 1991;101:1332–8.
8. Bergasa NV, Hoofnagle JH, Axiotis CA, Rabin L, Park Y, Jones EA. Oral methotrexate (MTX) for primary biliary cirrhosis (PBC): preliminary report. Gastroenterology. 1991;100:A720.
9. Buscher H-P, Zietzschmann Y, Gerok W. Positive responses to methotrexate and ursodeoxycholic acid in patients with primary biliary cirrhosis responding insufficiently to ursodeoxycholic acid alone. J Hepatol. 1993;18:9–14.
10. Poupon RE, Balkau B, Eschwège E, Poupon R, and the UDCA–PBC study group. A multicenter, controlled trial of ursodiol for the treatment of primary biliary cirrhosis. N Engl J Med. 1991;324:1548–54.
11. Heathcote EJL, Cauch K, Walker V et al. The Canadian multi-centre double blind randomized controlled trial of ursodeoxycholic acid in primary biliary cirrhosis. Hepatology. 1992;16:91A.
12. Lindor KD, Baldus WP, Jorgensen RA, Ludwig J, Murtaugh PA, Dickson ER. Ursodeoxycholic acid (UDCA) is beneficial therapy for patients with primary biliary cirrhosis (PBC). Hepatology. 1992;16:91A.
13. Leuschner U, Fischer H, Kurtz W et al. Ursodeoxycholic acid in primary biliary cirrhosis: results of a controlled double-blind trial. Gastroenterology. 1989;97:1268–74.
14. Matsuzaki Y, Tanaka N, Osuga T et al. Improvement of biliary enzyme levels and itching as a result of long-term administration of ursodeoxycholic acid in primary biliary cirrhosis. Am J Gastroenterol. 1990;85:15–23.
15. Poupon RE, Chrétien Y, Balkau B, Niard AM, Poupon R, and the UDCA-PBC study group. Ursodeoxycholic therapy for primary biliary cirrhosis: a four year controlled study. Hepatology. 1992;16:91A.
16. Hadziyannis SJ, Hadziyannis ES, Lianidou E, Makris A. Long-term treatment of primary

biliary cirrhosis with ursodeoxycholic acid: the third year of a controlled trial. In: Paumgartner G, Stiehl A, Gerok W, editors. Bile acids as therapeutic agents. From basic science to clinical practice. Dordrecht: Kluwer; 1990:287–96.

17. Perdigoto R, Wiesner RH. Progression of primary biliary cirrhosis with ursodeoxycholic acid therapy. Gastroenterology. 1992;102:1389–91.

18. Van de Meeberg PC, van Erpecum KJ, van Berge-Henegouwen GP. Therapy with ursodeoxycholic acid in cholestatic liver disease. Scand J Gastroenterol. 1993;28(Suppl.200):15–20.

19. Kaplan MM. The therapeutic effects of ursodiol and methotrexate are additive and well tolerated in primary biliary cirrhosis (PBC). Hepatology. 1992;16:92A.

20. Ludwig J, Dickson ER, McDonald GSA. Staging of chronic nonsuppurative destructive cholangitis (syndrome of primary biliary cirrhosis). Virchows Arch A Pathol Anat. 1978;379:103–12.

21. Flowers MA, Heathcote J, Wanless IR et al. Fulminant hepatitis as a consequence of reactivation of hepatitis B virus infection after discontinuation of low-dose methotrexate therapy. Ann Intern Med. 1990;112:381–2.

22. Brunner G, Klinge O. Ein der chronisch-destruierenden nicht-eitrigen Cholangitis ähnliches krankheitsbild mit antinukleären Antikörpern (Immunchlangitis). Dtsch Med Wochenschr. 1987;112:1454–8.

23. Michieletti P, Wanless IR, Katz A et al. Antimitochondrial antibody negative primary biliary cirrhosis: a distinct syndrome of autoimmune cholangitis. Gut. 1994;35:260–5.

24. Parmentier GG, Janssen GA, Eggermont EA, Eyssen HJ. C27 bile acids in infants with coprostanic acidemia and occurrence of a $3\alpha,7\alpha,12\alpha$-trihydroxy-5β-C29 dicarboxylic bile acid as a major component in their serum. Eur J Biochem. 1979;102:173–83.

25. Klein R, Klöppel G, Garbe W, Fintelmann V, Berg PA. Antimitochondrial antibody profiles determined at early stages of primary biliary cirrhosis differentiate between a benign and a progressive course of the disease. A retrospective analysis of 76 patients over 6–18 years. J Hepatol. 1991;12:21–7.

26. Wiesner RH, Ludwig J, Lindor KD et al. A controlled trial of cyclosporine in the treatment of primary biliary cirrhosis. N Engl J Med. 1990;322:1419–24.

27. Dickson ER, Grambsch PM, Fleming TR, Fisher LD, Langworthy A. Prognosis in primary biliary cirrhosis: model for decision making. Hepatology. 1989;10:1–7.

28. Weber P, Scheurlen M, Wiedmann K-H. Methotrexat in der Therapie der primären biliären Zirrhose. Dtsch Med Wochenschr. 1991;116:1347–52.

29. Rosenthal GJ, Germolec DR, Lamm KR, Ackermann MF, Luster MI. Comparative effects on the immune system of methotrexate and trimetrexate. Int J Immunopharmacol. 1987;9:793–801.

30. Miller LC, Dinarello CA. Methotrexate inhibits interleukin-1 activity. Arthritis Rheum. 1986;29:S86.

31. Miller LC, Cohen SE, Orencole SF, Dinarello CA. Interleukin 1B is structurally related to dihydrofolate reductase: effect of methotrexate on IL-1. Lymphokine Res. 1988;7:272A.

32. Asako H, Wolf RE, Granger DN. Leukocyte adherence in rat mesenteric venules: effects of adenosine and methotrexate. Gastroenterology. 1993;104:31–7.

33. Kaplan MM, Knox TA. Effective treatment of pre-cirrhotic primary biliary cirrhosis (PBC) with methotrexate (MTX): remission in some. Hepatology. 1989;10:585.

34. Roll J, Boyer JL, Barry D, Klatskin G. The prognostic importance of clinical and histological features in asymptomatic and symptomatic primary biliary cirrhosis. N Engl J Med. 1983;308:1–7.

35. Christensen E, Neuberger J, Crowe J et al. Beneficial effect of azathioprine and prediction of prognosis in primary biliary cirrhosis. Final results of an international trial. Gastroenterology. 1985;89:1084–91.

36. Gilbert SC, Klintmalm G, Menter A, Silverman A. Methotrexate-induced cirrhosis requiring liver transplantation in three patients with psoriasis: a word of caution in light of the expanding use of this 'steroid-sparing' agent. Arch Intern Med. 1990;150:889–91.

37. Zachariae H, Sogaard H. Methotrexate-induced liver cirrhosis: a follow-up. Dermatologica. 1987;175:178–82.

38. Walker AM, Funch D, Dreyer NA et al. Determinants of serious liver disease among patients receiving low-dose methotrexate for rheumatoid arthritis. Arthritis Rheum. 1993;36:329–35.

39. Lanse SB, Arnold GL, Gowans JDC, Kaplan MM. Low incidence of hepatotoxicity associated with long-term, low-dose oral methotrexate in treatment of refractory psoriasis, psoriatic arthritis, and rheumatoid arthritis. An acceptable risk/benefit ratio. Dig. Dis Sci. 1985;30:104–9.
40. Lewis JH, Schiff E. Methotrexate-induced chronic liver injury: guidelines for detection and prevention. Am J Gastroenterol. 1988;88:1337–45.
41. Searles G, McKendry RJR. Methotrexate pneumonitis in rheumatoid arthritis: potential risk factors. Four case reports and a review of the literature. J Rheumatol. 1987;14: 1164–71.

28
Colchicine treatment and prognostic value of cholangiography in primary sclerosing cholangitis

R. OLSSON, U. BROOMÉ, Å. DANIELSSON, I. HÄGERSTRAND, G. JÄRNEROT, L. LÖÖF, H. PRYTZ, B.-O. RYDÉN, S. WALLERSTEDT and M. ASZTELY

PROGNOSTIC VALUE OF CHOLANGIOGRAPHY

Different prognostic clinical and biochemical factors have been identified for survival in primary sclerosing cholangitis (PSC)[1-6] and prognostic models have been produced, based on clinical, histological and biochemical features[3,6,7]. Recently, it was reported from the Mayo Clinic that findings on cholangiograms are predictive of prognosis[8]. These authors furthermore observed that intrahepatic bile duct changes are better predictors of survival without liver transplantations than is extrahepatic bile duct disease[8].

We (R.O. and M.A.) have retrospectively studied the predictive value of the bile duct changes seen on the first diagnostic cholangiogram, not only for survival without liver transplantation but also for survival without jaundice, pruritus, upper right-sided abdominal pain, fever, variceal bleeding or ascites, respectively.

Material and methods

The material comprised 94 patients with PSC, who had been followed up in our clinic. The starting point for follow-up was the date of the first cholangiogram showing features characteristic of PSC. The end-points for follow-up were:

1. date of death or liver transplantation;
2. dates of first appearance of fever, pruritus, right upper quadrant pain, serum bilirubin >2 times the upper reference value, variceal bleeding and ascites;
3. the date 1 May 1992.

Table 1 Cholangiographic prognostic predictors of death/liver transplantation (OLT), fever, abdominal pain, jaundice, pruritus, ascites and variceal bleeding in patients with primary sclerosing cholangitis

Bilirubin >2 times ref. value	Grade I
Death/OLT	Grade I
Fever	Grade E, dilatation LD
Abdominal pain	Grade E, dilatation CBD
Pruritus	Grade E
Ascites	None
Variceal bleeding	Length, dilatation SEC

Abbreviations: I = intrahepatic, E = extrahepatic, CBD = common bile duct, LD = left main hepatic duct, SEC = secondary intrahepatic ducts

The cholangiograms were scored by M.A., without knowledge of the clinical findings and outcome, as described by Craig *et al.*[8], i.e. for intra- and extrahepatic grade of strictures (1–4), length of strictures (band, segmental, confluent), extent of strictures (localized, diffuse) and for degree of dilatation (none, mild, marked) of common duct, left and right main ducts and secondary intrahepatic ducts.

The correlation between a set of variables and the different end-points was tested by a survival test closely related to Mantel's test[9,10]. The end-point hazard functions were estimated as functions of the predictors by Poisson models[11].

Results

The mean follow-up time was 5 years (2 months–15 years). The 5-year survival rate was 72%. Taking into consideration that some of the variables in the radiological scoring are correlated to each other, we obtained the prognostic predictors of a poor outcome given in Table 1. The fact that death/liver transplantation as well as the appearance of a high serum bilirubin were predicted by the same bile duct changes, namely the grade of *intra*hepatic bile duct changes, is of interest in view of the fact that, in the different prognostic models that have been published[3,6,7], jaundice is the only symptom that has been associated with a poor prognosis in multivariate analysis.

The other PSC-associated symptoms (*viz.* fever, right upper quadrant pain and pruritus) were all related to the grade of *extra*hepatic duct obstruction.

We also estimated the end-point hazard functions as functions of the predictors by Poisson models, and on the basis of the hazard functions the probabilities of escaping an end-point during a period of 24 and 60 months were calculated. This is exemplified in Fig. 1, which illustrates the probability of survival without liver transplantation, and without jaundice, respectively, in relation to the grade of intrahepatic strictures.

EFFECT OF COLCHICINE

The main histological features in PSC are bile duct inflammation and fibrosis. Since colchicine is, among other things, also considered to have antifibrotic

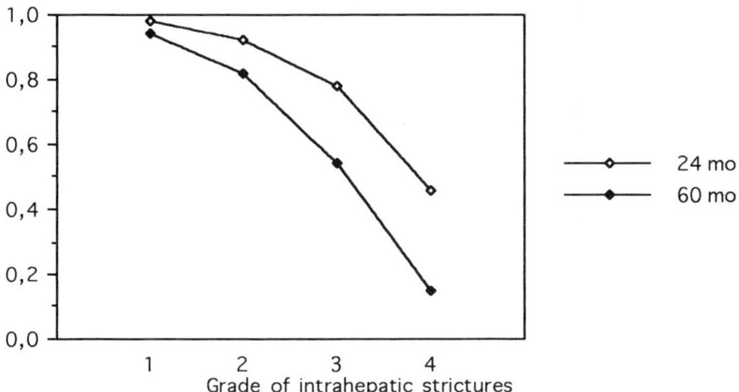

Fig. 1 Probability of survival for 24 and 60 months, respectively, without liver transplantation and without jaundice in relation to grade of intrahepatic bile duct obstruction in the first diagnostic cholangiogram

properties[12-15], we decided to perform a controlled study of this drug in PSC. At the time this study was planned, colchicine was reported to have promising effects on survival in primary biliary cirrhosis[16] and in other types of cirrhosis[17]. Furthermore, there was one case report that suggested a beneficial effect of colchicine in PSC[18].

Material and methods

In a multicentre study, performed by members of the Swedish Internal Medicine Liver Club, 84 patients (56 males, 28 women; 63 with concomitant inflammatory bowel disease, IBD) were randomized to 1 mg colchicine daily (44 patients), or placebo for 3 years. The assessment comprised:

1. Serum biochemistry every 6 months.
2. Histopathology of liver biopsies at the start and end of the study. A histopathologist (I.H.) blindly graded 10 different variables in the biopsies.
3. Patient's daily self-recording of PSC-associated symptoms (pain, fever, pruritus). The patients were asked to score the symptoms on a scale from 0 to 3.

The patients were well matched regarding sex, age, prevalence of IBD, serum biochemistry and histopathology. The only significant differences between the groups were higher scores for portal lymphocyte infiltration and bile duct destruction in the placebo group.

Results

Thirty-three patients in each group completed the study (Table 2). There were no differences in survival without liver transplantation between the groups (Fig. 2).

Table 2 Number of patients in the 3-year study of colchicine in PSC

	Colchicine	*Placebo*
Randomization	44	40
Drop-outs	8	2
Deaths	1	2
OLT	2	3
Completing the study	33	33

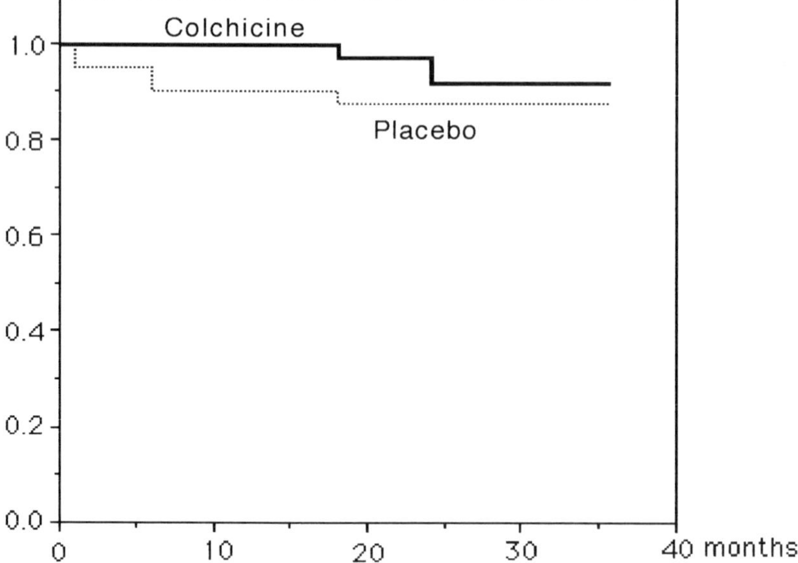

Fig. 2 Kaplan–Meier survival curves for colchicine- and placebo-treated patients

As to symptoms, patients on colchicine had more pain (Fig. 3). This difference is most likely fortuitous and due to randomization, by chance, of more patients with pain to the colchicine group. This assumption is supported by the results of a comparison of the summarizing judgements by the patients of the change in their condition during each 6-month period compared to before the study, since 16% of the colchicine patients and 13% of the placebo patients (p = n.s.) considered their condition to be worse or much worse than before the study.

There were remarkably small changes in the different biochemical variables, the only statistically significant differences between the groups being increased values of IgA at 6 and 36 months, IgM at 36 months, and α_1-antitrypsin at 36 months, compared to the changes in the control group (Fig. 4). There were no significant differences in the degree or frequency of histopathological changes between the groups at the end of the study, or between first and final biopsies (Fig. 5).

To summarize:

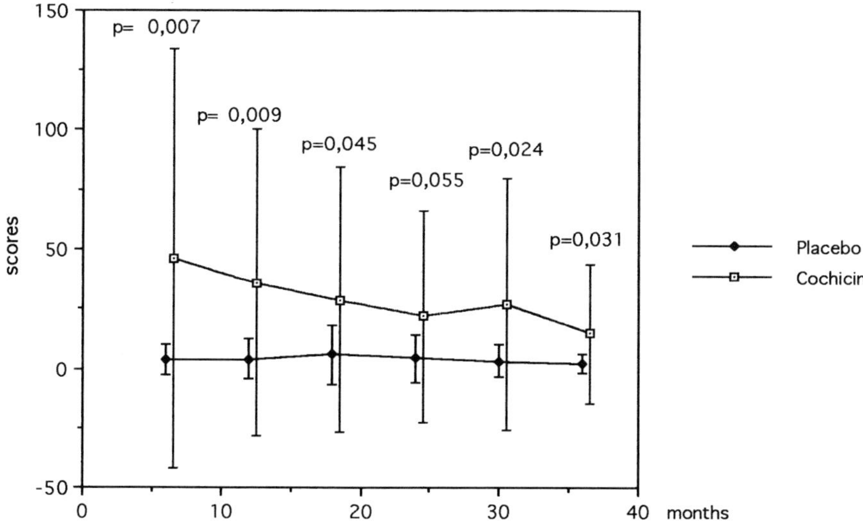

Fig. 3   Self-recorded scores for pain per 6-month period for patients on colchicine and placebo. Means with SD

1. severe *intra*hepatic bile duct obstruction at diagnosis predicts short survival without liver transplantation, and early jaundice;
2. severe *extra*hepatic bile duct obstruction predicts early pain, jaundice and fever;
3. colchicine, 1 mg daily for 3 years, does not influence the course of PSC.

References

1. Helzberg JH, Petersen JM, Boyer JL. Improved survival with primary sclerosing cholangitis. Gastroenterology. 1987;92:1869–75.
2. Lebovics E, Palmer M, Woo J, Schaffner F. Outcome of primary sclerosing cholangitis. Arch Intern Med. 1987;147:729–31.
3. Wiesner RH, Grambsch PM, Dickson ER *et al.* Primary sclerosing cholangitis: natural history, prognostic factors and survival analysis. Hepatology. 1989;10:430–6.
4. Porayko MK, Wiesner RH, LaRusso NF *et al.* Patients with asymptomatic primary sclerosing cholangitis frequently have progressive disease. Gastroenterology. 1990;98: 1594–602.
5. Ismail T, Angrisani L, Powell JE *et al.* Primary sclerosing cholangitis: surgical options, prognostic variables and outcome. Br J Surg. 1991;78:564–7.
6. Farrant JM, Hyallar KM, Wilkinson ML *et al.* Natural history and prognostic variables in primary sclerosing cholangitis. Gastroenterology. 1991;100:1710–17.
7. Dickson ER, Murtaugh PA, Wiesner RH *et al.* Primary sclerosing cholangitis: refinement and validation of survival models. Gastroenterology. 1992;103:1891–901.
8. Craig DA, MacCarty RL, Wiesner RH, Grambsch PM, LaRusso NF. Primary sclerosing cholangitis: value of cholangiography in determining the prognosis. Am J Roentgenol. 1991;957:959–64.
9. Merck C, Angervall L, Kindblom LS. Myxofibrosarcoma. A malignant soft tissue tumor of fibroblastic-histiocytic origin. Acta Pathol Microbiol Immunol Scand. Section A, 1983 (Suppl. 282), Vol. 81.

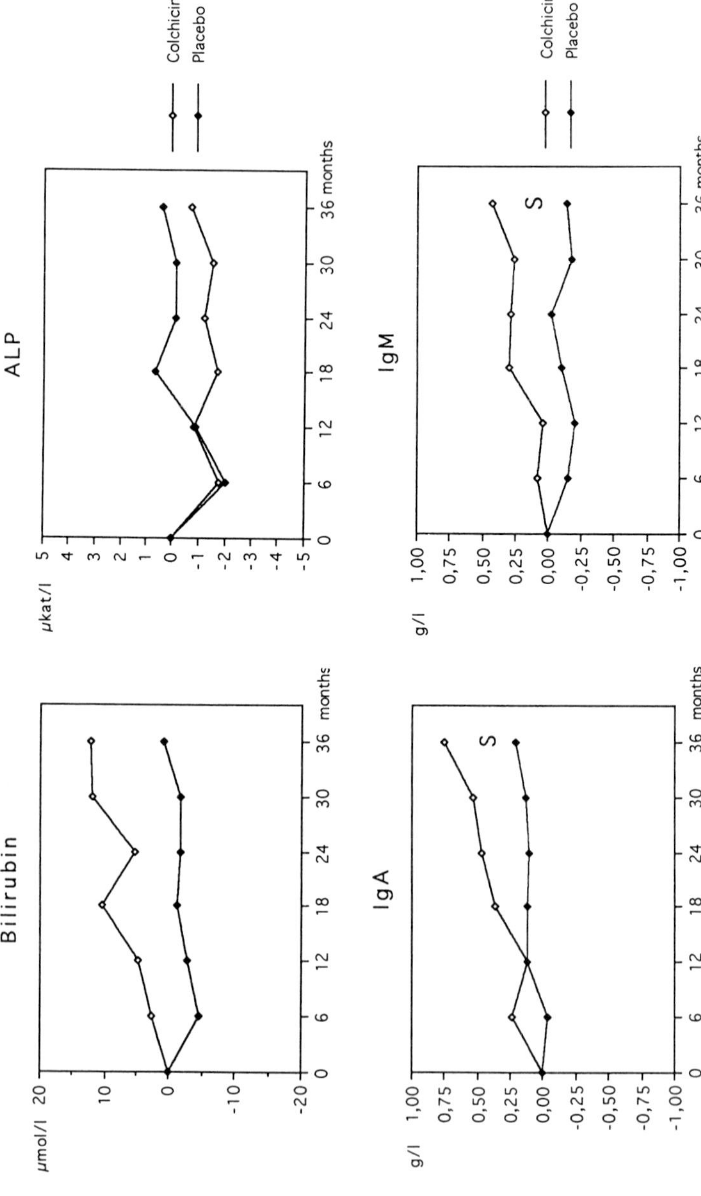

Fig. 4 Results of serum bilirubin, alkaline phosphatase (ALP), immunoglobulin A (IgA) and immunoglobulin M (IgM) determinations in the 33 colchicine- and 33 placebo-treated patients who completed the study. Means of differences from the start values. **S** = statistically significant

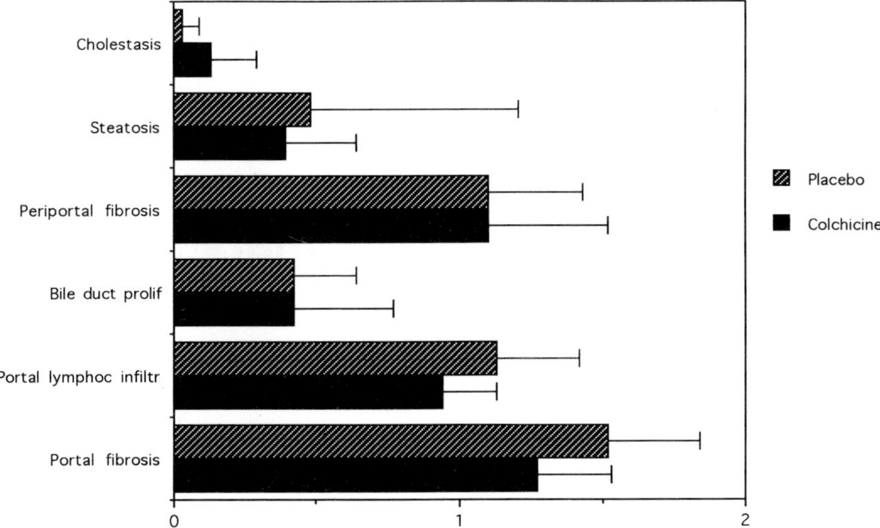

Fig. 5 Means (with 95% confidence intervals) of scores for six histological variables at the end of the study in the 31 colchicine- and 31 placebo-treated patients who completed the study and had liver biopsies of acceptable quality both at the start and end of the study

10. Mantel N. Chi-square test with one degree of freedom; extensions of the Mantel–Haenszel procedure. J Am Statist Assoc. 1963;58:690–700.
11. Breslow NE, Day NE. Statistical methods in cancer research, vol. II. Lyon: IARC Scientific Publications, 1987; No. 32:131–5.
12. Harris Ed Jr, Krane SM. Effects of colchicine on collagenase in cultures of rheumatoid synovium. Arthritis Rheum. 1971;14:669–84.
13. Diegelmann RF, Peterkofsky B. Inhibition of collagen secretion from bone and cultured fibroblasts by microtubular disruptive drugs. Proc Natl Acad Sci USA. 1972;69:892–6.
14. Ehrlich HP, Bornstein P. Microtubules in transcellular movement of procollagen. Nature (New Biol). 1972;238:257–60.
15. Rojkind M, Kersenobich D. Effect of colchicine on collagen, albumin and transferrin synthesis by cirrhotic rat liver slices. Biochim Biophys Acta. 1975;378:415–23.
16. Kaplan MM, Alling DW, Zimmerman HJ et al. A prospective trial of colchicine for primary biliary cirrhosis. N Engl J Med. 1986;315:1448–54.
17. Kersenobich D, Vargas F, Garcia Tsao G, Tamayo RP, Gent M, Rojkind M. Colchicine in the treatment of cirrhosis of the liver. N Engl J Med. 1988;318:1709–13.
18. Lieser A, Kadish U. Case report. Beneficial effect of colchicine in a case of sclerosing cholangitis. Am J Med Sci. 1986;291:416–18.

29
Medical treatment of primary sclerosing cholangitis

R. W. CHAPMAN

There is a wide range of medical, radiological, endoscopic and surgical therapies for primary sclerosing cholangitis (PSC). Assessment of efficacy of the treatment, however, has proved to be particularly difficult in PSC as the disease is relatively uncommon, and the natural history of the disease is fluctuant, variable and difficult to predict.

MEDICAL THERAPY

In primary biliary cirrhosis (PBC) and PSC the primary site of inflammation and damage is the biliary epithelium. In contrast to hepatocytes, which are the primary focus of injury in various parenchymal liver diseases, the bile ducts do not have the capacity to regenerate when severely damaged or destroyed. The number of bile ducts within the liver is finite and the natural history of PSC, like PBC, is that of a progressive loss of functioning intrahepatic bile ducts (ductopenia). The ductopenia leads to a progressive and ultimately irreversible failure of hepatic biliary excretion. In PSC, in contrast to PBC, the number of prospective randomized controlled trials has been very few, although a wide variety of agents including anti-inflammatory, anti-fibrogenic, cupruretic and immunosuppressive have been studied.

D-PENICILLAMINE

As in all cases of prolonged cholestasis, increased hepatic copper levels are found in PSC. This provided the rationale for the controlled trial of D-penicillamine performed by the Mayo Clinic[1]. Seventy patients were randomized to either D-penicillamine or placebo therapy for 36 months. Although the authors demonstrated an effective cupruresis with a concomitant reduction in hepatic copper concentrations, there appeared to be no benefit with regard to disease progression or survival. Moreover, there was a high incidence of toxicity due to side-effects from penicillamine which included pancytopenia and proteinuria[1].

CORTICOSTEROIDS

Although both systemic and topical corticosteroid therapy has been evaluated in PSC, most studies have been uncontrolled and only contain a small number of patients. In an uncontrolled pilot study in ten patients with PSC who had high elevations in aminotransferases, a beneficial response to oral prednisolone therapy was found with the majority of patients showing biochemical improvement[2].

However, these hopeful results were not confirmed in a study by Lindor *et al.*[3]. In this report, twelve patients were treated with a combination of low dose prednisone (10 mg daily) and colchicine (0.6 mg twice daily). The treated patients' clinical course was compared with a group of control patients, but the study was not randomized. After two years of therapy there were no significant differences in biochemistry, and the liver histology showed no significant differences between the two groups. There appeared to be no important benefit in disease progression or patient survival in the treatment group in this relatively small study[3]. Moreover, there was a strong suggestion that corticosteroid therapy in these patients was associated with an enhanced bone loss, leading to increased risk of developing compression fracture of the spine, which occurred even in young male patients. It remains surprising that there has been no long-term study of the effect of corticosteroid therapy on histological progression and survival in PSC. The development of new agents which may prevent bone loss in this group of patients may enable further larger controlled trials to be carried out. It should be stated, however, that large numbers of these patients have received short courses of corticosteroids for treatment of ulcerative colitis with no apparent beneficial effect on the course of their liver disease.

There has been a number of small studies regarding the use of topical corticosteroid therapy. The corticosteroids are normally administered through a nasobiliary drain left in situ following ERCP. Three small anecdotal studies have reported benefit[4-6]. However, a small controlled trial of nasobiliary lavage with corticosteroids from the Royal Free Hospital showed no benefit when compared with a placebo group[7]. Indeed, the treatment appeared to induce a higher incidence of bacterial cholangitis and in all patients their bile became rapidly colonized with enteric bacteria[7].

In conclusion, there is no direct evidence to suggest that either oral or topical corticosteroids are beneficial in PSC. Further studies of corticosteroids are indicated in patients with early disease.

METHOTREXATE

Following an apparent beneficial effect of oral pulse methotrexate in an open study, Knox and Kaplan have recently reported the findings of a double blind, randomized control trial, comparing oral pulse methotrexate 15 mg per week with a well-matched placebo group in PSC[8]. Twelve patients were entered into each treatment arm. It is noteworthy, however, that seven of the twelve patients in the treatment group and five of the twelve in the placebo group had cirrhosis representing an endstage group of patients. After two years of therapy the only significant biochemical improvement was observed in the serum alkaline phosphatase in the patients who received methotrexate. There was no significant improvement in the serum bilirubin, transaminases and albumin and liver histology did not improve. There were no significant differences in outcome of the two groups with regard to treatment failure or death[8]. Surprisingly, side-effects attributed to methotrexate were few and consisted of a transient decrease in white cell count following a bout of bacterial cholangitis. However, in the light of recent reports of severe lung damage occurring in patients with primary biliary cirrhosis receiving pulse methotrexate, and with the negative results of this controlled clinical trial, it is difficult to justify a larger controlled trial at the present time.

OTHER IMMUNOSUPPRESSIVE AGENTS

There has been a case report of two patients improving clinically on azathioprine[9] and one patient who experienced clinical deterioration[10]. No controlled trials of azathioprine in PSC have been reported. A randomized controlled trial has been performed by the Mayo Clinic evaluating the use of cyclosporin in the treatment of PSC[11]. Whilst cyclosporin appeared to have a role in reducing the symptoms of ulcerative colitis there appeared to be no benefit in the course or prognosis of PSC and the prevalence of side-effects was high[11]. Although the results of the immunosuppressant agents described above are disappointing, there have been few randomized controlled studies in patients with early disease containing adequate numbers of patients. There would appear to be little point in giving immunosuppressive therapy to patients with advanced liver disease, who have suffered irreversible bile duct loss and in whom the damaging process of chronic cholestasis is well established.

ANTI-FIBROGENIC AGENTS

A recent controlled trial from Sweden compared colchicine in a dose of 1 mg daily by mouth in 44 patients with PSC compared with 40 patients treated with placebo in a randomized control trial, who were then followed for three years[12]. Thirty-three patients in each group completed the trial. At three-year follow-up there were no differences in clinical symptoms, serum biochemistry, liver histology or survival in the two groups. Three patients died in the treated group and five in the placebo group[12].

URSODEOXYCHOLIC ACID (UDCA)

The hydrophilic bile acid has become widely used in the treatment of cholestatic liver disease of all causes. Ursodeoxycholic acid (UDCA) appears to exert three main effects which may all be beneficial in chronic cholestasis, viz. a choleretic effect by increasing bile flow; reducing the toxic intracellular effects of increased hydrophobic bile acids; and, thirdly, by producing an immunomodulatory effect. Ursodeoxycholic acid has been demonstrated to decrease class I expression on hepatocytes following long-term treatment in PBC patients[13] and, in addition, in PSC, UDCA has been shown to decrease HLA-DR expression on bile ducts[14]. In an open study by O'Brien et al., UDCA was evaluated in 12 patients with PSC on an open basis over 30 months[15]. The authors noted an improvement in fatigue, pruritus and diarrhoea and they also noted a significant improvement in hepatic enzymes, particularly alkaline phosphatase, during the UDCA treatment period[15].

A prospective randomized double-blind placebo-controlled trial of UDCA in PSC was performed by Beuers et al.[16] who compared six patients who received ursodeoxycholic acid 13–15 mg per kg body weight and eight patients who received placebo. Treatment was for one year and after six months significant improvements in alkaline phosphatase and aminotransferases were demonstrated. After 12 months a significant decrease in bilirubin was also noted. A reduction in liver inflammation was found in the UDCA group. However, amelioration[16] of symptoms was not significantly different from placebo.

Similar results were reported from Stiehl et al. who randomized 20 patients who received either UDCA 750 mg per day or placebo[17]. Although three studies have shown a decrease in liver inflammation after treatment with UDCA, there is no evidence that fibrosis or progression to cirrhosis is altered.

There is no evidence from these small studies that UDCA retards the progression of the disease, or prevents major complications, death or the need for liver transplantation. UDCA has proven to be a very safe drug; the only significant side-effect may be a dose-dependent diarrhoea which has been reported in two of 18 PSC patients in the study by Stiehl et al.[17]. A large randomized controlled trial is currently taking place at the Mayo Clinic over a six-year follow-up period and this study will provide useful information. Further studies are in progress testing larger doses of UDCA in PSC, namely 20 mg per kg. The results are not yet available.

CONCLUSION

There is no proven effective medical therapy for primary sclerosing cholangitis. Ursodeoxycholic acid appears the most promising agent, but further long-term studies are required to prove its efficacy. Randomized controlled trials of immunosuppressive agents in early PSC are needed and possibly new anti-fibrogenics may offer some hopeful therapy for patients with more advanced disease in the future. Liver transplantation remains the only therapeutic option for patients with advanced end-stage PSC.

References

1. LaRusso NF, Wiesner RH, Ludwig L, MacCarty RL, Beaver SJ, Zinsmeister AR. Prospective trial of penicillamine in primary sclerosing cholangitis. Gastroenterology. 1988;95:1036–42.
2. Burgert SL, Brown BP, Kirkpatrick RB, LaBrecque DR. Positive corticosteroid response in early primary sclerosing cholangitis (Abstract). Gastroenterology. 1984;86:1037.
3. Lindor KD, Wiesner RH, Colwell LJ, Steiner BL, Beaver S, LaRusso NF. The combination of prednisone and colchicine in patients with primary sclerosing cholangitis. Am J Gastroenterol. 1991;85:57–61.
4. Grijm R, Huibrejtse K, Bartelsman J, Mathus-Vliegan EMH, Dekker W, Tytgat GN. Therapeutic investigations in primary sclerosing cholangitis. Dig Dis Sci. 1986;31:792–8.
5. Jeffrey GP, Reed WD, Laurence BH, Shilkin KB. Primary sclerosing cholangitis: clinical and immunopathological review of 21 cases. J Gastroenterol Hepatol. 1990;5:135–40.
6. Craig PI, Williams SJ, Hatfield ARW, Ng M, Cotton PB. Endoscopic management of primary sclerosing cholangitis (Abstract). Gut. 1990;31:1182a.
7. Allison MC, Burroughs AK, Noone P, Summerfield JA. Biliary lavage with corticosteroids in primary sclerosing cholangitis: a clinical, cholangiographic, and bacteriologic study. J Hepatol. 1986;3:118–22.
8. Knox TA, Kaplan MM. Double-blind trial of methotrexate in the treatment of primary sclerosing cholangitis (Abstract). Gastroenterology. 1991;100:61a.
9. Javett SL. Azathioprine in primary sclerosing cholangitis. Lancet. 1971;1:810–11.
10. Wagner A. Azathioprine treatment in primary sclerosing cholangitis. Lancet. 1971;2:663–4.
11. Wiesner RH. Advances in therapy for primary sclerosing cholangitis. Eur J Gastroenterol Hepatol. 1992;4:276–82.
12. Olsson R, Broome U. A multicentre controlled trial of colchicine for the treatment of primary sclerosing cholangitis. Gastroenterology. 1994 [in press].
13. Poupon RE, Balkau B, Eschwege E, Poupon R, the UDCA-PBC study group. A multicenter, controlled trial of ursodiol for the treatment of primary biliary cirrhosis. N Engl J Med. 1991;324:1548–54.
14. Lo SK, Fleming K, Chapman RW. Ursodeoxycholic acid reduces aberrant bile duct HLA-DR expression in primary sclerosing cholangitis (abstract). Hepatol. 1992.
15. O'Brien CB, Senior JR, Arora-Mirchandani R, Batta A, Salen G. Ursodeoxycholic acid for the treatment of primary sclerosing cholangitis: a 30-month pilot study. Hepatology. 1991;14:838–47.
16. Beuers U, Spengler U, Kruis W *et al.* Ursodeoxycholic acid for treatment of primary sclerosing cholangitis: a placebo-controlled trial. Hepatology. 1992;16:707–14.
17. Stiehl A, Walker S, Stiehl L, Rudolph G, Hofman WJ, Theilmann L. Effect of ursodeoxycholic acid on liver and bile duct disease in primary sclerosing cholangitis. A 3 year pilot study with a placebo controlled study period. J Hepatol. 1994;20:57–64.

30
Treatment of primary sclerosing cholangitis with ursodeoxycholic acid

A. STIEHL

INTRODUCTION

Primary sclerosing cholangitis (PSC) is a cholestatic disease of unknown origin characterized by progressive obstruction of intra- and/or extrahepatic bile ducts. Fibrosing inflammation around the bile ducts leads to multiple strictures and stenoses. In general the disease leads to cirrhosis of the liver. In approximately 80–90% of patients the disease is associated with ulcerative colitis, and approximately 10–15% of patients with ulcerative colitis in addition have PSC. Up to now effective therapy was lacking. Previously, prednisolone, azathioprine, methotrexate and D-penicillamine have been evaluated as therapy in PSC. All these substances have been associated with severe toxicity. None of these treatment regimens has been associated with sustained clinical, biochemical or histological remission. Since PSC is characterized by multiple episodes of bacterial inflammation, immunosuppressive treatment may even be harmful.

In 1987 we started a study on the efficacy and tolerance of ursodeoxycholic acid (UDCA) in PSC[1,2]. In a 1-year UDCA treatment period which preceded the controlled study, UDCA treatment led to rapid improvement of liver enzymes, and was well tolerated in almost all our patients. In the meantime several uncontrolled[3–5] and another controlled study[6] on the effects of UDCA in PSC have been published.

UDCA IN PATIENTS WITH INFLAMMATORY BOWEL DISEASE

Since the majority of patients with PSC have additional ulcerative colitis the tolerability of UDCA in such patients was evaluated. The clinical colitis activity index in the treatment group was not different from the control group, indicating that UDCA is well tolerated in patients with PSC who also have ulcerative colitis[7]. Up to now only 2/53 patients did not tolerate a UDCA dose of 750 mg/day and responded with diarrhoea, which stopped

Table 1 Ursodeoxycholic acid in primary sclerosing cholangitis: results of placebo controlled studies

Author	Reference	n	AP, γ-GT, ALT, AST	Bilirubin	Histology
Stiehl	2, 7	20	improved	unchanged	favourable*
Beuers	6	14	improved	improved	favourable

*Favourable effect in comparison to pretreatment histology

on reduction of the dose to 500 or 250 mg UDCA/day. No other side-effects were noted.

EFFECT OF UDCA ON BIOCHEMICAL PARAMETERS

UDCA treatment leads to significant amelioration of AP, γ-GT, ALT and AST (Table 1). Serum bilirubin decreased in one controlled study[6] significantly, and was unchanged in the other one[7]. Serum cholesterol decreased in patients with elevated levels before treatment[7] and was unchanged in the others. No significant changes of IgA, IgM, and IgG were noted.

EFFECT OF UDCA ON FATIGUE AND PRURITUS

During treatment with UDCA, fatigue improved in almost half of the patients but, in comparison to placebo, the difference was not significant[7]. Similar results were obtained with respect to pruritus which decreased in almost half of the patients but, in comparison to placebo, the difference was not significant.

EFFECT OF UDCA ON LIVER HISTOLOGY

In PSC, inflammation around the bile ducts and ductular degeneration and proliferation are focally distributed over the liver and, therefore, single-liver biopsies are of only limited value in the evaluation of improvement and worsening induced by UDCA or placebo. In a controlled study, five biopsies on UDCA were compared to six on placebo. In comparison to placebo, the histological score was significantly better in the patients on UDCA[6]. The difference in the histological score was based mainly on the decrease of the cellular infiltrates in the portal fields[6]. In our own study, 14 liver biopsies of 10 patients after 1 and 2 years of UDCA treatment were compared to pretreatment histology[7]. Since, according to the ethical guidelines, the two-fold increase in serum transaminases during placebo treatment led to the discontinuation of the study 3 months after the beginning of placebo treatment, biopsies on placebo are not available. In comparison to the pretreatment histology, cellular infiltrates in the portal triads decreased significantly, whereas all other changes were not significant[7]. The changes

Table 2 Outcome in the treatment and dropout group

	Study group (n = 43)	Dropout group (n = 10)
Average treatment time (years)	3.1	3.2
Stage (Nu)		
1	10	1
2	16	
3	9	2
4	8	2
OLT (Nu, %)	0 (0%)	3 (30%)*
Deaths (Nu, %)	2[a] (4.6%)	1[b] (10%)

*$p < 0.01$
[a]Both deaths due to bile duct carcinoma
[b]Due to myocardial infarction

in liver histology observed during treatment of patients with PSC with UDCA are very similar to those reported in PBC.

MAJOR DUCT STENOSIS AND ENDOSCOPIC DILATATION

Cholangiographic alterations

We used cholangiography for evaluation of treatment success. So far, our study is the only one in which endoscopic cholangiography (ERC) was performed at yearly intervals to evaluate treatment success[7]. During treatment of 20 patients with UDCA, within 3 years progression of bile duct disease was noted in one patient[7]. In all other patients no changes were noted. Endoscopic dilatation led to a marked improvement of the stenosis and the laboratory parameters. In the meantime, of 43 patients treated since 1987 in our institution, seven patients developed stenosis of major bile ducts while being treated with UDCA. In 10 further patients dilatation of a stenosis of a major bile duct had to be performed at entry into the study. In all of these patients endoscopic dilatation was successful.

LIVER TRANSPLANTATION AND SURVIVAL

An interim analysis of our ongoing study indicates that of 43 patients treated with UDCA since 1987 in our institution, two patients died due to cholangiocarcinoma and none had to undergo liver transplantation[8]. The survival rate appears much better than the natural course of the disease. Of 10 patients who initially were included in our UDCA treatment group, and dropped out from the study for various reasons, three had to undergo liver transplantation, which is significantly more than that in our treatment group (Table 2).

CONCLUSION

UDCA treatment of PSC reduces the inflammatory process in the liver, but seems not to prevent development of major duct stenosis. Such patients need endoscopic management with repeated dilatations of the stenosis as soon as they reappear.

At present, treatment of PSC with UDCA, and in addition by endoscopic dilatations of major bile ducts whenever necessary, seems promising. Some of our patients have been treated with UDCA since 1987 with an average treatment time of approximately 3.5 years. In a study comparing outcome in patients treated with UDCA with that of patients dropping out from the study, fewer liver transplantations were performed in the treatment group. Furthermore, survival without liver transplantation was approximately two-fold better than the survival predicted from survival models. On the basis of available data it appears that, with the treatment regime used, the time until liver transplantation becomes necessary can be prolonged.

References

1. Stiehl A, Raedsch R, Kommerell B. The effect of ursodeoxycholate in primary sclerosing cholangitis. A comparison to primary biliary cirrhosis. Gastroenterology. 1988;94:595(abstr.).
2. Stiehl A, Raedsch R, Rudolph G, Theilmann L. Treatment of primary sclerosing cholangitis with ursodeoxycholic acid: first results of a controlled study. Hepatology. 1989;10:602(abstr.).
3. Hayashi H, Hihucchi T, Ichimiya H et al. Symptomatic primary sclerosing cholangitis treated with ursodeoxycholic acid. Gastroenterology. 1990;99:533–5.
4. Chazouilleres O, Poupon R, Capron J-P et al. Ursodeoxycholic acid for primary sclerosing cholangitis. J Hepatol. 1990;11:120–3.
5. O'Brien CB, Senior JR, Arora-Mirchandi R, Batta A, Salen G. Ursodeoxycholic acid for the treatment of primary sclerosing cholangitis: a 30 months pilot study. Hepatology. 1991;14:838–47.
6. Beuers U, Spengler U, Kruis W et al. Ursodeoxycholic acid for treatment of primary sclerosing cholangitis: a placebo controlled trial. Hepatology. 1992;16:707–14.
7. Stiehl A, Walker S, Stiehl L et al. Effects of ursodeoxycholic acid on liver and bile duct disease in primary sclerosing cholangitis. A 3 year pilot study with a placebo-controlled study period. J Hepatol. 1994;20:57–64.
8. Stiehl A, Walker S, Rudolph G, Sauer P, Theilmann L. Survival in patients with PSC treated with ursodeoxycholic acid and by endoscopic dilatations of common duct stenosis: a controlled study. Hepatology. 1993;18:219A(abstr.).

31
Liver transplantation for cholestatic liver diseases

J. B. OTTE and J. LERUT

INTRODUCTION

Patients afflicted with cholestatic diseases are a significant proportion of the potential candidates to liver transplantation. These diseases include biliary atresia, ductular paucity (Alagille syndrome), familial cholestasis (Byler's disease) and sclerosing cholangitis in children. In adults, cholestatic diseases which may lead to transplantation include primary biliary cirrhosis, primary sclerosing cholangitis, secondary biliary cirrhosis, biliary atresia (late sequelae) and graft-versus-host disease.

CHILDREN

Childhood ends with puberty; teenagers aged >15 years should be listed with adults and not with children, as often adopted by several groups, to avoid bias in interpreting age-specific management and survival rates. Due to the epidemiology of paediatric liver diseases, most children are diseased and doomed to death in early childhood. Many reports in the field of paediatric liver transplantation fall short of relevance because age distribution is not given, and teenagers sometimes up to 21 years old are included.

Biliary atresia

Biliary atresia is the most frequent cause of chronic cholestasis in infants, affecting 1:8000 to 1:12000 live births[1,2]. It is a panbiliary disease affecting both the intra- and extrahepatic biliary tree, which is probably the end-result of a destructive inflammatory process leading to fibrosis and obliteration of the biliary tract[3] with development of secondary biliary cirrhosis. The condition most likely has an acquired aetiology. Although biliary atresia is usually an isolated lesion, associated congenital malformations which are part of the 'polysplenia syndrome' occur in approximately 10% of the affected children[4-7]; this observation led some authors[4] to question the theory of the acquired pathogenesis of biliary atresia. When left untreated, the condition leads to death from liver insufficiency in early childhood, with an average survival of 12–19 months and less than 10% surviving beyond 3 years[5-7].

The majority of patients have a complete atresia up to the porta hepatis; in the minority, atresia can be limited either to the hepatic duct with a patent gallbladder and common duct or to the distal common duct (the latter type constituted in the past the correctable type, with the first successful correction reported by Ladd[8] in 1929).

In the very young infant, histology of the residual tissue of the porta hepatis discloses ductular remnants which have been shown to communicate with intrahepatic bile ducts[9]. Later, these minute luminal structures disappear, to be replaced by fibrous tissue; total obliteration is usually completed by the age of 3–4 months[10]. Most Western authors consider that the intrahepatic bile ducts are involved primarily by the disease process[11,12].

The modern therapeutic approach to biliary atresia relies on a sequential strategy with portoenterostomy as a first step and, in case of failure, liver transplantation[13].

Portoenterostomy

Portoenterostomy was devised by Kasai for the uncorrectable type of biliary atresia[14] and it has become the standard operative procedure worldwide. Its principle consists of excising the fibrous remnant of the extrahepatic bile ducts up to the porta hepatis. A Roux-en-Y loop is anastomosed around the transected end of the fibrous cone in the hilum of the liver. The remaining luminal structures drain bile into the bowel loop, acting as internal biliary fistulae. Operative mortality is less than 5% in experienced centres.

There is a wide spectrum of results regarding jaundice disappearance rate. In reports from Western centres it varies from 25% to 65%[15-20] to reach 81% in a recent series (1987–91) from Kasai's group at the Tohoku University Hospital[2]. The short-term results regarding disappearance of jaundice depend on age at surgery, with the best results being obtained in patients operated before 45 days (Gauthier F *et al.*, unpublished observations, May 1993) or even before 30 days[7].

Other prognostic factors that are partly related to age are a favourable portal hilar histology (size of biliary remnants) and the degree of liver fibrosis at the initial operation; the surgeon's experience is also of paramount importance. Infants with biliary atresia should be treated by paediatric surgeons who specialize in hepatobiliary surgery.

The main complication of portoenterostomy is cholangitis, with a reported incidence ranging from 40% to 60%[2]; its occurrence can result in cessation of bile flow early in the postoperative period, while repeated attacks can cause a progressive deterioration of hepatic function leading to biliary cirrhosis and late failure[20]. In order to prevent cholangitis, several modifications to the original Kasai portoenterostomy have been devised. Those consisting of complicated Roux loop techniques or venting procedures with a skin stoma have been proved inefficient[2]; moreover their presence is a source of technical complications during subsequent liver transplantation[21,22]. These techniques should therefore be abandoned, with the exception of hepatic portocholecystostomy (gallbladder Kasai) and antireflux valve, which are associated with the lowest incidence of cholangitis[2,7].

Portal hypertension is an early complication of biliary atresia. Bleeding from oesophageal varices is common in children with a failed Kasai operation. It is also a significant hazard for non-jaundiced patients. In patients who have bled from oesophageal varices, endoscopic sclerotherapy is at present the treatment of choice[23]; the transjugular intrahepatic portosystemic shunt (TIPSS) is still in development in children (the youngest child successfully treated with this modality in our institution was 5 years old). It is better to avoid shunt surgery, which could interfere with subsequent liver transplantation.

In most Western series the long-term survival rate after portoenterostomy is between 47% and 60% at 5 years[7,20,24], and around 30% at 10 years[7,25]. An exceptional 10-year survival rate of 65% has been reported in 181 infants operated on after 1971 in Sendai[2]; the rate of survival was 82% in patients with successful operation and 10% in patients with failed hepatic portoenterostomy. Seven patients older than 20 years and still in good health (the oldest being 34 years) were followed by Kasai et al. in 1989[26]. However, the 10-year survival rate in a collective review of 2013 patients operated in 49 institutions in Japan before 1978 was only 15.9%[27].

The contribution of portoenterostomy to the treatment of biliary atresia can be summarized as follows. As an optimistic estimate no more than 20–30% of patients will live jaundice-free, reach adult life and hopefully will be cured of their disease, even though their liver histology often remains abnormal. Another one-third will be palliated and have extended survival; these patients will become candidates for liver transplantation in later childhood (2–15 years) because of persistent or relapsing cholestasis, intractable pruritus, repeated cholangitis, failure to thrive, hepatopulmonary syndrome, bleeding and finally liver insufficiency. The remaining 30–40% will not benefit from Kasai operation, and will die of liver failure in infancy if they are not transplanted.

Liver transplantation

Taking into account the incidence and natural history of biliary atresia, and the limited therapeutic benefit of the portoenterostomy, the annual need for liver transplantation has been estimated to be about one case per million people both in France[12] and in the USA[28]. Biliary atresia is the main indication for liver transplantation in children in the largest series of the world literature: 53.5% of the 334 children included in the first 1000 liver recipients treated in Pittsburgh under cyclosporin–steroid therapy and reported by S. Iwatsuki et al. in 1988[29], 53.8% of the 438 paediatric patients reported by T. E. Starzl and A. J. Demetris in 1990[30], 51% of the first 100 paediatric recipients of the Cambridge and King's College Hospital series[31], 48% of the first 200 children transplanted between 1986 and 1991 in Bicêtre and Cochin Hospitals in Paris[32] and 66% of our own series of 322 children

(1984–93). Biliary atresia represents a sizeable proportion of the total population of patients needing a liver transplant: 16.4% of 1469 adult and paediatric patients referred to Pittsburgh[30] and 6.9% of the 8622 patients reported to the European Liver Transplant Registry between January 1988 and December 1992. To the best of our knowledge there is no evidence that biliary atresia might recur in a liver transplant.

Main series from the literature

Few reports deal specifically with biliary atresia. In 1987, at the European Symposium on Liver Transplantation in children, Starzl *et al.*[33] reported a 64% 5-year survival rate in 137 biliary atresia patients, which was about 10% lower than for other paediatric recipients; this difference was ascribed to 'the greater difficulty in treating patients with biliary atresia after extensive prior operations for the performance of portoenterostomy or revision of such procedures'. A similar difference was noted by Starzl and Demetris[30] when they updated the Pittsburgh experience with 235 cases of biliary atresia in 1990. Andrews *et al.* reported the Dallas experience with 37 patients transplanted for biliary atresia between 1984 and 1988[34]. The 1-year survival rate of their entire group of 80 transplanted children was 75%, but they did not give specific data for biliary atresia patients. In 1989 Kalayoglu *et al.*, reporting on their first 25 paediatric recipients including 16 with biliary atresia, showed that patients with prior abdominal surgery had longer operations with greater blood loss[35]; overall patient survival was 88%. A detailed analysis of the Omaha experience was reported by Wood *et al.* in 1990[36] comparing 48 children transplanted for biliary atresia with 35 children transplanted for other liver diseases. The trend in all the intraoperative parameters was that the transplant procedure was more difficult in biliary atresia patients, particularly in those who had undergone a portoenterostomy with a stoma.

Lynch *et al.* reported in 1992[37] the Brisbane experience of 52 children transplanted for biliary atresia. Actuarial survival at 1 year was 78%; it was 83% for 12 children less than 1 year of age at transplantation. The nutritional condition of the recipients had a major impact on their results. Results obtained in Cincinnati in 37 patients treated between 1986 and 1992 were reported by Ryckman *et al.* in 1993[38]. The actuarial survival was 80% at 2 years without statistically significant difference in the incidence of surgical complications comparing biliary atresia and non-biliary atresia patients. Meister *et al.*[39] have recently reviewed their experience with 42 transplants for biliary atresia to determine if the complication rate was increased by a previous portoenterostomy with or without a stoma. A greater morbidity was observed, consisting of increased operative time and number of reoperations, whether or not the stoma had been closed prior to transplantation. Vacanti *et al.*[19] analysed the results in 28 infants treated between 1981 and 1988 by surgeons who performed both the portoenterostomy and liver transplantation. Fifty-seven per cent achieved total biliary drainage after portoenterostomy; 32% had undergone liver transplantation, 89% were alive, 92% of those alive being jaundice-free.

Table 1 Indications ($n = 322$)

Cholestatic diseases	237	*Miscellaneous*	36
Biliary atresia	215	Cryptogenic cirrhosis	7
Ductular paucity	14	Acute liver failure	17
Sclerosing cholangitis	3	Neonatal hepatitis	1
Cholestatic cirrhosis	5	Cong. hepatic fibrosis	3
		Tumours	6
Metabolic diseases	*51*		
Byler's disease	16	*Combined liver & kidney*	7
Wilson	9		
α_1-antitrypsin def.	6		
Crigler–Najjar	5		
Glycogenosis	2		
Tyrosinaemia	6		
Hypercholesterolaemia	1		
Oxalosis	3		
Fructosaemia	1		
Methylmalonic aciduria	1		
Mitochondr. respir. chain. def.	1		

Personal experience

Between 1984 and 1993 we have transplanted 215 children for biliary atresia; the vast majority had undergone a Kasai portoenterostomy or one of its various modifications. They represented 66% of the total number of 322 children transplanted during that 10-year period (Table 1); at the time of transplantation, about 80% of these children were younger than 3 years, and had a mean weight of less than 10 kg; only 9% were older than 6 years (but <15 years).

One-fourth of the patients were transplanted urgently because of very advanced liver failure with very poor synthetic function, bleeding diathesis and intractable ascites. Many of the 39 infants transplanted under the age of 1 year fell into this category with an extremely poor nutritional status. Forty-five per cent of the transplants used were full-size grafts and 55% were technical variants including reduced, partial and split grafts[40,41].

The actuarial (Kaplan–Meier) survival rate of the 215 children was 83% at 1 year and 78% at 5 years (to be compared with 83% and 79% respectively for the total population of 322 transplanted children, and with 93% and 91% respectively for the 51 children transplanted for a metabolic disease).

The incidence of major complications was similar in biliary atresia patients and in patients transplanted for other indications regarding arterial thrombosis (11.1% and 8.3%), portal vein thrombosis (2.5% and 1%), primary non-function (6% and 6.2%), biliary complications (13.1% and 13.5%) and retransplantation rate (17.6% and 17.7%).

Paucity of intrahepatic bile ducts

Intrahepatic cholestasis associated with a paucity of interlobular bile ducts (observed in >50% of the portal triads) may occur without associated developmental anomalies[42]. Cholestatic jaundice with hepatomegaly is frequently present in the neonatal period. Total serum bile acids and cholesterol are often markedly elevated. Pruritus and skin xanthomas are frequently seen. The non-syndromic type has a very poor prognosis[43] with death from liver failure in childhood or near-adolescence; therefore indication of liver replacement is based on signs of liver insufficiency. Of the five patients we have transplanted for this entity, two (one with combined liver and kidney transplant for a renal disease of unknown aetiology) are alive more than 4 years after transplantation, and three died shortly after surgery. Two of these deaths were directly related to surgery; the third one had a progressive downhill course with multiple problems.

In the syndromic type (arteriohepatic dysplasia or Alagille syndrome), paucity of the interlobular ducts is associated with at least three of the following congenital developmental anomalies: unusual facies, vertebral arch defects (butterfly vertebrae, hemivertebrae and decrease in the interpedicular distance), posterior embryotoxon, peripheral pulmonary stenoses and, occasionally, short stature, mental retardation and hypogonadism[44].

The syndromic type of the disease is very rarely responsible for liver failure and death, and was considered by Alagille[43] himself never to be an indication for liver transplantation; such a negative opinion was also expressed by A-Kader *et al.*[45]. We disagree with this strong assertion, because some of these patients have a very poor quality of life due to the unresponsiveness of cholestasis to any therapy with intractable pruritus, debilitating xanthomas on hands and feet, poor school performance and poor growth. We agree with Whitington *et al.*[46] that liver transplantation should be offered to these debilitated children whose life is not threatened, although long-term outcome after liver transplantation has not been recorded in enough patients to determine whether growth resumes and school performance improves. Our series comprises nine children transplanted for Alagille syndrome. Pathological examination of the liver disclosed cirrhosis in three, fibrosis in two and ductular paucity without cirrhotic changes in four; all had severe cholestasis with elevated bilirubin (between 4.7 mg% and 29.2 mg%), severe pruritus and, in most cases, multiple xanthomas. Six were less than 4 years old, and three were between 6 and 13 years old. Seven became long-term survivors with a follow-up between 6 months and 9 years.

Primary sclerosing cholangitis

Primary sclerosing cholangitis is being increasingly recognized in childhood. In a quarter of cases no associated disorder can be found. The disease may start as a neonatal cholestatic syndrome and strictures of the bile ducts are recognized secondarily[47]; other cases can be associated with inflammatory bowel disease and coeliac disease, histiocytosis X, immune deficiencies and autoimmune hepatitis[48]. The treatment of primary sclerosing cholangitis is medical; when the stage of cholestatic cirrhosis has been reached the only therapeutic option is liver transplantation[49].

Only three (0.6%) of 481 children from eight different centres reported to the First International Symposium on Liver Transplantation in Children had been operated for this indication[49].

We have transplanted three children for this disease because of the severity of cholestasis. One child who had a long-standing and severely debilitating disease, most likely of autoimmune origin, died of septic complications. The other two patients suffering from sclerosing cholangitis associated with histiocytosis X became long-term survivors.

Byler's disease

Familial intrahepatic cholestasis is the result of an uncharacterized genetic–metabolic disorder which progresses from fibrosis to cirrhosis and liver failure. Once the stage of cirrhosis has been reached, life expectancy does not exceed 2 years; indication for transplantation is based on liver failure, portal hypertension and, in some patients, poor quality of life related to intractable pruritus which interferes with sleeping and schooling attendance[50].

We have transplanted 16 children suffering from Byler's disease with liver fibrosis in seven and cirrhosis in nine (seven had signs of liver failure); five had bled from oesophageal varices and six had refractory ascites. The age at transplantation was under 2 years in three, between 2 and 6 years in seven, between 6 and 10 years in three and between 10 and 14 years in three. All became long-term survivors with a follow-up between 4 months and 8 years and full rehabilitation.

ADULTS

The main cholestatic diseases which can lead to liver transplantation are primary biliary cirrhosis and primary sclerosing cholangitis; secondary biliary cirrhosis of various origin and late failure after Kasaï portoenterostomy for biliary atresia can also become indications for liver transplantation in adult age.

Primary biliary cirrhosis (PBC)

This is the most frequent indication for liver transplantation in adults, next to posthepatitic and alcoholic cirrhosis; it represented 11% of the 8622 liver transplants reported to the European Liver Transplant Registry from 1988 to 1992. In this collective series the mean age at transplantation was 51.8 years; the 1- and 5-year survival rates were 79.2% and 72%, respectively. The main issue which still remains controversial is the timing of transplantation.

Our own experience includes 36 patients transplanted for PBC among 276 patients (13%) who were grafted between 1984 and 1993 (Table 2). Clinical characteristics are given in Table 3. This series includes a rather high proportion of modified (bilirubin < 4 mg%: A; 4–10 mg%; B; > 10 mg%; C) Child–Pugh class B (52.8%) and class C patients (30.6%). Three patients had no antimitochondrial antibodies at the time of transplantation. The main indication for liver transplantation was variceal bleeding in 10 patients,

Table 2   UCL – adult liver transplantation – indications

Chronic liver diseases (213 = 77.2%)	
Hepatocellular	156 (56.5%)
Cholestatic	46 (16.6%)†
Vascular	1 (0.4%)
Toxic	1 (0.4%)
Metabolic diseases	9 (3.26%)
Hepatobiliary tumours (36 = 13%)	
Malignant	34 (12.3%)‡
Benign	2 (0.8%)
Acute liver failure (non-cirrhotic liver)	27 (9.8%)

†PBC, 35 (12.7%); PSC, 7 (2.5%); SBC, 4 (1.4%)
‡One PBC and one PSC patient included

Table 3   PBC and liver transplantation: clinical characteristics

Study period	May 1984–December 1993
Patients	36/276 (13%)
Age	51 years median (26.3–68.4)
Gender	5 male (13.9%); 31 female (86.1%)
Negative antimitochondrial antibodies	4/36 (11.1%)
Blood group	O, 10 (30.5%); A, 21 (58.3%); B, 3 (8.3%); AB, 1 (2.7%)
Modified Child–Pugh	A, 6 (16.6%); B, 19 (52.8%); C, 11 (30.6%)
Elective/urgent liver transplantation	4/32 patients (12.5%)
Technical variants	2 patients
Follow-up	36 patients; 72 months median (4–103)

intractable pruritus in eight patients, severe jaundice (bilirubin > 10 mg%) in three patients, poor general condition with severe denutrition in five patients, severe jaundice with poor general condition with severe denutrition in five patients, severe jaundice with poor general condition in five patients, severe jaundice and intractable pruritus in two patients, severe jaundice with painful hepatomegaly, intractable pruritus with poor general condition and hepatocellular carcinoma in one patient each. Five patients (13.8%) were retransplanted for primary non-function ($n = 3$), acute rejection exacerbated by ABO incompatibility ($n = 1$) or chronic rejection ($n = 1$). Six patients died early (less than 3 months post-OLT) from haemorrhage ($n = 2$) or haemorrhage and sepsis ($n = 4$). Four more patients (11.1%) died later than 3 months post-OLT from sepsis (6 months), recurrence of HCCA (13 months), suicide (17 months) and lymphoproliferative disorder (79 months). The actuarial survival rates are 79%, 75.8% and 75.5% at 1, 3 and 5 years respectively. There was a close relationship between early mortality and modified Child–Pugh class at the time of transplantation with no mortality in six class A patients, one death in 19 class B patients (5.2%) and five deaths in 11 class C patients (45.5%); the long-term survival is 96% in 25 class A or B patients.

Quality of life in 30 long-term survivors was judged as excellent in 18 (60%), moderate in 5 (16.6%) because of fatigue and/or mood swing, poor in 3 (10%) because of HCV graft cirrhosis, cerebrovascular accident or osseous disease and bad in 4 patients (13.3%) because of complications leading to death (sepsis, recurrent HCCA, severe depression or lymphoproliferative disorder). Thirteen of 36 patients (36%) had associated systemic diseases (arthritis: 5; thyroiditis: 2; sarcoidosis: 1; coeliac disease: 1; breast cancer: 1; Sicca syndrome: 1; cardiomyopathy: 1; glomerulonephritis: 1). Post-transplantation, the Sicca syndrome persisted in one patient as well as thyroiditis in another patient and coeliac disease in one patient. Moreover, arthritis, goitre and mammary adenoma appeared *de novo* in one patient each. Antimitochondrial antibodies disappeared in only two of 27 patients having this marker pretransplant (7.4%).

As stated earlier, the main issues which are still controversial regarding liver transplantation in PBC are the selection of patients to be transplanted and the timing of the procedure.

Mathematical models, predicting survival for individual patients with PBC, have been developed in Europe and in the USA. By contrast with the Yale model[51] and the European model[52], the Mayo model, derived from the data from 312 Mayo Clinic patients[53], does not require liver biopsy; it is based on clinical and biochemical variables which are easily obtainable; age, total bilirubin, albumin, prothrombin time (in seconds) and oedema. When cross-validated on an independent set of 106 Mayo Clinic patients, the model predicted survival accurately for the individual PBC patients[53]; this model has been further validated with the European model and with other intramural and extramural independent data sets, and has been found to be generalizable and applicable to a broad spectrum of PBC patients[54]. Three more studies have been conducted in which multivariate analysis of Cox regression hazard modelling has been used to determine independent risk factors to estimate survival for the individual patient with PBC[55-57]. In each prognostic model the serum level of bilirubin is the most heavily weighted variable. Indeed, Shapiro *et al.*[58] observed that patients with PBC typically have a long and stable course followed by an accelerated preterminal phase, during which time serum levels of bilirubin frequently rise above 10 mg/dl. In these patients the mean survival time was determined to be 1.4 year.

To assess the efficacy of liver transplantation in PBC, Wiesner *et al.* from the Mayo Clinic[59,60] compared the Kaplan–Meier estimated survival of 161 PBC patients who had undergone liver transplantation at the University of Pittsburgh and at Baylor University in Dallas with the estimated survival of those same patients if they had been treated conservatively without liver transplantation. The results revealed that, 6 months after liver transplantation, the Kaplan–Meier survival probabilities in liver transplant patients were significantly higher than the Mayo model estimated survival probabilities without liver transplantation ($p < 0.001$). Furthermore, the study showed that early post-transplantation survival was better for all risk scores, including the lowest risk score (those having a better prognosis without transplantation). These findings have been confirmed in reports from the Nordic countries[61], the Netherlands[62] and the United Kingdom[63]. On the basis of these studies it appears clearly that maximum early survival with liver transplantation can be achieved if PBC patients undergo early transplantation, i.e. when they develop a Mayo PBC risk score between 8 and 9. Moreover, the Mayo investigators have shown that optimal timing of liver transplantation in PBC patients may not only decrease mortality related to liver transplantation, but may also significantly decrease morbidity and cost of the procedure[60]. It might be added that these mathematical models do not take into account the patient's quality of life (e.g. related to intractable pruritus), a factor which most clinicians feel is extremely important in making the decision for liver transplantation in an individual patient.

The second controversial issue regarding liver transplantation in PBC is the radicality of the cure achieved by OLT: does PBC recur after OLT? Quite evidently this important question cannot be answered from biochemical markers; indeed the persistence of high levels (although often lower than pre-OLT) of antimitochondrial antibodies and of IgM is the rule after OLT which is easily explained by the non-organ specificity of AMA.

The diagnosis of recurrence of PBC can be made only on histological criteria, but even this approach is controversial because each of the autoimmune diseases (PBC, PSC, chronic active hepatitis) can show overlap histologically, with rejection, chronic viral hepatitis, drug reactions, graft-versus-host disease, particularly in the case of vanished bile duct syndrome and damage of the large bile ducts caused by ischaemia (preservation sequelae, arterial thrombosis, etc.) or other causes (bacterial cholangitis, cytomegalovirus infection, etc.). Most studies that failed to find recurrence of PBC after OLT[63-68] had few patients with long-term histological follow-up. The Cambridge–King's College group was the first to report evidence that the disease might recur in the grafted liver[69]: three patients who received transplants 3.5–4.5 years earlier had each developed, after an initial asymptomatic period of 2 years, a mild cholestatic jaundice with histological appearances of the liver characteristic of, or compatible with, recurrent PBC. At least in one patient, who was retransplanted 10 years later in another centre by one of the authors (J.L.), the final histological diagnosis was chronic rejection. In 1989 the same group[70] reported updated data on 23 patients who survived > 1 year (including the three patients reported in 1992). In 10 of these patients, who had liver biopsies more than 1 year after OLT, nine had histological features consistent with PBC-like ductular proliferation, lymphocytic aggregates, breaks in the basement membrane of the bile ducts, copper-associated protein in the absence of cholestasis and paucity of bile ducts; granulomas were noted only in three patients and granulomatous duct destruction was not reported. The Birmingham[71] and Innsbruck[72] groups have also reported recurrent PBC after OLT. As stressed recently by the Mayo group[73], *the hallmark of PBC is the florid duct lesion* which is typically seen in early stages of PBC (stages 1 and 2); all other histological features of PBC can also be seen in hepatic allograft rejection, as well as in several non-rejection processes that may affect allografts. Specifically, *the portal inflammation* typical of PBC is also seen in cellular rejection, viral hepatitis and drug reactions. *Lymphocytic bile duct destruction,* common in PBC, is also seen in cellular rejection and can be found in conjunction with hepatitis C[74]; *granulomas* are found in several infections and drug reactions. *Duct loss* (ductopenia) typical of late-stage PBC is also seen in the vanished bile duct syndrome which is typical of irreversible, chronic rejection. *Copper deposition* is noted in a variety of cholestatic conditions and *ductular proliferation* is common in intrahepatic and extrahepatic biliary obstruction.

Until recently, biliary reconstruction was routinely done in Cambridge with a biliary conduit using the donor liver gallbladder; this type of biliary reconstruction technique has since been abandoned because of the prohibitively high complication rate (it is noteworthy that eight of the 23 PBC patients surviving >1 year, who were reported in 1989[70], had recurrent cholangitis or biliary obstruction requiring medical or surgical treatment).

The hallmark of PBC (the florid bile duct lesion) was detected by the Mayo investigators in five of their 60 patients given transplants for PBC and in whom histological follow-up of at least 1 year was available[73].

Undoubted disease recurrence in two patients transplanted for PBC under FK506 were reported by the King's group[75]. Liver biopsies performed at 10 months post-OLT in the first patient (because of recurrence of pruritus, *de-novo* appearance of the sicca syndrome and marked elevation of γ-GT) and at 12 months in the second patient (protocol biopsy) displayed the florid histological abnormalities, namely dense lymphocytic and plasma cell infiltrates with granuloma formation in the portal tracts closely associated with damaged interlobular bile ducts; these lesions were considered by the authors to be strongly suggestive, if not diagnostic, of PBC; all other diagnoses able to mimic some of the histological features were excluded.

On the basis of these reports the possibility of recurrence of PBC after OLT could hardly be denied. The risk of recurrence is evaluated to a minimum of 8% by the Mayo group[71]. The short-term prognosis of recurrent PBC seems quite good because the quite slow natural evolution of the disease could even be slowed down by immunosuppression. The rather early (<1 year) recurrence in two cases treated with FK506 led the King's group to speculate about the possibility that FK506 has less of an action in PBC than cyclosporin A.

In our series we have not observed proven recurrence until now.

Primary sclerosing cholangitis (PSC)

Primary sclerosing cholangitis is an infrequent indication for liver transplantation in European countries. Only 367 of the 8622 patients (4.2%) reported to the European Liver Transplant Registry between 1988 and 1992 were transplanted for PSC.

In our own series of 276 adult patients transplanted over a 10-year period (1984–93), only eight (3.3%) received a transplant for PSC. The median age was 42 years (28.4–71.2); there were six males and two females. Inflammatory bowel disease, portal vein thrombosis and cholangiocarcinoma were associated with PBC in three, three and one patient respectively. The indication for liver replacement was recurrent cholangitis in four patients, progressive liver insufficiency in two patients, uncontrollable variceal bleeding and poor clinical condition in one patient each. One patient who had recurrent cholangitis induced by a biliary endoprosthesis and a Crohn disease was found to have cholangiocarcinoma on the operative specimen; he died from sepsis 33 days after OLT. The remaining seven patients (87.5%) are alive with a median follow-up of 37 months (17–86); recurrence was not documented in any case. Both patients with inflammatory bowel disease who are alive had exacerbation of their IBD after steroid withdrawal; one patient had to be converted to FK506 because of threatening chronic rejection.

The natural history of PSC is less well understood as compared with PBC. As for PBC, a mathematical model allowing prediction of survival would help to make a decision for an individual patient regarding selection and timing of transplantation. A first model was developed at the Mayo Clinic from the prospective evaluation of 174 patients[76]. The mean follow-up for this group of PSC patients was 6 years, during which time 34% died. The median survival from time of diagnosis of PSC was estimated to be 11.9 years.

More recently, the patient database from the Mayo Clinic study on the natural history of PSC was expanded to 426 PSC patients by adding patients from four additional medical centres throughout the world, all having a major interest in PSC[77].

In this new model, multivariable analysis revealed the following variables to be independent predictors of survival: total serum bilirubin, age, histological stage and the presence of absence of splenomegaly. Although prospective evaluation of this model will be needed, such a model will be helpful in patient counselling and in patient selection and timing for liver transplantation.

To provide control data for evaluating the efficacy of OLT in improving survival for patients with advanced PSC, the Mayo PSC natural history model[76-78] was mathematically applied to the combined population of patients who underwent hepatic replacement for PSC at the University of Pittsburgh and Mayo Medical Center (total number: 286 patients with a mean post-OLT follow-up of 34 ± 25 months). Actual survival after transplantation was compared with the survival estimated with the use of the Mayo model. Within 6 months the Kaplan–Meier survival probability after OLT (89%) was already higher than predicted by the Mayo model (83%). At 5 years, actuarial survival with OLT was 73% compared with 28% predicted by the Mayo model. The overall increased survival rate with transplantation was statistically significant ($p < 0.001$), although the entire transplant population had more advanced disease than the patients used to build the natural history Mayo model. At all risk stratifications, OLT significantly improved survival, including the low-risk patients. Patients with concomitant inflammatory intestinal disease, or who underwent biliary or portal surgery, tended to have a less favourable survival after OLT, but the difference was not statistically significant.

There is a significant risk, for patients with PSC, of developing cholangiocarcinoma, which is evaluated to be 7–10%[78] but has been found to be as high as 50% in the 49 patients transplanted out of the total series of 392 patients who served to build the Mayo model. Incidental cholangiocarcinoma significantly reduces the life expectancy after OLT[79].

Inflammatory bowel disease does not influence the evolution of the liver disease. On the contrary, liver transplantation itself seems to have a beneficial influence on the further evolution of the IBD; this effect is probably due in part to the enhanced post-transplant immunosuppression.

References

1. Alagille D. Extrahepatic biliary atresia. Hepatology. 1984;4:7S–10S.
2. Ohi R, Ibrahim M. Biliary atresia. Semin Pediatr Surg. 1992;1:115–24.
3. Landing BH. Considerations on the pathogenesis of neonatal hepatitis, biliary atresia and choledochal cyst. The concept of infantile obstructive cholangiopathy. In: Bill AH, Kasai M, editors. Progress in pediatric surgery, vol. 6. Baltimore, MD: University Park Press; 1974:113–39.
4. Karrer FM, Hall RJ, Lilly JR. Biliary atresia and the polysplenia syndrome. J Pediatr Surg. 1991;26:524–7.
5. Adelman S. Prognosis of uncorrected biliary atresia: an update. J Pediatr Surg. 1978;13: 389–91.
6. Hays D, Snyder WH. Life-span in untreated biliary atresia. Surgery. 1963;64:373–5.
7. Karrer FM, Lilly JR, Stewart BA, Hall RJ. Biliary atresia registry, 1976 to 1989. J Pediatr Surg. 1990;25:1076–81.
8. Ladd WE. Congenital atresia and stenosis of the bile ducts. JAMA. 1929;91:1082–5.
9. Kasai M, Ohi R, Chiba T. Intrahepatic bile ducts in biliary atresia. In: Kasai M, Shiraki K, editors. Cholestasis in infancy. Baltimore, MD: University Park Press, 1980:181–8.
10. Ohi R, Shikes RH, Stellin GP, Lilly JR. In biliary atresia, duct histology correlates with bile flow. J Pediatr Surg. 1984;19:467–70.
11. Altman RP, Chandra R, Lilly JR. Ongoing cirrhosis after successful portoenterostomy. J Pediatr Surg. 1975;10:685–91.
12. Alagille D. Liver transplantation in children. Indications in cholestatic states. Transplant Proc. 1987;29:3242–8.
13. Otte JB, de Ville de Goyet J, Reding R et al. Sequential treatment of biliary atresia with Kasaï portoenterostomy and liver transplantation. A review. Hepatology. 1994;20:41S–48S.
14. Kasai M, Kimura S, Asakura Y, Suzuki Y, Taira Y, Obashi E. Surgical treatment of biliary atresia. J Pediatr Surg. 1968;3:665–75.
15. Grosfeld JL, Fitzgerald JF, Predaina R et al. The efficacy of hepatoportoenterostomy in biliary atresia. Surgery. 1989;106:692–701.
16. Schweizer P. Treatment of extrahepatic bile duct atresia: results and long-term prognosis after hepatic portoenterostomy. Pediatr Surg Int. 1986;1:30–6.
17. Caccia G, Dessanti A, Alberti D. Clinical results in 90 patients with biliary atresia. In: Ohi R, editor. Biliary atresia. Tokyo: Professional Postgraduate Services; 1987:281–6.
18. Gauthier F, Laurent J, Bernard O, Valayer J. Improvement of results after Kasai operation: the need for early diagnosis and surgery. In: Ohi R, editor. Biliary atresia. Tokyo: Icom Associates; 1991:91–5.
19. Vacanti JP, Shamberger RC, Eraklis A, Lilleley CW. The therapy of biliary atresia combining the Kasai portoenterostomy with liver transplantation: a single center experience. J Pediatr Surg. 1990;25:149–52.
20. Houwen RHJ, Zwierstra RP, Severijnen RS et al. Prognosis of extrahepatic biliary atresia. Arch Dis Childh. 1989;64:214–18.
21. Iwatsuki S, Shaw BW, Starzl TE. Liver transplantation for biliary atresia. World J Surg. 1984;8:51–6.
22. Otte JB, Eucher P, Latour JP et al. Liver transplantation for biliary atresia: indications and results. Z Kinderchir. 1988;43:99–105.
23. Sokal E, Van Hoorebeeck N, Van Obbergh L, Otte JB, Buts JP. Upper gastrointestinal tract bleeding in cirrhotic children candidates for liver transplantation. Eur J Pediatr. 1992;151:326–8.
24. Howard ER. Biliary atresia: aetiology, management and complications. In: Howard ER, editor. Surgery of liver disease in infancy. London: Butterworth: 1991:39–59.
25. Laurent J, Gauthier F, Bernard O et al. Long-term outcome after surgery for biliary atresia. Gastroenterology. 1990;99:1795–7.

26. Kasai M, Ohi R, Chiba T, Hayashi Y. A patient with biliary atresia who died 28 years after hepatic portojejunostomy. J Pediatr Surg. 1988;23:430–1.
27. Ohi R. Biliary atresia: long-term results of hepatic portoenterostomy. In: Howard ER, editor. Surgery of liver diseases in infancy. London: Butterworth; 1991:60–71.
28. Whitington PF, Balistreri WF. Liver transplantation in pediatrics: indications, contraindications and pretransplant management. J Pediatr. 1991;118:169–77.
29. Iwatsuki S, Starzl TE, Todo S et al. Experience in 1,000 liver transplants under cyclosporine–steroid therapy: a survival report. Transplant Proc. 1988;20:498–504.
30. Starzl TE, Demetris AJ. Candidacy, original disease and outcome in liver transplantation: a 31-year perspective. Chicago, IL: Year Book Medical Publishers; 1990:119–36.
31. Salt A, Noble-Jamieson G, Barnes ND et al. Liver transplantation in 100 children: Cambridge and King's College Hospital series. Br Med J. 1992;304:416–21.
32. Bernard O. Transplantation hépatique chez l'enfant. Indications et résultats. Pediatrie. 1991;48:133–7.
33. Starzl TE, Esquivel C, Gordon R, Todo S. Pediatric liver transplantation. Transplant Proc. 1987;29:3230–5.
34. Andrews WS, Wanek E, Fyolk B, Gray S, Benser M. Pediatric liver transplantation: a 3-year experience. J Pediatr Surg. 1989;24:77–82.
35. Kalayoglu M, Stratta RJ, Sollinger HW et al. Liver transplantation in infants and children. J Pediatr Surg. 1989;24:70–6.
36. Wood RP, Langnas AN, Stratta RJ et al. Optimal therapy for patients with biliary atresia: portoenterostomy ('Kasaï' procedures) versus primary transplantation. J Pediatr Surg. 1990;25:153–62.
37. Lynch SV, Akiyama T, Ong Th et al. Transplantation in children with biliary atresia. Transplant Proc. 1992;24:186–8.
38. Ryckman F, Fisher R, Pederson S et al. Improved survival in biliary atresia patients in the present era of liver transplantation. J Pediatr Surg. 1993;28:382–6.
39. Meister RK, Esquivel CO, Cox KL et al. The influence of portoenterostomy with stoma on morbidity in pediatric patients with biliary atresia undergoing orthotopic liver transplantation. J Pediatr Surg. 1993;28:387–90.
40. Otte JB, de Ville de Goyet J, Sokal E et al. Size reduction of the donor liver is a safe way to alleviate the shortage of size match organs in pediatric liver transplantation. Ann Surg. 1990;211:38–49.
41. de Ville de Goyet J, Hausleithner V, Reding R, Lerut J, Janssen M, Otte JB. Impact of innovative techniques on the waiting list and the results in pediatric liver transplantation. Transplantation. 1994;56:1130–6.
42. Ahrens EHJ, Harris RC, McMahon HE. Atresia of the intrahepatic bile ducts. Pediatrics. 1951;8:628.
43. Alagille D. Liver transplantation in children. Indications in cholestatic states. Transplant Proc. 1987;29:3242–8.
44. Alagille D, Odievre M, Gauthier M, et al. Hepatic ductular hypoplasia associated with characteristic facies, vertebral malformations, retarded physical, mental and sexual development and cardiac murmur. J Pediatr. 1975;86:63.
45. A-Kader HH, Ryckman FC, Balistreri WF. Liver transplantation in the pediatric population: indications and monitoring. Clin Transplant. 1991;5:161–7.
46. Whitington PF, Emond JC, Black DD et al. Indications for liver transplantation in pediatric patients. Clin Transplant. 1991;5:156–60.
47. Amedee-Manesme O, Bernard O, Brunelle F et al. Sclerosing cholangitis with neonatal onset. J Pediatr. 1987;111:225–9.
48. Sokal EM. Diseases of the biliary tract. In: Buts JP, Sokal EM, editors. Management of digestive and liver disorders in infants and children. Amsterdam: Elsevier; 1993:631–9.
49. Otte JB, Starzl TE, Ascher N, Vacanti JP, Klintmalm G, Andrews W. Liver transplantation in children. Transplant Proc. 1987;29:3229–380.
50. Mowat A. Liver disorders in children: the indications for liver replacement in parenchymal and metabolic disorders. Transplant Proc. 1987;21:3236–41.
51. Roll J, Boyer JL, Barry D, Klatskin G. The prognostic importance of clinical and histological features in asymptomatic and symptomatic primary biliary cirrhosis. N Engl J Med. 1983;308:1–7.

52. Christensen E, Neuberger J, Crowe J et al. Beneficial effect of azathioprine and prediction of prognosis in primary biliary cirrhosis. Final results of an international trial. Gastroenterology. 1985;312:1011–15.
53. Dickson ER, Grambsch PM, Fleming TR, Fisher LD, Langworthy A. Prognosis in primary biliary cirrhosis: model for decision making. Hepatology. 1989;10:1–7.
54. Grambsch PM, Dickson ER, Kaplan M, Lesage G, Fleming TR, Langworthy AL. Extramural cross-validation of the Mayo primary biliary cirrhosis survival model establishes its generalizability. Hepatology. 1989;10:846–50.
55. Rydning A, Schrumpf E, Abdelmoor M, Elgio K, Jenssen E. Factors of prognostic importance in primary biliary cirrhosis. Scand J Gastroenterol. 1990;25:119–26.
56. Goudie BM, Burt AD, Malfarlane GJ et al. Risk factors and prognosis in primary biliary cirrhosis. Am J Gastroenterol. 1989;84:713–16.
57. Jeffrey GP, Reed WA, Shilkin KB. Natural history and prognostic variables in primary biliary cirrhosis. Hepatology. 1990;12:955(abstr.).
58. Shapiro JM, Smith H, Schaffner F. Serum bilirubin: a prognostic factor in primary biliary cirrhosis. Gut. 1979;20:137–40.
59. Makkus BH, Dickson ER, Grambsch PM et al. Efficacy of liver transplantation in patients with primary biliary cirrhosis. N Engl J Med. 1989;320:1709–13.
60. Wiesner RH, Porayko MK, Dickson ER et al. Selection and timing of liver transplantation in primary biliary cirrhosis and primary sclerosing cholangitis. Hepatology. 1992;16:1290–9.
61. Keiding S, Ericzon GB, Eriksson S et al. Survival after liver transplantation of patients with primary biliary cirrhosis in the Nordic countries. Scand J Gastroneterol. 1990;25: 11–18.
62. Bonsel GJ, Klompmaker IJ, van de Veer F, Habbema JD, Slooff MJ. Use of prognostic models for assessment of value of liver transplantation in primary biliary cirrhosis. Lancet. 1990;335:493–7.
63. Neuberger JM, Gunson BK, Buckels JP, Elias E, McMaster P. Referral of patients with primary biliary cirrhosis for liver transplantation. Gut. 1990;31:1069–72.
64. Esquivel CO, Van Thiel DH, Demetris AJ et al. Transplantation for primary biliary cirrhosis. Gastroenterology. 1988;94:1207–16.
65. Haagsma EB, Manns M, Klein R et al. Subtypes of antimitochondrial antibodies in primary biliary cirrhosis before and after orthotopic liver transplantation. Hepatology. 1987;7: 129–33.
66. Hart J, Busuttil RW, Lewin KJ. Disease recurrence following liver transplantation. Am J Surg Pathol. 1990;14(Suppl. 1):79–91.
67. Demetris AJ, Markus BH, Esquivel C et al. Pathologic analysis of liver transplantation for primary biliary cirrhosis. Hepatology. 1988;8:939–47.
68. Samuel D, Gugenheim J, Mentha G et al. Liver transplantation for primary biliary cirrhosis. Transplant Proc. 1990;22:1497–8.
69. Neuberger J, Portmann B, MacDougall BRD, Calne RY, Williams R. Recurrence of primary biliary cirrhosis after liver transplantation. N Engl J Med. 1982;306:1–4.
70. Polson RJ, Portmann B, Neuberger J, Calne RY, Williams R. Evidence for disease recurrence after liver transplantation for primary biliary cirrhosis. Gastroenterology. 1989;97:715–25.
71. Hubscher SG, Buckers JAC, Elias E, Mayer AD, McMaster P, Neuberger JM. Does primary biliary cirrhosis recur after liver transplantation? Hepatology. 1992;16:545(abstr.).
72. Dietze O, Vogel W, Margreiter R. Primary biliary cirrhosis after liver transplantation. Transplant Proc. 1990;22:1501–2.
73. Balan V, Batts KP, Porayoko MK, Krom RAF, Judwig J, Wiesner RH. Histological evidence for recurrence of primary biliary cirrhosis after liver transplantation. Hepatology. 1993;18:1392–8.
74. Scheuer PJ, Ashrafzadeh P, Sherlock S, Brown D, Dusheiko GM. The pathology of hepatitis C. Hepatology. 1992;15:567–71.
75. Wong PYN, Portmann B, O'Grady JG et al. Recurrence of primary biliary cirrhosis after liver transplantation following FK 506-based immunosuppression. J Hepatol. 1993;17: 284–7.
76. Wiesner RH, Grambsch PM, Dickson ER et al. Primary sclerosing cholangitis: natural history, prognostic factors, and survival analysis. Hepatology. 1989;10:430–6.
77. Dickson ER, Murtaugh PA, Grambsch PM et al. Primary sclerosing cholangitis: refinement

and validation of survival model. Gastroenterology. 1992;103:1893–901.
78. Abu-Elmagd KM, Malinchoc M, Dickson ER *et al*. Efficacy of hepatic transplantation in patients with primary sclerosing cholangitis. Surg Gynecol Obstet. 1993;177:335–44.
79. Rosen CB, Nagorney DM, Wiesner RH, Coffey RJ, LaRusso NF. Cholangiocarcinoma complicating primary sclerosing cholangitis. Ann Surg. 1990;213:21–5.

32
Large bile duct strictures in primary sclerosing cholangitis patients developing ductopenic rejection after liver transplantation; does this represent recurrence of PSC?

B. VAN HOEK, R. H. WIESNER, L. SANCHEZ-URDAZPAL,
J. LUDWIG and R. A. F. KROM

INTRODUCTION

Chronic (ductopenic) rejection (DR) occurs in about 8% of first orthotopic liver allografts when using immunosuppression based on cyclosporin and prednisone[1], and recurs in 90% of subsequent allografts if similar immunosuppression is used[2]. DR is more frequent if no azathioprine is added to cyclosporin and prednisone[3]. Primary sclerosing cholangitis (PSC) as the underlying liver disease is an independent risk factor for the development of DR of the allograft[4]. We hypothesized that this might reflect our inability to distinguish DR from recurrent PSC in the allograft. Apart from the changes of interlobular and septal bile ducts, including ductopenia, as may be seen in liver biopsies, PSC before liver transplantation is usually characterized by intra- and extrahepatic large bile duct strictures. After liver transplantation, non-anastomotic large bile duct strictures (LBS) can occur in a variety of settings[5], such as prolonged cold ischaemia time (especially beyond 11 h)[6-11], ABO blood group incompatibility[12-14], hepatic artery thrombosis[1,15], bacterial cholangitis, possibly cytomegalovirus infection, and DR[15]. Repeated percutaneous dilatation of these strictures is often successful[15], although graft survival may be reduced[7].

In order to test the hypothesis that DR after liver transplantation for PSC might represent recurrent PSC in the allograft, we related the presence of non-anastomotic large bile duct strictures in patients developing DR after liver transplantation to the underlying liver disease.

PATIENTS AND METHODS

Patients

From 1985 through 1990, 278 orthotopic liver transplantations (OLT) were performed at the Mayo Clinic; 236 were first OLT, 42 retransplantations. In the 206 patients receiving a first OLT with graft survival of 3 months or more 17 developed DR. The underlying liver diseases in these patients were: eight PSC, three chronic active hepatitis (CAH), two primary biliary cirrhosis (PBC), two fulminant hepatic failure (FHF), two other (one venoocclusive disease, one a haemangioendothelioma). In these 17 patients 11 retransplants were performed, all for DR: seven second OLT, three third OLT, and one fourth OLT. Therefore in these 17 patients 28 allografts could be examined for the development of non-anastomotic large bile duct strictures.

Methods

DR was defined as described, and included the loss of more than 50% of interlobular and septal bile ducts on subsequent liver biopsies[16]. Protocol liver biopsies were performed on days 7 and 21, at 3, 6 and 12 months and then yearly. Routine cholangiograms were performed at day 10 and at 3 months. Additional investigations were performed as indicated. Routine immunosuppression consisted of cyclosporin A, prednisone and, from OLT 90 on, azathioprine. Twice-weekly routine rapid 'shell-vial' blood cultures for cytomegalovirus (CMV) were performed. Liver biopsies were stained for CMV detection. Thrice-weekly cultures were taken from all sites, including from bile. In patients with PSC a Roux-en-Y biliodigestive anastomosis, and in most other patients a bile duct-to-bile-duct anastomosis had been performed.

RESULTS

In six out of the 17 patients with DR non-anastomotic large bile duct strictures (LBS) were detected on serial cholangiograms. An example cholangiogram from one of these patients is shown in Fig. 1. In three out of these six patients LBS occurred in the first allograft; in the three other patients LBS occurred in the second allograft (in one of these patients LBS developed in the third allograft as well). Out of the eight patients with DR after OLT for PSC, five developed LBS as well, while this was the case in only one out of nine patients with DR after OLT for other underlying liver diseases ($p < 0.05$). Out of the six patients with both DR and LBS, five had PSC and one had CAH as underlying liver disease. Cold ischaemia time was less than 11 h in the five PSC patients and was close to 12 h in the CAH patient. No hepatic artery thrombosis and no bacterial cholangitis occurred in this group, and no relation to CMV infection was found. One patient who underwent OLT for PSC experienced DR in his first, second and third allograft, with LBS in the second and third transplant liver; in this patient neither DR nor

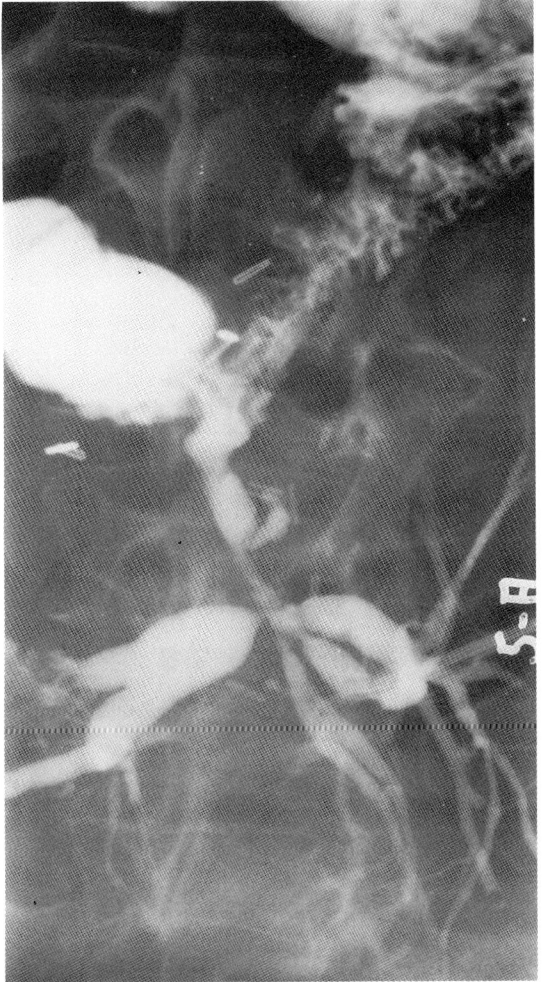

Fig. 1 Cholangiogram with non-anastomotic large bile duct stricturing in a hepatic allograft with ductopenic rejection developing after liver transplantation for primary sclerosing cholangitis. Recurrence of PSC?

LBS recurred in his fourth liver allograft when FK506 and prednisone were used as immunosuppression. The first time rejection was detected by liver biopsy was median 8 days after OLT (range 7–126 days), ductopenia was diagnosed at a median $2\frac{3}{4}$ months (range $1\frac{1}{2}$–14 months) after OLT. On the serial cholangiograms LBS were detected median $3\frac{1}{2}$ months (range $\frac{3}{4}$–10 months) after OLT.

Table 1 Timing of histology of rejection, of ductopenia, and of non-anastomotic biliary stricturing after liver transplantation in six patients (seven grafts) developing ductopenic rejection coinciding with non-anastomotic stricturing of large bile ducts

Patient, graft number	Rejection (days after OLT)	Ductopenia (days after OLT)	Biliary strictures (months after OLT)
A, 2	7	109	2
B, 1	7	61	3.5
C, 2	8	109	10
D, 2	126	419	8
D, 3	14	105	1.5
E, 1	8	42	3.5
F, 1	8	42	3
Median	8	105 ($2\frac{3}{4}$ months)	$3\frac{1}{2}$
Range	7–126	42–419 ($1\frac{1}{2}$–14 months)	$\frac{3}{4}$–10

CONCLUSIONS

We previously showed that PSC as the underlying liver disease is an independent risk factor for development of DR after liver transplantation. We now show that non-anastomotic strictures of the large bile ducts can develop in patients with DR after OLT, and that such a combination of DR and large bile duct strictures is strongly correlated to PSC as the underlying liver disease. In the one patient with CAH as the underlying liver disease a prolonged ischaemia time may have caused the bile duct strictures. Furthermore, while histology compatible with rejection preceded biliary stricturing in all patients, histology of ductopenia occurred simultaneously with biliary stricturing. Thus, histology of DR, especially in combination with non-anastomotic strictures of larger bile ducts after OLT for PSC, may very well represent recurrence of PSC in the allograft. Immunologically mediated arteriopathy leading to ischaemia of bile ducts may, at least in part, be responsible for these lesions[17,18] and possibly also for PSC. Protocol liver biopsies and cholangiograms may add to early detection of this complication[16,19], allowing for early percutaneous, endoscopic or surgical treatment[15,20–22]. Especially when steroid-resistant rejection or biliary stricturing after OLT for PSC develop, this may represent recurrent PSC, and early augmented immunosuppression (e.g. early conversion to FK 506) should be considered.

References

1. Wiesner RH, Ludwig J, van Hoek B, Krom RAF. Current concepts in cell-mediated hepatic allograft rejection leading to ductopenia and liver failure. Hepatology. 1991;14:721–9.
2. van Hoek B, Wiesner RH, Ludwig J, Paya C. Recurrence of ductopenic rejection in liver allografts after retransplantation for vanishing bile duct syndrome. Transplant Proc. 1991;23:1442–3.
3. van Hoek B, Wiesner RH, Ludwig J, Gores GJ, Moore SB, Krom RAF. Combination immunosuppression with azathioprine reduces the incidence of ductopenic rejection and

vanishing bile duct syndrome after liver transplantation. Transplant Proc. 1991;23:1403–5.
4. van Hoek B, Wiesner RH, Krom RAF, Ludwig J, Moore SB. Severe ductopenic rejection following liver transplantation: incidence, time of onset, risk factors, treatment, and outcome. Semin Liver Dis. 1992;12:41–50.
5. Klein SA, Savader S, Burdick JF *et al.* Reduction of morbidity and mortality from biliary complications after liver transplantation. Hepatology. 1991;14:818–23.
6. Sanchez-Urdazpal L, Gores GJ, Ward EM *et al.* Ischemic-type biliary complications after orthotopic liver transplantation. Hepatology. 1992;16:49–53.
7. Sanchez-Urdazpal L, Gores GJ, Ward EM *et al.* Clinical outcome of ischemic-type biliary complications after orthotopic liver transplantation. Transplant Proc. 1993;25:1107–9.
8. Sanchez-Urdazpal L, Gores GJ, Ward EM *et al.* Diagnostic features and clinical outcome of ischemic-type biliary complications after liver transplantation. Hepatology. 1993;17:605–9.
9. Colonna JO, Skaked A, Gomes AS *et al.* Biliary strictures complicating liver transplantation. Incidence, pathogenesis, management and outcome. Ann Surg. 1992;216:344–52.
10. Sankary HN, McChesney L, Hart M, Foster P, Williams J. Identification of donor and recipient risk factors associated with nonanastomotic biliary strictures in human hepatic allografts. Transplant Proc. 1993;25:1964–7.
11. Adam R, Bismuth H, Diamond T *et al.* Effect of extended cold ischemia with UW solution on graft function after liver transplantation. Lancet. 1992;340:1313–16.
12. Sanchez-Urdazpal L, Sterioff S, Janes C, Schwerman L, Rosen C, Krom RAF. Increased bile duct complications in ABO incompatible liver transplant recipients. Transplant Proc. 1991;23:1440–1.
13. Gugenheim J, Samuel D, Reynes M, Bismuth H. Liver transplantation across ABO blood group barriers. Lancet. 1990;336:519–23.
14. Worster AS, Ghent CN. Cholangiographic appearances of ductular rejection of ABO-incompatible liver transplants. J Clin Gastroenterol. 1992;15:222–4.
15. Ward EM, Kiely MJ, Maus TP, Wiesner RH, Krom RAF. Hilar biliary strictures after liver transplantation: cholangiography and percutaneous treatment. Radiology. 1990;177:259–63.
16. Wiesner RH, Ludwig J, Krom RAF, Hay JE, van Hoek B. Hepatic allograft rejection: new developments in terminology, diagnosis, prevention and treatment. Mayo Clin Proc. 1993;68:69–79.
17. Oguma S, Belle S, Starzl TE, Demetris AJ. A histometric analysis of chronically rejected human liver allografts: insights into the mechanisms of bile duct loss: direct immunologic and ischemic factors. Hepatology. 1989;9:204–9.
18. Wiesner RH, van Hoek B, Ludwig J *et al.* Foam cell arteriopathy in hepatic allografts: incidence, relationship to severe ductopenic rejection, and the sensitivity of needle biopsy for diagnosis. Hepatology. 1992;16:292A(abstr.).
19. van Hoek B, Wiesner RH, Ludwig J, Krom RAF. The role of protocol liver biopsies in diagnosis and treatment of early cellular rejection after orthotopic liver transplantation. Hepatology. 1990;12:866 (abstr.).
20. Ward EM, Wiesner RH, Hughes RW, Krom RAF. Persistent bile leak after liver transplantation: biloma drainage and endoscopic retrograde cholangiopancreatographic sphincterotomy. Radiology. 1991;179:719–20.
21. Zajko AB, Campbell WL, Bron KM *et al.* Cholangiography and interventional biliary radiology in adult liver transplantation. Am J Roentgenol. 1985;144:127–33.
22. Langnas AN, Stratta RJ, Wood RP, Ozaki CF, Bynon JS, Shaw BW. The role of intrahepatic cholangiojejunostomy in liver transplant recipients after extensive destruction of the extrahepatic biliary system. Surgery. 1992;112:712–18.

Section V
Gallbladder and bile duct stones: epidemiology and treatment

33
Epidemiology of gallstone disease

E. RODA, D. FESTI, S. SOTTILI, A. SANGERMANO, A. COLECCHIA,
M. ORSINI and the M.I.COL. GROUP*

In spite of several studies published in recent decades on the epidemiology[1], pathophysiology, diagnosis and treatment of gallstone disease[2], the natural history and risk factors of this disorder are still not fully understood. The difficulty in drawing a definitive conclusion is mainly due to the lack of standardized methods, definitions and selection of patients in the presently available studies. Thus, prognosis of gallstone patients represents a difficult problem to resolve. The introduction of ultrasonography (US) as a sensitive and accurate diagnostic tool for gallstone recognition has allowed cross-sectional and longitudinal studies on the general population that opened a new era in gallstone epidemiology. Previous approaches to gallstone disease using clinically diagnosed cases or necroscopy data, although useful in performing historical comparisons of gallbladder disease rates, and in identifying ethnic/racial differences, were unable to evaluate the true prevalence of the disease in the general population, and suffered from potential referral bias and from the underestimation of clinically 'silent stones'[3].

This chapter discusses the preliminary results of the Multicenter Italian Study on Cholelithiasis (M.I.COL.) compared with those obtained in the previous epidemiological studies realized in the earlier 1980s in Italy, the GREPCO[4] and Sirmione[5] studies, since the M.I.C.O.L. study had a similar experimental model, e.g. cross-sectional and longitudinal phases, use of ultrasonography and dietary investigation, but was performed on a larger population.

The M.I.COL. study was designed to obtain a broad representative general population sample which would permit an overview of gallstone disease in Italy. This study involves 18 operative units covering almost all Italian regions; each operative unit enrolled 2000 males and 1300 females aged from 30 to 69 years, using electoral rolls in cities and from the Municipal Census in smaller towns. The screening protocol included a questionnaire, a US investigation of the upper abdomen, a physical examination and a blood

---

*For the composition of the M.I.COL. Group, see Appendix.

Table 1 M.I.COL.: prevalence of gallstone disease

Patients	Number	Percentage
Normals	25 453	86.0
Gallstones	2 472	8.3
Cholecystectomized	1 617	5.5
Biliary sludge	53	0.2
Total	29 595	100

Table 2 M.I.COL.: frequency of biliary pain (percentages) ($n = 29\,595$)

Subjects	Normal	Gallstone	Cholecystectomized
Symptomatic	6.2	14.2	64.4
Asymptomatic	93.8	85.8	35.6

sample taken in the fasting condition. The precoded questionnaire inquired about social and demographic data, medical and family history, and dietary habits. The cross-sectional phase was carried out in 1985–86 and the longitudinal one is ongoing. From 54 040 individuals of both sexes a total of 33 494 subjects were examined, of whom 29 595 were suitable for statistical analysis. Four operative units were excluded from analysis due to their low attendance rate (<60%). A quality control programme on all biochemical analyses was implemented under the supervision of the Biochemical Laboratory of the National Institute of Health. The inter- and intra-observer variation in the US detection of gallstones was assessed by means of a reliability study[6].

To date overall prevalence of gallstone disease is 13.8% (8.3% with gallstones, 5.5% with previous cholecystectomies for gallstones) (Table 1). The prevalence was higher in females (18.8%) than in males (9.5%) and increased linearly with age in both sexes.

Parity, familiality, obesity and serum levels of triglycerides proved to be significantly associated with gallstone disease, while the use of oral contraceptives and cholesterol serum levels appeared to be inversely related.

Since high energy intake is associated with an increased risk of gallstone disease[1], the precoded questionnaire included a list of 38 food items, and subjects were asked how often they consumed each item. A commonly used unit of portion size was identified. The preliminary results do not confirm that high energy intake is associated with an increased risk of gallstone; low carbohydrate and protein intake, high fibre and moderate alcohol consumption seem to be factors protecting against gallstones[7].

According to previous epidemiological studies[4,5] specific biliary symptoms were defined as a pain in the right hypochondrium and/or epigastrium, lasting more than $\frac{1}{2}$ h. Other digestive symptoms such as bloating, fatty food intolerance, etc., were considered non-specific biliary symptoms since, in agreement with previous studies, their frequency was similar in normals and gallstone patients. Table 2 shows biliary pain frequency in normals, gallstone and cholecystectomized patients, and confirms that the majority of gallstone patients are asymptomatic (up to 80%); cholecystectomized patients presented

Table 3 M.I.COL: frequency of biliary pain and awareness in gallstone patients (percentages) ($n = 2472$)

	Asymptomatic	Symptomatic
Aware	72.8	27.2
Unaware	90.3	9.7

a very high frequency of specific biliary symptoms (72.5%) before surgery.

Awareness seems to be an important factor for the presence of biliary pain: gallstone patients aware of having gallstones report biliary pain more frequently, as shown in Table 3. However, these data show that frequency of biliary pain in aware patients is lower (27.2%) than that reported in the Sirmione study (63.0%)[8].

In order to obtain information regarding gallbladder function and physico-chemical characteristics of gallstones, US-positive subjects underwent oral cholecystography. In 21.2% the gallbladder was not visualized; in 78.8% the gallbladder was visualized. Radiolucent gallstones accounted for 66.6% and mixed gallstones for 21.3%. From these data we observe a high prevalence of mixed gallstones in our population even if radiolucent gallstones are the most frequent ones.

The longitudinal phase of the M.I.COL. study is ongoing, and will finish in late 1995. However, preliminary results regarding incidence rate and natural history are currently available for one operative unit (Brisighella). The cumulative incidence rate after 8 years is 4.8% (0.6%/year).

Natural history shows that in symptomatic gallstone patients the recurrence rate of biliary pain after 4 years is 53.3%, and during the next 4 years it decreases to 33.3%; in asymptomatic patients the rate of developing biliary pain after 4 years is 23.3%, and it increases to 32.5% in the following 4 years. These preliminary results are in agreement with those observed in Sirmione[8], confirming that the natural history of asymptomatic patients is benign, and suggesting that the natural history of symptomatic patients is better than previously expected.

In conclusion, epidemiological studies, performed on a very large population, such as M.I.COL., show that prevalence of gallstone disease is higher if compared to the clinically expected one, and confirm that this disease may be considered a 'mass disease', like obesity, diabetes and atherosclerosis. Furthermore these data indicate the possible existence of environmental and behavioural causes.

Cross-sectional studies cannot identify those relationships which can be evaluated by longitudinal studies. The identification of risk factors for the disease could allow the planning of preventive programmes in the near future.

One of the aims of the epidemiological studies is to evaluate the frequency of symptoms in the natural history of the disease. This knowledge is extremely important in clinical decision-making. As far as gallstone disease is concerned, epidemiological studies have clearly shown that the majority of patients are without specific biliary symptoms, i.e. biliary colic.

The available evidence indicates that the natural history of asymptomatic gallstone patients is benign; consequently these patients need no therapy. For symptomatic gallstones the choice of treatment should focus on two different goals: (a) preventing biliary pain, (b) preventing future biliary complications or death. Based on these considerations, clinicians may consider a spectrum of alternatives for symptomatic gallstone patients: expectant management, bile acid therapy alone or with lithotripsy for the best candidates, and open or laparoscopic cholecystectomy, but only when the surgeon's experience is well established. The results of ongoing studies on a large number of subjects, such as the M.I.COL. study, will probably answer most of the unsolved questions related to epidemiology, prevention and overall management of this disease in the near future.

Appendix: Composition of the research group of the Italian Multicenter Study on Epidemiology of Cholelithiasis

Operative Unit of Bari
III Clinica Medica, Università di Bari. *Directors*: O. Albano, G. Palasciano; *Principal investigators*: G. Calò Gabrieli, P. Portincasa, S. Tardi; *Biochemical staff*: G. Vendemiale, A. Velardi; *Field staff*: V. Vinciguerra, G. Baldassarre, C. Origilia, V. Palmieri, N. Morelli, A. Belfiore.

Operative Unit of Bologna I
Clinical Medica I, Università di Bologna. *Director*: L. Barbara; *Principal investigator*: E. Roda; *Biochemical staff*: M. S. Benassi, M. Forni; *Field staff*: C. Sama, D. Festi, A. M. Morselli-Labate, M. C. Nacchiero, S. Parro, G. Pollini, M. Rossi, A. G. Rusticali, G. Tassinari, G. Canè, B. Crinò, O. Masiello, D. Panuccio, A. Romani, R. Romanelli

Operative Unit of Bologna II
Istituto di Patologia Speciale Medica II e Medicina del Lavoro; *Cattedra di Gastroenterologia, Università di Bologna. *Directors*: A. Gaddi, E. Roda*; *Principal investigators*: A. Dormi, D. Festi*; *Biochemical staff*: Z. Sangiorgi, G. Copparoni, R. Mambelli; *Field staff*: B. Benassi, M. D. Ceccardi, S. D'Addato, G. De Simone, L. Finazzo, C. Mussoni, D. Pomata, S. Rimondi, N. Scoz, C. Alberghini, L. Lolli, Y. Piazzi, E. Stagni, M. Nanni, S. Bagnoli, F. Bonafé, M. Fedeli, A. Sangermano*, M. Orsini*, S. Sottili*, A. Colecchia*

Operative Unit of Bologna III
Cattedra di Gastroenterologia; *Dipartimento di Scienze Statistiche, Università di Bologna. *Directors*: E. Roda, I. Scardovi; *Supervisor*: A. Menotti. *Principal investigators*: P. Monari*, D. Festi; *Field staff*: A. Cazzola*, S. Mignani*, A. Montanari*, R. Miglio*, A. Sangermano, A. Colecchia, M. Orsini, S. Sottili, A. M. Morselli Labate.

Operative Unit of Bolzano
Divisione di Gastroenterologia, Ospedale General Regionale, Bolzano. *Director*: G. Dobrilla; *Principal investigators*: M. Valentini, G. De Pretis; *Biochemical staff*: U. Gaspa; *Field staff*: S. Amplatz, S. Benvenuti, I. Bresolin.

Operative Unit of Cagliari
Divisione di Medicina Interna, Centro per la Lotta contro l'Arteriosclerosi, Ospedale Brotzu, Cagliari. *Director*: S. Muntoni; *Principal investigator*: F. Pintus; *Biochemical staff*: F. Pintus; *Field staff*: P. Pintus, P. Mascia, E. Ganga, R. Ganga, P. Tronci, G. Cabiddu

Operative Unit of Castellana Grotte
Ospedale Spec. in Gastroenterologia, IRCCS, Castellana Grotte. *Director*: I. Giorgio; *Principal investigator*: G. Misciagna; *Biochemical staff*: C. Messa, V. Mangini; *Field staff*: G. Angelelli, S. Elba, A. Mossa, M. Noviello, J. Petruzzi

Operative Unit of Como
Divisione di Medicina Interna, Ospedale Niguarda, Milano. *Director:* G. Ideo; *Principal investigators:* G. Ideo, B. Caspani; *Biochemical staff:* M. Cavalleri; *Field staff:* B. Caspani, A. Molteni, A. Stefini, G. B. Molteni, D. Albonico, G. Alfieri, D. Gola, M. Guanziroli, G. Carrara, L. Snider, G. Restelli

Operative Unit of Ferrara
Istituto di Clinica Medica, Università di Ferrara e I Divisione Medicina Arcispedale S. Anna, Ferrara. *Director:* V. Alvisi; *Principal investigator:* P. Pazzi; *Biochemical staff:* G. Guerra, D. Frenzé; *Field staff:* F. Pavani, M. Massari, S. Putinati, M. Vincenzi, A. Laterza, D. Ferraresi, I. Caberletti, C. Andreati, L. Trevisani, G. Bozzolani, A. Zangirolami, D. Sighinolfi, G. Stabellini, A. D'Ambrosi

Operative Unit of Firenze
Istituto Clinica Medica IV, Università di Firenze. *Director:* P. Gentilini; *Principal investigators:* G. Buzzelli, F. Curradi; *Biochemical staff:* C. Ignesti; *Field staff:* P. Bandini, L. La Villa, U. Arena, C. Smorlesi, C. Bonechi, D. Coletta, D. Mondenelli, G. Parronchi, L. Mondelli, E. Calabresi

Operative Unit of Milano
Clinical Medica III, Università di Milano. *Director:* M. Podda; *Principal investigator:* M. Zuin; *Biochemical staff:* U. Alieri; *Field staff:* P. M. Battezzati, E. Bertolini, A. Crosignani, C. De Fazio, G. Grandinetti, A. Camisasca, C. Caserta, M. L. Petroni, P. Roccucci

Operative Unit of Modena I
Istituto di Clinica Medica I, Università di Modena. *Director:* N. Carulli; *Principal investigators;* P. Loria, D. Menozzi; *Biochemical staff:* G. Grossi; *Field staff:* G. Medici, A. Tripodi, L. Roncucci, M. Montanari, P. Di Donato, M. Iori, A. Digrisolo, R. Iori, V. Boraldi, D. Gollini, C. Sacche

Operative Unit of Modena II
Istituto Clinica Medica, Università di Modena. *Director:* G. Salvioli; *Principal investigator:* R. Lugli; *Biochemical staff:* A. Carbonieri, E. Gaetti; *Field staff:* G. Basi, E. Tondelli, V. Boccaletti, A. Frignani, J. Pradelli

Operative Unit of Napoli
Istituto di Medicina Interna e Malattie Metaboliche, II Facoltà, Università di Napoli. *Director:* M. Mancini; *Principal investigators:* E. Farinaro, F. Contaldo; *Biochemical staff:* G. De Biase; *Field staff:* N. Maturo, A. Cecere, G. Fusco, G. Di Biase

Operative Unit of Padova
Istituto di Medicina Interna, Università di Padova. *Directors:* L. Okolicsanyi, G. Crepaldi; *Principal investigators:* A. Burlina, C. Zacchi, G. Rampazzo; *Biochemical staff:* G. De Franchis, N. Di Vitofrancesco; *Field staff:* G. Nassuato, F. Angelini, A. Fragasso, R. M. Iemmolo, M. Muraca, R. Orlando, D. Passera, M. Strazzabosco

Operative Unit of Pietra Ligure
Ospedale Santa Corona, Divisione di Medicina Generale, Pietra Ligure. *Director:* G. Marenco; *Principal investigator:* G. Marenco; *Biochemical staff:* L. Santorirella; *Field staff:* P. Colombo, A. Artom, A. Giudici Cipriani, U. Forlo

Operative Unit of Roma I
II Cattedra di Gastroenterologia, Clinica Medica III, Università di Roma "La Sapienza". *Director:* L. Capocaccia; *Principal investigator:* A. F. Attili; *Biochemical staff:* G. Pinto; *Field staff:* A. De Santis, S. Ginanni Corradini, C. De Luca, A. Romiti, E. Scafato, D. Porto, R. Capri, A. Cantagalli, E. Giuliani, F. Giambenedetti, A. Rosati, S. Gualandi, P. Pallotto

Operative Unit of Roma II
Istituto di Terapia Medica Sistematica, Università di Roma "La Sapienza". *Director:* G. Ricci; *Principal investigator:* L. Lalloni; *Biochemical staff:* R. Antonini, R. Cantini, S. Ciocca, B.

Mazzarella, F. Pacioni, A. Zucca; *Field staff:* G. Argento, A. Azzarri, L. Azzarri, L. Bava, A. Bucci, R. Conti, I. De Felici, D. Degano, G. Graziani, L. Martini, A. Montali, P. Palombo, F. Pelliccia, G. Prosperi, B. Quattrini, P. Ricci, F. Ricciardi, G. Santoboni, A. Scarno, M. Valeo

Operative Unit of Roma III
Laboratorio di Epidemiologia e Biostatistica, Istituto Superiore di Sanità Roma. *Director:* A. Menotti; *Principal investigators:* R. Capocaccia, S. Mariotti, F. Taroni, F. Valente

Operative Unit of Roma IV
Laboratorio di Biochimica Clinica, Istituto Superiore di Sanità, Roma. *Director:* G. Morisi; *Principal investigator:* G. Morisi; *Biochemical staff:* A. M. Buongiorno

Operative Unit of Verona
Istituto di Clinica Medica, Università di Verona. *Directors:* L. A. Scuro, G. Angelini; *Principal investigator:* G. Angelini; *Biochemical staff:* M. Zatti; *Field staff:* G. Antolini, A. Bonioli, E. Bottona, A. Castagnini, G. Degani, G. Di Stefano, A. Fratta Pasini, E. Lavarini, G. Montagnoli, S. Perbellini, G. Pisani, L. Rigo, P. Rizzini, T. Sandrini, M. Sciortino, N. Tallon, D. Zordan

References

1. Capocaccia L, Ricci G, Angelico F, Angelico M, Attili AF, Lalloni L, editors. Recent advances in the epidemiology and prevention of gallstone disease. Dordrecht: Kluwer; 1991.
2. Diehl AK. Epidemiology and natural history of gallstone disease. Gastroenterol Clin N Am. 1991;20:1–19.
3. Gracie WA, Ransohoff DF. The natural history of silent gallstones. The 'innocent' gallstone is not a myth. N Engl J Med. 1982;307:798–800.
4. Rome Group for the Epidemiology and Prevention of Cholelithiasis (GREPCO). Prevalence of gallstone disease in an Italian adult female population. Am J Epidemiol. 1984;119: 796–805.
5. Barbara L, Sama C, Morselli-Labate AM *et al.* A population study on the prevalence of gallstone disease: the Sirmione study. Hepatology. 1987;7:913–17.
6. Festi D, Lalloni L, Taroni F and the M.I.COL. Study Group. The inter- and intra-observer variation in ultrasonographic detection of gallstones: the Multicenter Italian Study on Epidemiology of Cholelithiasis (M.I.COL.). Eur J Epidemiol. 1989;5:1:51–7.
7. Attili AF, Marchioli R, Scafato E, Marfisi RM and the M.I.COL. Group. Dietary habits and gallstones (GS) in the M.I.COL. study. Gastroenterology. 1993;104(Suppl. 4):A873(abstr.).
8. Sama C, Barbara L, Festi D *et al.* Natural history of gallstone disease: the Sirmione study. In: Capocaccia L, Ricci G, Angelico F, Angelico N, Attili AF, Lalloni L, editors. Recent advances in the epidemiology and prevention of gallstone disease. Dordrecht: Kluwer; 1991:51–5.

34
Duodenal diverticula are associated with pancreatic, biliary and intestinal anomalies

J. P. VAN BASTEN, P. CAENEPEEL, R. ZEIJEN and
R. W. STOCKBRÜGGER

INTRODUCTION

The existence of duodenal diverticula (DD) was first described by Chomel in 1710 and Morgagni in 1762[1,2]. A prevalence of DD of 11–22% has been reported from post-mortem results[3,4]. The prevalence of DD detected by endoscopic retrograde cholangiopancreatography (ERCP) varies from 5% to 23%[5–8]. Several studies indicate that the presence of DD increases with age[5,6].

In 1970 Pinotti et al. described an association between DD and pancreato-biliary (PB) disorders[7]. In 1981 Osnes et al. reported an increased frequency of biliary calculi, especially common bile duct stones (CBDS), in the presence of DD[8]. Also in 1981 Loveit et al. reported a predominance of pigment stones in the common bile ducts of patients with DD, while cholesterol calculi were more frequent in patients without DD[9,10].

Earlier, in 1966, Maki stated that pigment stones were associated with ascending infections of the biliary tract, caused by β-glucuronidase-producing bacteria[11]. Hydrolysing bilirubineglucuronidate bacterial contamination of the bile duct in patients with DD has also been demonstrated by Loveit et al.; Escherichia coli was the predominant species found in this study[12–14]. In 1986 Skar et al. performed bacterial cultures from bile of patients with CBDS, comparing these with bacterial cultures from duodenal aspirate in the same patients[13,14].

The bacteria cultured from bile were similar to those cultured from duodenal fluid and were frequently β-glucuronidase-producing[13,14]. This finding suggests reflux of β-glucuronidase-producing bacteria from the duodenum into the biliary tract. Periampullary diverticula, interfering with the function of the sphincter of Oddi, could facilitate such reflux. Loveit et al. and Kubota et al. independently reported (after performing manometric studies of the Oddi's sphincter) DD to be associated with papillary dysfunction[15,16].

Endoscopic papillotomy (EPT) has the consequence of papillary insufficiency, and in this way may also cause ascending biliary infection. In the study of Skar *et al.* bacterial growth in the duodenum and in the bile of patients with common bile duct calculi treated with EPT was studied, and the same type of bacteria were found in duodenum and bile[17].

Another hypothesis suggests stasis of duodenal contents and bezoar formation in DD, with resulting papillitis and cholestasis, as an aetiological factor in gallstone formation[18]. Kimura *et al.* studied the relationship between histological changes of the papilla of Vater and DD. No significant relationship was found between DD and the histology of the papilla of Vater[19].

If DD predispose to the occurrence of biliary calculi, recurrence of gallstones should be more frequent in cholecystectomized patients. This hypothesis was corroborated by Loveit *et al.*, who reported that patients with juxtapapillary DD more frequently developed recurrent biliary calculi after cholecystectomy than did patients without DD[20].

While the association between biliary calculi and DD is accepted, the association of DD and pancreatic disorders is still a matter of controversy[18,21]. With regard to duodenal inflammation and the presence of DD, no association was found by Van der Spuy[22].

This retrospective study was performed to further evaluate the association of DD with pancreatobiliary (PB) disorders diagnosed by ERCP, and to study the relationship, if any, between DD and duodenal mucosal pathology.

METHODS

Retrospectively all reports on complete endoscopic retrograde cholangiopancreaticographies (ERCP), for the years 1991 and 1992 at the University Hospital Maastricht, were reviewed for the presence of DD and concomitant PB or upper gastrointestinal pathology. From patient records the following data were recorded: age, sex, medical history, endoscopic findings, presence or absence of DD and their relationship to the papilla of Vater. If an ERCP examination was performed more than once in a patient, only the first results were reported.

For statistical analysis the SPSS V3.1 was used. The chi-square test, corrected for data size (Yate's correction), was used to test differences in frequencies. The *t*-test was used in the analysis of age in the relationship to duodenal diverticula. All tests used were two-tailed.

RESULTS

The mean age of the 273 patients was 64 (SD $\pm$ 15) years, with a range of 19–93 years and a male:female ratio of 1:1.9. Cannulation of the common bile duct failed in 19 cases (7%) (three of them had DD), and in 31 cases

Table 1 ERCP findings 1991–92 ($n = 273$), Academic Hospital, Maastricht

Duodenal diverticula	Present ($n = 49$)	Absent ($n = 224$)	p
Mean age ($\pm$ SD)	69 ± 12	63 ± 15	0.008
Male : female ratio	1 : 2	1 : 1.9	0.950
Previous cholecystectomy ($n = 58$)	11 (22.4)	47 (21.0)	0.820
Previous papillotomy ($n = 51$)	2 (28.6)	49 (17.7)	0.808
Biliary pathology			
Gallbladder stones ($n = 38$)	8 (16.3)	30 (13.4)	0.862
Common duct stones ($n = 75$)	26 (53.1)	49 (21.9)	0.000
Dilated bile ducts ($n = 95$)	27 (55.1)	68 (30.4)	0.004
Pancreatic pathology			
Dilated duct ($n = 17$)	4 (8.2)	13 (5.8)	0.367
Irregular duct ($n = 24$)	6 (12.2)	18 (8.0)	0.267
Intestinal pathology			
Duodenitis ($n = 23$)	8 (16.3)	15 (6.7)	0.056
Duodenal ulcer ($n = 11$)	7 (14.3)	4 (1.8)	0.000

Figures in parentheses are percentages.

(11.4%) the pancreatic duct was not visualized (eight of these patients had DD). In 49 patients (18%) DD were seen: in 30 cases (61%) the diverticulum was localized juxtapapillary, and in 18 cases (37%) the papilla of Vater was located within the diverticulum (circumpapillary). One patient (2%) had both types. The mean age of patients having a DD was significantly higher than that of patients without DD (69 vs 63 years, t-test; $p < 0.05$). Gender did not predispose to developing DD (Table 1).

The prevalence of biliary concrements was higher in patients with DD than in those without. There was a significant increase in CBDS in patients with DD compared to those without (53% versus 22%; $p < 0.05$). With regard to gallbladder stones no difference was seen between patients with and without DD. Eighteen patients had gallbladder stones as well as concomitant CBDS.

Although CBDS appeared more frequently in patients with circumpapillary DD (68.8%), than in those with juxtapapillary DD (50%), this difference was not significant ($p = 0.363$).

In the group of cholecystectomized patients ($n = 58$) CBDS were diagnosed in two patients with and in three patients without DD; figures too small for statistical analysis.

In this study a previous papillotomy was not related to biliary calculi ($p = 0.693$ for CBDS; $p = 0.703$ for gallbladder stones).

Pancreatic pathology ($n = 41$) was more frequently present in patients with DD, but this result did not reach significance ($p = 0.441$).

Duodenitis and duodenal ulcers ($n = 31$) were significantly more frequent in patients with DD ($n = 15$) than in those without ($n = 19$) (16.3% versus 6.7% for duodenitis, $p = 0.05$; 14.3% versus 1.8% for duodenal ulcers, $p < 0.05$).

DISCUSSION

In this retrospective study 273 ERCP examinations were reviewed for the presence of DD and concomitant pancreatobiliary and duodenal pathology. The prevalence of DD was 18%. The presence of CBDS was significantly related to the presence of DD. No significant association between DD and pancreatic anomalies could be established. DD were also associated with duodenal inflammation. Previous endoscopic papillotomy was not related to the presence of biliary calculi.

The prevalence of DD in this patient group is in agreement with previous ERCP studies[5,24]. A higher prevalence was found in post-mortem studies. As the prevalence of DD seems to increase with age this factor may also account for the difference of DD prevalence in ERCP and post-mortem studies[3-5,24].

In agreement with previous reports this study showed that there was a positive relationship between CBDS and DD, but gallbladder stones were not related to DD[24,25]. This fact supports the assumption that, in patients with DD, calculi in the common bile duct might have an aetiological background other than gallbladder concrements.

Contrary to the findings in earlier reports we could not establish the recurrence of bile stones in the common bile duct after cholecystectomy in patients with DD, but perhaps the number of patients in this study was too small to draw firm conclusions[20,26].

We have not found any significant association between the presence of DD and pancreatic pathology as had been previously suggested, but not confirmed in more recent reports[18,21-23].

In our study a significant relationship was present between duodenal inflammation, duodenal ulcers and the presence of DD. Formerly, as far as we know, this relationship was studied only by Van der Spuy; in that study 111 patients with endoscopically proven duodenal ulcers were screened for DD. DD were present in three cases (2.1%)[22]. However, this study is not in disagreement with our finding that duodenal ulcers were significantly associated with DD.

We hypothesize that stasis of food remnants in the diverticulum may cause pressure on the duodenal wall, disturbing the mucosal circulation and leading to inflammation. Bacterial overgrowth in DD may be another aetiological factor in duodenal ulcer formation. CBDS in patients with DD may also contribute to a diminished flow of bicarbonate-containing pancreatic fluids, impairing neutralization of gastric acid in the duodenum.

Because it was suggested in other studies that EPT (as well as DD) might facilitate the reflux of duodenal contents into the biliary tract, and thus predispose to biliary calculi, we studied the relationship between EPT, biliary calculi and dilated bile ducts. There was no significant association between EPT and biliary pathology[13,17].

In conclusion, this study confirms the relationship between DD and CBDS. We report a significant relationship between DD and duodenal inflammation. The relationship between DD and duodenal ulcers needs further examination. Therefore it is important to report the presence of DD and/or duodenal inflammation at ERCP examinations.

References

1. Chomel JBL. Histoire de l'Academie Royale. Paris: L'Institute de France; Academie des Sciences; 1710–37.
2. Morgagni GB, De sedibus et causi morborum. Epist. 34:Par. 17. Naples, 1762.
3. Baldwin WM. Duodenal diverticula in man.,Ann Rec. 1911;5:121–39.
4. Ackerman W. Diverticula and variations of the duodenum. Ann Surg. 1943;117:403–13.
5. Kennedy RH, Thompson MH. Are duodenal diverticula associated with choledocholithiasis? Gut. 1988;29:1003–6.
6. Skar V, Loveit T, Osnes M. Juxtapapillary duodenal diverticula predispose to common bile duct stones. Scand J Gastroenterol. 1989;24:202–4.
7. Pinotti HW, Talca M, Pontes JF, Betarello A. Juxta-ampullary duodenal diverticula as cause of biliopancreatic disease. Digestion. 1971;4:353–61.
8. Osnes M, Loveit T, Larsen S, Aune S. Duodenal diverticula and their relation to age, sex, and biliary calculi. Scand J Gastroenterol. 1981;16:103–7.
9. Loveit T, Foss OP, Osnes M. Biliary pigment and cholesterol calculi in patients with and without juxtapapillary duodenal diverticula. Scand J Gastroenterol. 1981;16:241–4.
10. Loveit T. The composition of biliary calculi in patients with juxtapapillary duodenal diverticula. Scand J Gastroenterol. 1982;17:653–6.
11. Maki T. Pathogenesis of calcium bilirubinate gallstones: Role of *E. coli*, beta-glucuronidase and coagulation by inorganic ions, polyelectrolytes and agitation. Ann Surg. 1966;164:90–9.
12. Loveit T, Osnes M, Aune S. Bacteriologic studies of the common duct bile in patients with gallstone disease and juxtapapillary duodenal diverticula. Scand J Gastroenterol. 1978;13:93–5.
13. Skar V, Skar AG, Midtvedt T, Loveit T, Osnes M. Beta-glucuronidase-producing bacteria in bile from the common bile duct in patients treated with endoscopic papillotomy for gallstone disease. Scand J Gastroenterol. 1986;21:253–6.
14. Skar V, Skar AG, Bratlie J, Osnes M. Beta-glucuronidase activity in bile of gallstone patients both with and without duodenal diverticula. Scand J Gastroenterol. 1989;24:205–12.
15. Loveit T, Osnes M, Aune S, Larsen S. Studies of the choledocho-duodenal sphincter in patients with and without juxtapapillary duodenal diverticula. Scand J Gastroenterol. 1980;15:875–80.
16. Kubota K, Itoh T, Shibayama K, Shimada K, Nomura Y, Idezuki Y. Papillary function of patients with juxtapapillary duodenal diverticulum. Consideration of pathogenesis of common bile duct stones. Scand J Gastroenterol. 1989;24:140–4.
17. Skar V, Skar AG, Midtvedt T, Osnes M. Bacterial growth in the duodenum and in the bile of patients with gallstone disease treated with endoscopic papillotomy. Endoscopy. 1986;18:10–13.
18. Gudjonsson H, Gamelli RL, Kaye MD. Symptomatic biliary obstruction associated with juxtapapillary duodenal diverticulum. Dig Dis Sci. 1988;33:114–21.
19. Kimura W, Nagai H, Kuroda A, Muto T. No significant correlation between histologic changes of the papilla of Vater and juxtapapillary diverticulum. Special reference to the pathogenesis of gallstones. Scand J Gastroenterol. 1992;27:951–6.
20. Loveit T, Osnes M, Larsen S. Recurrent biliary calculi. Duodenal diverticula as predisposing factor. Ann Surg. 1982;196:30–2.
21. Shemesh E, Friedman E, Czerniak A, Bat L. The association of biliary and pancreatic anomalies with periampullary duodenal diverticula. Arch Surg. 1987;122:1055–7.
22. Van der Spuy S. The relation between juxtapapillary diverticula and biliary calculi. An endoscopic study. Endoscopy. 1979;3:197–202.
23. Manny J, Muga M, Eyal Z. The continuing clinical enigma of duodenal diverticulum. Am J Surg. 1981;142:596–600.
24. Hagége H, Berson A, Pelletier G *et al.* Association of juxtapapillary diverticula with choledocholithiasis but not with cholecystolithiasis. Endoscopy. 1992;24:248–51.
25. Hall RI, Ingoldby CJ, Denyer ME. Periampullary diverticula predispose to primary rather than secondary stones in the common bile duct. Endoscopy. 1990;22:127–8.
26. Kirk AP, Summerfield JA. Incidence and significance of juxtapapillary diverticula at endoscopic retrograde cholangiopancreatography. Digestion. 1980;20:31–5.

35
Pathogenesis of gallbladder stones and strategies for their prevention

R. H. DOWLING, S. H. HUSSAINI, S. P. PEREIRA, J. A. H. WASS and G. M. MURPHY

INTRODUCTION

To develop strategies for preventing the development of gallbladder stones (GBS), one *probably* needs to understand all the mechanisms involved in their pathogenesis. One then needs to weigh their relative importance, and decide if they can be manipulated, to counter their adverse effects. Thus, in the pathogenesis of cholesterol-rich GBS, we now recognize[1] that there is at least a triple defect:

1. Supersaturation of gallbladder bile with cholesterol $(CH)^2$,
2. A nucleation defect with an imbalance between promoters and inhibitors of CH microcrystal precipitation[3] and
3. Stasis of bile within the gallbladder.

These abnormalities are often depicted as a Venn diagram with three overlapping circles (Fig. 1). However, there are several variations on this triple defect theme. Carey, for example, has suggested that there is really a quintuple, rather than a triple, defect. He has proposed that the abnormalities should be represented, graphically, by five overlapping circles – like the rings of the Olympic symbol[4]. Thus, in addition to impaired gallbladder emptying (which is found in some[5,6], but not all[7-9], patients with cholesterol GBS), Carey has proposed that the gallbladder mucosa is covered by a mucus glycoprotein (MGP) gel which traps precipitated CH microcrystals. Indeed, the synthesis of MGP by the gallbladder mucosa is increased in CH-GBS disease[10]. The excess MGP not only forms a layer of crystal-trapping gel; it is also secreted into the bulk phase of bile. MGP is a potent promoter of CH microcrystal precipitation[11,12].

Although we suggested that one probably needs to understand *all* the pathogenetic mechanisms in gallstone formation, if it were possible to identify a final common pathway in the stone-forming process it might *not* be necessary to understand all the preceding steps. In other words, if one could

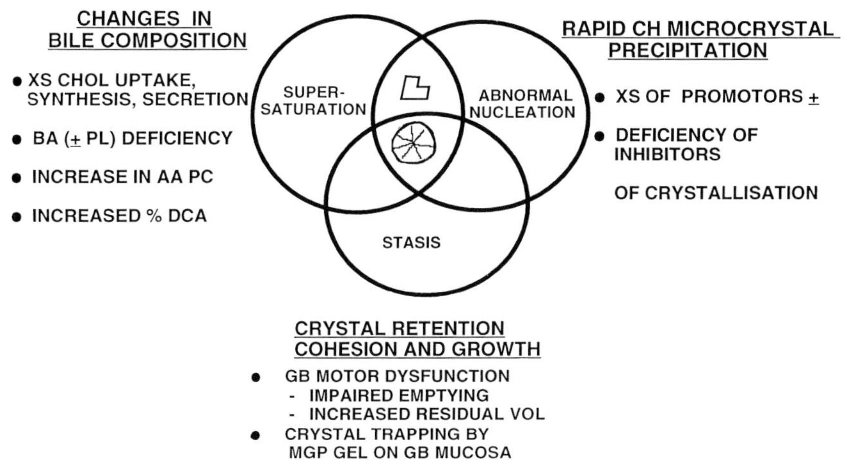

Fig. 1 Venn diagram illustrating, schematically, the triple defect in the pathogenesis of cholesterol-rich gallbladder stones (GBS). The symbols in the centre of the diagram represent a rhomboid-shaped cholesterol microcrystal with its notch and a gallstone with spoke-like, radiating fissures. XS = excess; GB = gallbladder; CHOL = cholesterol; BA = bile acids; PL = phospholipids; AA PC = arachidonic acid rich phosphatidyl choline; DCA = deoxycholic acid; Vol = volume; MGP = mucus glycoprotein

stimulate gallbladder emptying and ensure that any crystals which had precipitated would be expelled through the cystic duct[13,14], the presence of supersaturated gallbladder bile, and of a defect in CH microcrystal nucleation (or both), might not be important.

In addition to the defects already proposed there may be yet another abnormality – that of prolonged intestinal transit[15,16] – which, in theory, could be countered more easily than gallbladder hypomotility. This chapter deliberately emphasizes this abnormality – in part to make the point – although the relative importance of this defect, as opposed to the other two to four defects, is not yet clear.

Our own studies of GBS pathogenesis are based on two groups of patients at high risk of forming stones:

1. Acromegalic patients treated long term with octreotide – of whom up to 60% develop GBS within 2 years (primary stone formation)[17];
2. Those whose GBS were dissolved (with oral bile acids ± extra-corporeal shockwave lithotripsy (ESWL), or with contact solvents such as methyl tert-butyl ether (MTBE) or removed (by percutaneous cholecystolithotomy: PCCL), after which approximately 50% of patients develop recurrent stones (secondary gallstone formation) within 5 years[18-27].

THE PATHOGENESIS OF OCTREOTIDE-INDUCED GALLBLADDER STONES (OT-GBS)

Background

Octreotide (OT), a somatostatin analogue, is an effective treatment for acromegaly. It acts by suppressing the secretion of both growth hormone and insulin-like growth factor-I (IGF-I). However, it also inhibits meal-stimulated cholecystokinin (CCK) release from the intestine[28,29] and post-prandial gallbladder contraction[28-32] and, as noted above[17], it induces GBS in up to 60% of patients treated with daily OT for 2 years or more.

In theory, before cholesterol GBS can develop, all three (or more) components of the triple defect must coexist. In practice, it was believed that occasionally one of the three components could predominate and induce stone formation on its own[33]. Given the fact that OT virtually abolishes meal-stimulated gallbladder emptying[28-32], it was assumed that gallbladder stasis alone was enough to explain the high incidence of OT-GBS. However, the effects of somatostatin, and its analogue octreotide, on bile composition and physical chemistry had been largely ignored – despite a few earlier studies in animals[34-37] and man[38-42].

Methods

Therefore, in a series of experiments we: (a) extended previous studies of GBS prevalence and incidence during OT treatment[17,43]; (b) studied the composition of OT-associated GBS using both direct and indirect methods[44]; (c) examined bile composition (bile lipid, bile acid and phospholipid species) and physical chemistry (biliary CH saturation, the distribution of CH between vesicles and micelles, the stability/instability of the vesicles – as judged by the CH:PL molar ratio – and the CH microcrystal nucleation time)[45-51], in fresh samples of gallbladder bile obtained by ultrasound-guided fine-needle puncture[52,53], and (d) assessed the dissolvability of the OT-GBS with oral ursodeoxycholic acid[44]. Having found an increased percentage of biliary deoxycholic acid in gallbladder bile from these patients, we also measured both small and large bowel transit times[16].

Results

Prevalence and incidence

Most of the published data on the prevalence and incidence of OT-GBS were summarized in an earlier review of this subject[17]. The results of this survey showed that after 4–51 months of OT treatment in a dose of 100–1500 μg/day (mainly 300–600 μg/day), the crude prevalence figures for OT-GBS were around 30%. This was true for the majority of studies in which the absence of stones before OT treatment was not established, and for the smaller number where it was. However, the results of actuarial studies suggest that the true prevalence rate of OT-induced GBS is around 50% by 1–2 years, although in our own series[43], the rate was as high as 60%.

Composition of OT-associated GBS

It is widely believed that OT-induced gallstones are cholesterol-rich and dissolvable with oral bile acid treatment. In our experience[44], this is true for most, but by no means all, OT-associated stones. In common with 'conventional' GBS (unrelated to acromegaly or OT treatment), OT-induced stones are usually mixed in composition – even if the majority is cholesterol-rich.

Bile composition and physical chemistry

Compared to stone-free acromegalics untreated with OT ($n = 8$), gallbladder bile from disease controls with conventional GBS disease ($n = 11$), and from acromegalic patients with OT-associated GBS ($n = 6$) had:

1. Higher cholesterol saturation indices (CSI: $1.52 \pm$ SEM 0.17 and 1.32 ± 0.14 vs 0.90 ± 0.05; $p < 0.002$ and 0.01, respectively);
2. A greater percentage of total biliary cholesterol in the vesicular fraction – arbitrarily defined as < 1.06 g/ml sucrose after density gradient ultracentrifugation (61.2 ± 4.5 and 67.7 ± 7.2 vs $37.7 \pm 3.5\%$; $p < 0.003$ and 0.009);
3. Higher molar ratios of CH:PL in the vesicular fraction (an index of vesicle stability/instability) (0.97 ± 0.12 and 0.81 ± 0.16 vs 0.52 ± 0.05; $p < 0.02$ and 0.08);
4. More rapid cholesterol microcrystal nucleation times (medians of < 5 days and < 5 days vs > 18 days; $p < 0.001$ and 0.003);
5. A higher proportion of deoxycholic acid (DCA) conjugates in bile (22.8 ± 2.4 and 23.6 ± 4.8 vs $13.9 \pm 1.4\%$ of total bile acids; $p < 0.02$ and 0.05) with reciprocal changes in the percentage of the parent bile acid, cholic acid (CA).

Thus, in addition to gallbladder stasis, acromegalic patients with OT-GBS have similar changes in bile composition and physical chemistry to those seen in non-acromegalic individuals with conventional gallstone disease[2,3,54–56].

These changes seem to be induced by OT treatment – rather than secondary to the presence of gallstones. Thus, in paired before-and-during treatment studies of five acromegalic patients, the proportion of biliary DCA increased from 13.3 ± 2.1 to $24.9 \pm 2.7\%$ ($p < 0.03$) while the CSI rose from 0.89 ± 0.06 to 1.12 ± 0.03 ($p < 0.02$) after a mean of 8 months (range 3–24) OT treatment in a dose of 300–400 µg/day. Furthermore, there was a 34% reduction in the mean nucleation time ($p < 0.003$) – largely as a result of a fall in the nucleation time from 21 days to 1 day in a 59-year-old woman who developed new stones after only 3 months OT treatment.

The results of these, and other[57–59], studies support the hypothesis that the percentage DCA conjugates in bile is a major factor in the pathogenesis of GBS. Thus, we found[50] that there was a significant linear relation between the percentage DCA conjugates and:

1. The moles % cholesterol ($n = 35$; $y = 5.79 + 0.15x$; $r = 0.57$; $p < 0.001$) and
2. The CSI ($n = 35$; $y = 0.85 + 0.018x$; $r = 0.50$; $p < 0.01$) in gallbladder bile.

Moreover, there was a significant ($p < 0.05$) difference between the percentage DCA conjugates in bile from patients with pathologically rapid microcrystal nucleation times (<5 days; $n = 18$; $23.4 \pm 1.1\%$) and that from those with normally prolonged nucleation times (>10 days; $n = 11$; $17.3 \pm 1.9\%$)[46,50].

Mechanism for the changes in biliary bile acid composition

Given the fact that the increases in the percentage biliary DCA seen during OT treatment were accompanied by reciprocal decreases in the moles % CA, we can infer that the mechanism for the increased proportion of DCA must be due to a greater than normal conversion of CA to DCA. In turn, this increased conversion could, theoretically, be due to:

1. Prolongation of intestinal transit – thereby allowing more time for bacterial deconjugation and 7α-dehydroxylation of CA to form DCA (without necessarily changing the absolute numbers or species of intestinal bacteria or their enzyme activities);
2. Induced changes in the intestinal flora with greater than normal numbers of bacteria capable of 7α-dehydroxylation;
3. No change in the numbers or species of intestinal micro-organisms, but an up-regulation of their enzymatic activity;
4. Increased enterohepatic cycling of the bile acid pool as a result of functional exclusion of a paralysed, adynamic gallbladder, with repeated exposure of the bile acids to deconjugating and dehydroxylating intestinal bacteria;
5. Any combination of 1–4.

The effects of OT on small and large bowel transit

There is strong direct and indirect evidence to suggest that OT-induced prolongation of intestinal transit is an important mechanism for the increased percentage DCA in bile. Thus, in control subjects given a single injection of $50\,\mu g$ OT, 30 min before a liquid test meal containing lactulose, the mouth-to-caecum transit time (as measured by the breath hydrogen technique) increases by 200–300%[15,60–63].

Until recently there was no information about the effects of OT on small and large bowel transit in acromegalic patients on long-term treatment – as opposed to control subjects given a single injection. Therefore, in a randomized, double-blind, placebo-controlled (saline injections) trial[16], we examined the effects of a single $50\,\mu g$ dose of OT, given 30 min before a fat-rich liquid meal (250 ml 'Ensure', which stimulates the release of regulatory peptides that are prokinetic to both gut and gallbladder) containing 20 ml lactulose, on the mouth-to-caecum transit time in six non-acromegalic controls and eight acromegalic patients who had not been treated with OT.

The major intestinal site for the conversion of CA to DCA is the colon – rather than the small bowel[64]. Therefore, in addition to measuring small bowel transit, we used radio-opaque marker shapes[65] to compare large bowel transit times (LBTT) in 10 non-acromegalic controls and seven acromegalic patients who had not previously received OT.

Our results[16] showed that, before OT treatment, both the MCTT (171 ± 17.9 min) and the LBTT (38 ± 10 h) were greater in acromegalic patients than in controls (108 ± 22.9 min; $p < 0.005$ and 22.4 ± 4.6 h; n.s., respectively). We confirmed that OT markedly increased the MCTT – both in control subjects (to 230 ± 20.4 min; $p < 0.008$) and in acromegalic patients (to more than 300 min in all six individuals; $p < 0.003$). As yet, the data on colonic transit in acromegalic patients, studied before and during *chronic* OT treatment, are incomplete. There is some evidence[66] that OT affects small bowel, more than large bowel, transit but it is generally believed that prolongation of small bowel transit is usually accompanied by corresponding changes in the colon.

INTERPRETATION/DISCUSSION

We still need to test the other possible mechanisms advanced to explain the increased proportions of DCA in the bile of our OT-treated patients. Nonetheless, our results to date support the concept that OT induces gallstone formation not only by inhibiting fasting[29], and meal-stimulated[28-32], gallbladder contraction, but also by slowing intestinal transit. This interim conclusion, based on studies of OT-treated acromegalic patients, supports a recent observation by Heaton and colleagues[15] in normal-weight women with GBS who had no other risk factors for gallstone formation. These authors showed, by direct measurement and indirect calculation, that the whole gut transit time (due mainly to large bowel transit) in the women with stones ($82 \pm$ SD 25 h) was significantly ($p < 0.05$) longer than that in age-matched controls (63 ± 16 h; $p < 0.05$). Furthermore, the stool output in the women with stones (74 ± 54 g/24 h) was significantly less than that in controls (141 ± 56 g; $p < 0.02$). Put simply, the normal-weight women with gallstones seemed to be suffering from slow transit constipation.

Based on this, as yet incomplete, story, and on tunnel-vision selection of a few scattered observations from the literature, it would be mischievous to imply that gallstones form mainly as a consequence of disordered intestinal transit. Nonetheless, given the invitation to speculate about strategies for their prevention, it seems reasonable to ask what lessons can be learned from these results.

1. Do induced changes in intestinal transit affect biliary bile acid and bile lipid composition? If so, what is the most cost-effective way of accelerating transit and reducing biliary cholesterol saturation?
2. Should we consider the use of bran or hydrophilic bulking agents, to stimulate intestinal transit?

3. Alternatively, should we use synthetic disaccharides, such as lactulose, prokinetic drugs such as cisapride, or the non-antibiotic analogues of erythromycin, which are motilin agonists?
4. Is there a place for recommending time-honoured laxatives such as senna or even phenolphthalein?
5. Could prokinetic regulatory peptides, such as cholecystokinin (CCK), be given with the hope of stimulating both gallbladder emptying and intestinal transit?

The answers to most of these rhetorical questions are not known, but they are/will be the subject of current/future research.

Logically, preventative strategies should be based on the results of carefully conducted, prospective trials. As yet, however, there is only fragmentary short-term evidence to support these conjectures. Thus, when Thornton and Heaton gave lactulose to patients with supersaturated bile[67], they were able to accelerate intestinal transit and reduce biliary cholesterol saturation significantly. Similarly, in patients given total parenteral nutrition, there is a high incidence of sludge and gallstone formation, but Roslyn et al.[13] and Sitzmann et al.[14] showed that daily injections of CCK, which provoke gallbladder emptying, completely prevented the stone and sludge formation which would otherwise have occurred. The presumption is that the exogenous CCK prevented the sludge and stone formation by stimulating gallbladder emptying. However, CCK is also pro-kinetic to the gut. Could it be, therefore, that the CCK injections in these patients acted on the gut – as well as the gallbladder – and that the prevention of GBS was, in part, due to the action of CCK on intestinal transit? However, CCK is expensive and must be given parenterally. At present, therefore, it cannot be proposed as a *practical* approach for long-term prevention of gallstones – even in high-risk patients.

PATHOGENESIS OF RECURRENT STONES AFTER GALLBLADDER CLEARANCE BY GBS DISSOLUTION OR PCCL

Prevalence and incidence

The prevalence of recurrent GBS has been defined in a number of reports[18-27]. The consensus of these studies is that the incidence of recurrence is approximately 10–15% per annum. The actuarial (life-table) rate of recurrence increases linearly with time, but seems to reach a plateau of around 50% by 5 years. The published figures for this apparent plateau vary from under 40% to over 70% by $3\frac{1}{2}$–7 years. However, in all these studies, the number of patients 'at risk' by 5 years is small, with the result that confidence about the predicted actuarial rate at this time is low. As a result, the detection of one or two further recurrences after 5 years of follow-up, influences the results disproportionately.

Nonetheless, patients with 'post-stone gallstone disease'[68] are at high risk of developing new stones. Therefore, *provided* that the mechanisms involved in the pathogenesis of the secondary (recurrent) stones are the same as those of primary (original) stones, studies of gallstone pathophysiology and prevention of recurrence in these patients should yield invaluable results. It should also be possible to apply this information to trials of prevention in patients at risk of developing primary stones. Given the impact of laparoscopic cholecystectomy, however, the number of GBS patients being treated 'medically' has fallen dramatically. Therefore, the present cohort of patients rendered stone-free by dissolution or clearance, is an invaluable resource which may not be readily available for study in the future.

Do GBS recur true-to-type?

Before reviewing what is known about recurrence or persistence of pathogenetic abnormalities in post-clearance patients, we should first address the question – do gallstones recur 'true-to-type'[69]? In other words, if the primary GBS were single – as opposed to multiple – will the recurrent stones also be solitary? Moreover, if the original stones were radio- and CT-lucent (and, therefore, presumably cholesterol-rich), will the recurrent stones also be lucent or will they be radio-opaque, CT-dense and calcium-containing?

These questions are important, since the pathogenesis of cholesterol-rich stones is different from that of calcium- and pigment-containing non-cholesterol stones. Therefore, measures designed to prevent cholesterol stone formation may not be appropriate for non-cholesterol stones.

Several groups[70–72] have shown that the nucleation time for cholesterol crystal precipitation and detection is different in patients with solitary stones, from that in those with multiple stones. Thus, the nucleation time is rapid in patients with multiple stones but slow in those with solitary stones. Since the best lithotripsy results are obtained in patients with solitary stones, this may explain why there are lower recurrence rates in GBS patients treated with lithotripsy[23,73,74], than in those managed by other 'non-surgical' methods[18–27]. We[26], and others[22], have shown that the mean cumulative recurrence rate, in patients who originally had solitary stones, is approximately one-third of that in patients who, before treatment, had multiple primary stones.

In a preliminary report, Pereira et al.[69] described 20 patients who developed gallstone recurrence some 2 years after being rendered stone-free with oral bile acids, ESWL + adjuvant bile acids, contact solvents or PCCL. They showed that, in individual patients, the number of recurrent stones was different from that of primary stones in 40% of patients. Thus, before treatment, four patients had had solitary stones and 16 had had multiple stones. On recurrence, however, all four patients with solitary stones developed multiple recurrent stones, while four of the 16 who originally had had many primary stones, developed solitary recurrence.

There were also discrepancies between the maximum CT attenuation scores of the primary, and recurrent, stones – especially in the patients treated by PCCL. Thus as a result of selection, all 14 patients treated with one of the dissolution options had had radiolucent primary stones with maximum CT attenuation scores of <100 Hounsfield Units (HU). On recurrence, the maximum HU scores were unchanged in six, decreased in three and increased in five – two of whom developed calcium-containing stones. Conversely, all six patients treated with PCCL had started with radio-opaque stones with high HU scores but, on recurrence, only one of the six developed calcified stones (HU 140). In the remaining five, the recurrent stones were radiolucent with maximum HU scores of < 100. Overall, therefore, the number and composition of the recurrent stones differed from that of the originals in 65% of the patients.

These results suggest that the pathogenetic factors cannot be constant. Nonetheless, all 13 patients with recurrent stones treated with oral bile acids showed ultrasonographic evidence of partial or complete GBS dissolution. This implies that, independent of their original composition, recurrent GBS are usually radio- and CT-lucent, presumed cholesterol-rich and dissolvable with oral bile acid therapy. For this reason, the remaining discussion emphasizes the pathogenesis of cholesterol gallstones, and possible ways of countering their recurrence.

The role of supersaturated bile

We have known for 20 years[75,76] that when GBS have been dissolved and oral bile acid treatment is withdrawn, the bile, which had been rendered unsaturated in cholesterol during oral therapy, almost always reverts to its supersaturated state in 1–3 weeks[77]. This seems to be the time required for *de-novo* hepatic bile acid synthesis to displace the CDCA-rich or UDCA-rich bile which occurs during treatment with these two agents. Put simply, recurrence of supersaturated gallbladder bile is (almost) invariable, but recurrence of gallstones affects only 50% of patients. Therefore, the presence of supersaturated bile has low value in predicting GBS recurrence. However, given the fact that many gallstone-free subjects also have supersaturated fasting gallbladder bile[3] (especially if they are obese[78]), this lack of predictive value could perhaps have been foreseen 20 years ago. Nonetheless, there are no good data to show whether the *degree* of supersaturation is a better discriminant between those who will, and those who will not, develop recurrent stones. Intuitively, one suspects that an individual with a CSI of 2.50 is more likely to develop GBS than someone with a lesser degree of supersaturation – say a CSI of around 1.25.

This rather dated discussion ignores the fact that cholesterol microcrystal precipitation occurs when a high percentage of the total biliary cholesterol is present in vesicles – rather than micelles – particularly if the vesicles are unstable with a high cholesterol:phospholipid molar ratio[79]. There is no uniformly acceptable, 'non-invasive' way of separating vesicles (and other non-micellar cholesterol carriers) from micelles. However, most agree that attempts to do so, and to measure nucleation times, should be based on aliquots of fresh gallbladder bile – and not on bile-rich duodenal aspirates (Strasberg, personal communication: Holzbach, personal communication) or on bile samples obtained at ERCP[80]. For this reason, there are few data on the distribution of biliary cholesterol between vesicles and micelles in patients with post-stone gallstone disease. Since these patients opted for 'medical' treatment of their GBS as an alternative to cholecystectomy, few subsequently come to laparotomy when it might be possible to sample their gallbladder bile directly by fine-needle puncture.

Recently, however, we have used the technique of ultrasound-guided, percutaneous, transhepatic, fine-needle puncture of the gallbladder[52,53] to study bile composition and physical chemistry in a small number of post-dissolution patients[81]. We confirmed that all had supersaturated bile (CSI values of >1.0). We also showed that they had a high proportion of the excess biliary cholesterol transported in vesicles (isolated by sucrose density gradient ultracentrifugation), and that all had high vesicular cholesterol: phospholipid molar ratios. Moreover, the mean percentage DCA in the bile of these patients was almost twice that of stone-free controls, although the difference was not statistically significant. However, measurement of cholesterol microcrystal nucleation times did show a variable pattern (see below).

The efficacy of reducing biliary cholesterol saturation on gallstone recurrence

Apart from rare occasions when there is resistance[82,83], or acquired tolerance[83], to the desaturating effects of oral UDCA and/or CDCA, continued full-dose treatment with these bile acids should ensure that the gallbladder bile remains unsaturated in cholesterol and, therefore, that GBS recurrence is prevented indefinitely. However, cost, and possible side-effects of bile acid therapy, mean that long-term, full-dose treatment is not a practical long-term management option to prevent recurrence.

The results of most, but not all, studies suggest that low-dose oral bile acid treatment does not effectively prevent gallstones from developing or re-forming. Thus, in the American National Cooperative Gallstone Study[84], CDCA in a dose of 375 mg/day (half the so-called full dose) did not significantly affect the GBS recurrence rate – when compared with placebo-treated controls.

In the randomized prospective double-blind placebo-controlled British/ Belgian trial[26], UDCA in one-third the full therapeutic dose (3 mg/kg^{-1} day^{-1}) slowed and reduced, but did not prevent, GBS recurrence. As a result of randomization and stratification, there was an imbalance in risk factors between the three treatment groups. When this imbalance was adjusted, retrospectively, the 'corrected' recurrence rate in the UDCA-treated patients was only half that of the other two groups. Even so, this difference was not statistically significant – perhaps a type II error because of relatively small patient numbers. Certainly, studies of duodenal bile composition and the use of a steady-state marker perfusion technique, showed that this small dose of UDCA (mainly 200 mg and only occasionally 300 mg/day) was adequate to reduce biliary cholesterol secretion and to desaturate fasting gallbladder bile[85].

Furthermore, in a study from Italy[22], UDCA in a dose of 300 mg/day did reduce the gallstone recurrence rates – even if this effect was age-dependent and the conclusions were based on a retrospective clinical analysis, rather than on a prospective planned trial.

The most convincing evidence that UDCA may prevent stones from developing comes not from post-dissolution trials but from a preliminary report[86] of primary GBS development in a high-risk group – obese persons undergoing acute weight reduction as a result of low (520 kcal/day) calorie dieting. In this study, 22.6% of the placebo-treated group developed GBS over the 16-week period of the trial – compared with only 6% of those treated with 150 mg UDCA twice daily (300 mg/day; $p < 0.001$). Moreover, this prevention of gallstone formation by UDCA was dose-dependent. Thus, only 2.8% of those taking 600 mg/day, and 1.6% of those taking 1200 mg/day, developed stones.

UDCA prevention of recurrent or primary stone formation may not only be due to the desaturating effect of the treatment. It could be due, in part or in whole, to prolongation of the cholesterol microcrystal nucleation time[87,88]. Thus, the evidence that bile acid treatment will prevent GBS formation is mixed and controversial. However, measures designed to accelerate intestinal transit, thereby reducing the conversion of cholic to deoxycholic acid, lowering biliary cholesterol secretion and saturation and prolonging the cholesterol microcrystal nucleation time, may prove to be a cost-effective alternative way of preventing CH-GBS formation and recurrence (see below).

The role of cholesterol microcrystal precipitation/detection (nucleation time)

Several lines of evidence suggest that studies of nucleation time may be particularly important in the pathogenesis of recurrent stones.

First, as noted above, recurrence of supersaturated bile is almost invariable within weeks of withdrawing oral dissolution therapy[75-77]. Furthermore, the gallbladder motor dysfunction, which characterizes GBS patients, persists unchanged for at least 1 year after stone clearance by lithotripsy and adjuvant oral bile acid therapy[89]. Since GBS do *not* recur in approximately 50% of patients, it follows that measurements of biliary CH saturation and gallbladder emptying have little value in predicting who will, and who will not, develop recurrent stones. By implication, therefore, studies of the third component of the triple defect in GBS pathogenesis – nucleation time – may provide the missing link.

Second, very few patients whose gallbladders have been cleared of stones with dissolution therapy or by percutaneous stone removal (PCCL), come to surgery when fresh samples of gallbladder bile might be obtained for studies of bile physical chemistry and measurement of nucleation time. Since nucleation times cannot be measured, reliably, in duodenal bile or in bile-rich duodenal fluid, until recently there were no data on nucleation times measured in fresh gallbladder bile from post-dissolution/clearance patients. With the application of the ultrasound-guided percutaneous fine-needle puncture technique[52,53], however, we have studied gallbladder bile[81] in a small group of patients with 'post-stone gallstone disease'[68]. Of these, roughly half had normal and half pathologically rapid nucleation times. Since approximately 50% of the post-dissolution/clearance patients will, ultimately, develop recurrent stones, it is tempting to speculate that it is the patients with the rapid nucleation times who are destined to re-form stones. However, we would need to study a larger number of patients, and follow them for at least 5 years, to prove or disprove this speculative prediction.

Third, as noted above we[26], and the Bologna group[22], showed that in patients who, before medical treatment, had solitary stones, the recurrence rate is approximately one-third that in patients who, initially, had had multiple stones. Furthermore, as noted earlier, the nucleation time in patients with single stones is much less abnormal than that in individuals with multiple stones[70–72]. It seems likely that there is a cause-and-effect relationship between these two observations.

Fourth, is the series of observations in experimental animals and in man, showing that aspirin or non-steroidal anti-inflammatory drugs (NSAIDs) inhibit gallbladder mucosal mucus glycoprotein (MGP) synthesis[90,91] and secretion[92,93], and prevent primary[94] or recurrent[95] stone formation. MGP is a potent pronucleator[96] and the implication is that, by inhibiting gallbladder mucosal cyclo-oxygenase activity, aspirin and NSAIDs reduce MGP synthesis and secretion by the gallbladder, and prevent stone formation/recurrence. However, O'Donnell et al.[97] have shown that indomethacin also promotes meal-stimulated gallbladder emptying. It may, therefore, prevent stone formation/recurrence by this mechanism – instead of (or as well as), inhibiting MGP production.

In prairie dogs fed a lithogenic diet the gallbladder mucosa responds to the resultant supersaturation of bile by increasing its MGP synthesis and secretion, *before* crystals and stones appear[98]. Furthermore, aspirin treatment of these animals inhibits the increase in MGP production and prevents the stone formation which would otherwise occur[92].

As discussed earlier, obese patients undergoing acute weight reduction by dieting are at risk of developing cholesterol microcrystals, microstones and gallstones[86,94]. However, Broomfield and colleagues[94] showed that treatment of these patients with aspirin, in a dose of 1300 mg/day, largely prevented the crystal and stone formation. Furthermore, in a retrospective survey of 75 post-dissolution patients, Hood et al.[95] showed that none of the 12 who regularly took NSAIDs developed recurrent stones, while no less than 20 of 63 patients who never (or only rarely) took NSAIDs, re-formed stones ($p < 0.02$). Finally, Rhodes et al.[91] showed that treatment of patients scheduled for elective cholecystectomy with 300 mg aspirin per day for 1 week before surgery, halved the rate of MGP synthesis by the mucosa of their freshly excised gallbladders.

CONCLUSIONS

The proposal to use prokinetic drugs, such as 5-HT$_3$ and 5-HT$_4$ agonists, may represent an oversimplified approach, since the effects of these agents are complex. They have differing effects on intestinal motility during fasting and after food. They also have variable effects on different parts of the gastrointestinal tract – such as the gallbladder, small bowel and colon.

The number of patients who are at risk of gallstone formation as a result of chronic OT treatment is tiny – in relation to the overall problem of gallstone disease. However, we need to learn much more about the mechanisms whereby OT affects intestinal transit. Are they mediated solely by inhibition of meal-stimulated secretion of prokinetic peptides – such as CCK – or are there additional effects of OT on receptors in the smooth muscle of the gut? Whether or not the basic physiological mechanisms of action can be defined, we still need to know if drugs, such as cisapride or other prokinetic agents, can overcome the inhibitory effects of OT, or its new long-acting derivatives, on intestinal transit.

Despite our ignorance about these matters, clinical research in gallstone pathogenesis has come a long way since the concept that supersaturated bile was the major, if not the sole, abnormality[2]. It seems likely that the solution to the problem will come only with a multifaceted approach to the many mechanisms involved in gallstone development. The answers to most of these rhetorical questions are not known. They are the subject of current and future research. Only when we are armed with the results of these studies will we be in a position to propose logical, preventative treatments which can then be tested in carefully conducted, prospective trials.

References

1. Dowling RH, Gleeson D, Ruppin DC, Murphy GM. Gallstone recurrence and post-dissolution management. In: Paumgartner G, Stiehl A, Gerok W, editors. Enterohepatic circulation of bile acids and sterol metabolism. Lancaster: MTP Press; 1984:361–70.
2. Admirand WH, Small DM. The physico-chemical basis of cholesterol gallstone formation in man. J Clin Invest. 1968;47:1043–52.
3. Holan KR, Holzbach RT, Hermann RE *et al.* Nucleation time; a key factor in the pathogenesis of cholesterol gallstone disease. Gastroenterology. 1979;77:611–17.
4. Carey MC. Formation of cholesterol gallstones: the new paradigms. In: Paumgartner G, Stiehl A, Gerok W, editors. Trends in bile acid research. Dordrecht: Kluwer; 1989:259–81.
5. Fisher RS, Stelzer F, Rock E, Melmud LS. Abnormal gallbladder emptying in patients with gallstones. Dig Dis Sci. 1982;27:1019–24.
6. Forgacs IF, Maisey MN, Murphy GM, Dowling RH. Influence of gallstones and ursodeoxy-cholic acid on gallbladder emptying. Gastroenterology. 1984;87:299–307.
7. Thompson JC, Fried GM, Ogden WD *et al.* Correlation between release of cholecystokinin and contraction of the gallbladder in patients with gallstones. Ann Surg. 1982;195:670–5.
8. Pomeranz IS, Shaffer EA. Abnormal gallbladder emptying in a subgroup of patients with gallstones. Gastroenterology. 1985;88:787–91.
9. Van Erpecum KJ, Van Berge Henegouwen GP, Stolk MFJ, Hopman WPM, Jansen JBMJ, Lamers CBHW. Fasting gallbladder volume, postprandial emptying and cholecystokinin release in gallstone patients and normal subjects. J Hepatol. 1992;14:194–202.
10. Lee SP, LaMont JT, Carey MC. Role of gallbladder mucus hypersecretion in the evolution of cholesterol gallstones. Studies in the prairie dog. J Clin Invest. 1981;67:1712–23.
11. Gallinger S, Taylor RD, Harvey PRC, Petrunka CN, Strasberg SM. Effects of mucous glycoprotein on nucleation time of human bile. Gastroenterology. 1985;89:648–58.
12. Smith BF. Human gallbladder mucin binds biliary lipids and promotes cholesterol crystal nucleation in model bile. J Lipid Res. 1987;28:1088–97.
13. Roslyn JJ, DenBesten L, Pitt HA, Kuchenbecker SL, Polarek JW. Effects of cholecystokinin on gallbladder stasis and cholesterol gallstone formation. J Surg Res. 1981;30:200–4
14. Sitzmann JV, Pitt HA, Steinborn PA, Pasha ZR, Sanders RC. Cholecystokinin prevents

parenteral nutrition induced biliary sludge in humans. Surg Gynecol Obstet. 1990;33:4–9.
15. Heaton KW, Emmett PM, Symes CL, Braddon FEM. An explanation for gallstones in normal-weight women: slow intestinal transit. Lancet. 1993;341:8–10.
16. Hussaini SH, Pereira SP, Kennedy C *et al.* The role of intestinal transit in the pathogenesis of octreotide-induced gallbladder stones (GBS). Gut. 1994;35(Suppl. 2):S57(abstr.).
17. Dowling RH, Hussaini SH, Murphy GM, Besser GM, Wass JAH. Gallstones during octreotide therapy. Metabolism Clin Exp. 1992;41(Suppl. 2):22–33.
18. Ruppin DC, Dowling RH. Is recurrence inevitable after gallstone dissolution by bile acid treatment. Lancet. 1982;1:181–5.
19. Lanzini A, Jazrawi RP, Kupfer RM, Maudgal DP, Joseph AE, Northfield TC. Gallstone recurrence after medical dissolution: an over-estimated threat? J Hepatol. 1986;3:241–6.
20. O'Donnell LDJ, Heaton KW. Recurrence and re-recurrence of gallstones after medical dissolution; long term follow up. Gut. 1988;29:655–8.
21. Scholz DG, McCullough JE, Peterson BT, Thistle JL. Gallstone recurrence following complete dissolution with bile acid therapy or methyl tert-butyl ether. Hepatology. 1988;8:A1372.
22. Villanova N, Bazzoli F, Taroni F *et al.* Gallstone recurrence after successful oral bile acid treatment. Gastroenterology. 1989;97:726–31.
23. Sackmann M, Ippisch E, Sauerbruch T, Holl J, Brendel W, Paumgartner G. Early gallstone recurrence rate after successful shock-wave therapy. Gastroenterology. 1990;98:392–6.
24. Darzi A, McCollum P, Leahy A, Tanner WA, Keane FBV. Gallstone recurrence after successful shock wave lithotripsy. Br J Surg. 1990;77:A703(abstr.).
25. Petroni M, for the British/Italian Gallstone (BIG) Group. Intermittent bile acid therapy for cholesterol gallstones: a 5-year prospective multicentre trial. Gastroenterology. 1992;102:A328(abstr.).
26. Hood KA, Gleeson D, Ruppin DC, Dowling RH and the British–Belgian Gallstone Study Group. Gallstone recurrence and its prevention: the British/Belgian gallstone study group's post-dissolution trial. Gut. 1993;34:1277–88.
27. Donald JJ, Cheslyn-Curtis S, Gillams AR, Russell RCG, Lees WR. Percutaneous cholecystolithotomy: is gallstone recurrence inevitable? Gut. 1994;34:692–5.
28. van Liessum PA, Hopman WP, Pieters GF. Postprandial gallbladder motility during long term treatment with the long-acting somatostatin analog SMS 201-995 in acromegaly. J Clin Endocrinol Metab. 1989;69:557–62.
29. Stolk MFJ, van Erpecum KJ, Koppeschaar HPF *et al.* Postprandial gallbladder motility and hormone release during intermittent and continuous subcutaneous octreotide therapy in acromegaly. Gut. 1993;34:808–13.
30. Hussaini SH, Pereira SP, Kennedy C *et al.* Meal-stimulated gallbladder (GB) emptying in acromegaly: the effect of octreotide (OT) treatment. Gut. 1994;35(Suppl. 2):S57(abstr.).
31. Lembcke B, Creutzfeldt W, Schleser S *et al.* Effect of somatostatin analogue Sandostatin (SMS 201-995) on gastrointestinal, pancreatic and biliary function, and hormone release in normal men. Digestion. 1987;36:108–24.
32. Mitsukawa T, Takemura J, Nishizono F, Nakatsuru K, Ogho S, Matsukura S. Effects of atropine, proglumide and somatostatin analogue (SMS 201-995) on bombesin-induced gallbladder contraction and CCK secretion in humans. Am J Gastroenterol. 1989;84:1371–4.
33. Carey MC, Cahalane MJ. Whither biliary sludge? Gastroenterology. 1993;95:508–23.
34. Ricci GL, Fevery J. Cholestatic action of somatostatin in the rat: effect on the different fractions of bile secretion. Gastroenterology. 1981;81:552–62.
35. Lewis MH, Baker AL, Moossa AR. Effects of somatostatin on determinants of bile flow in unanesthetized dogs. Ann Surg. 1982;195:97–103.
36. Hanks JB, Kortz WJ, Andersen DK, Jones RS. Somatostatin suppression of canine fasting bile secretion. Gastroenterology. 1983;84:130–7.
37. Rene E, Danzinger RG, Hofmann AF, Nakagaki M. Pharmacologic effect of somatostatin on bile formation in the dog. Gastroenterology. 1983;84:120–9.
38. Magnusson I, Einarsson K, Angelin BO *et al.* Effects of somatostatin on hepatic bile formation. Gastroenterology. 1989;96:206–12.
39. Marteau P, Chretien Y, Calmus Y, Parc R, Poupon R. Pharmaceutical effect of somatostatin on bile secretion in man. Digestion. 1989;42:16–21.
40. Cucchiaro G, Branum GD, O'Dorisio T, Meyers WC. Effect of somatostatin and its

analogue sandostatin on biliary lipid composition. Gastroenterology. 1990;98:A246(abstr.).
41. Buscail LE, Puel-Bousquet C, Harris AG *et al.* Effets sur la lithogenese biliaire du traitement au long cours par octreotide (SMS 210-995) chez des patients acromegales. Gastroenterol Clin Biol. 1991;15:800–4.
42. Ahredt SA, McGuire GE, Pitt HA, Lillemoe KD. Why does somatostatin cause gallstones? Am J Surg. 1991;161:177–83.
43. Catnach SM, Anderson JV, Fairclough PD *et al.* The effect of octreotide on gallstone prevalence and gallbladder motility in acromegaly. Gut. 1993;34:270–3.
44. Hussaini SH, Pereira SP, Murphy GM *et al.* The composition of octreotide-associated gallbladder stones: response to oral ursodeoxycholic acid. Gut. 1994;35(In press).
45. Hussaini SH, Murphy GM, Kennedy C, Wass JAH, Besser GM, Dowling RH. Pathogenesis of octreotide (OT)-associated gallbladder stones (GBS) in acromegaly. Gut. 1992;33:S26(abstr.).
46. Hussaini SH, Maghsoudloo M, Murphy GM, Kennedy C, Wass JAH, Dowling RH. Octreotide (OT) increases the proportion of deoxycholic acid (DCA) in gallbladder (GB) bile – the prime mover in the pathogenesis of OT-induced gallbladder stones (GBS)? Gut. 1992;33:S57(abstr.).
47. Hussaini SH, Maghsoudloo M, Murphy GM, Kennedy C, Wass JAH, Dowling RH. The roles of biliary deoxycholic acid (DCA) and vesicular cholesterol (CH) in the pathogenesis of CH gallbladder stones (GBS). Gut. 1992;33:S57(abstr.).
48. Hussaini SH, Pereira SP, Murphy GM, Kennedy C, Wass JAH, Dowling RH. Chronic octreotide treatment of acromegaly induces changes in gallbladder bile composition which predispose to gallstones. Gastroenterology. 1993;104:A365(abstr.).
49. Pereira SP, Hussaini SH, Cassell TB, Murphy GM, Wass JAH, Dowling RH. Octreotide increases the proportions of arachidonic acid-rich phospholipids in gallbladder bile. Gut. 1993;34:S32(abstr.).
50. Hussaini SH, Pereira SP, Murphy GM, Dowling RH. Biliary deoxycholic acid (DCA) influences the partitioning of biliary cholesterol (CH) between micelles and vesicles. Clin Sci. 1993;85:12P.
51. Hussaini SH, Murphy GM, Kennedy C, Besser GM, Wass JAH, Dowling RH. The role of bile composition and physical chemistry in the pathogenesis of octreotide-associated gallbladder stones. Gastroenterology. 1994;107(In press).
52. Swobodnik W, Hagert N, Janowitz P, Wenk H. Diagnostic fine-needle puncture of the gallblader with US guidance. Radiology. 1991;178:755–8.
53. Hussaini SH, Kennedy C, Pereira SP, Wass JAH, Dowling RH. Ultrasound-guided percutaneous fine needle puncture of the gallbladder for studies of bile composition. Br J Radiol. (in press).
54. Holzbach RT, Marsh M, Olszewski M, Holan K. Cholesterol solubility in bile. Evidence that supersaturated bile is frequent in healthy man. J Clin Invest. 1973;52:1467–79.
55. Metzger AL, Adler R, Heymsfield S. Diurnal variations in biliary lipid composition. N Engl J Med. 1973;288:333–6.
56. Carey MC, Small DM. The physical chemistry of cholesterol solubility in bile. Relationship to gallstone formation and dissolution in man. J Clin Invest. 1978;61:998–1026.
57. Low-Beer TS, Nutter S. Colonic bacterial activity, biliary cholesterol saturation, and pathogenesis of gallstones. Lancet. 1978;2:1063–5.
58. Carulli N, Loria P, Bertolotti M *et al.* Effects of acute changes in bile acid pool composition on biliary lipid secretion. J Clin Invest. 1985;74:616–24.
59. Marcus SN, Heaton KW. Deoxycholic acid and the pathogenesis of gallstones. Gut. 1988;29:522–33.
60. Fuessl HS, Carolan G, Williams G, Bloom SR. Effect of a long-acting somatostatin analogue (SMS 201-995) on postprandial gastric emptying of ^{99m}Tc-tin colloid and mouth-to-caecum transit time in man. Digestion. 1987;36:101–7.
61. Lembcke B, Creutzfeldt W, Schleser S *et al.* Effect of somatostatin analogue Sandostatin (SMS 201-995) on gastrointestinal, pancreatic and biliary function, and hormone release in normal men. Digestion. 1987;36:108–24.
62. Møller N, Petrany G, Cassidy D *et al.* Effects of the somatostatin analogue SMS 201-955 (sandostatin) on mouth-to-caecum transit time and absorption of fat and carbohydrates in normal man. Clin Sci. 1988;75:345–50.

63. O'Donnell LDJ, Watson AJM, Cameron D, Farthing MJG. Effect of octreotide on mouth-to-caecum transit time in healthy subjects and in the irritable bowel syndrome. Aliment Pharmacol Ther. 1990;4:177–82.
64. Samuel P, Saypol GM, Meilman E, Mosbach EH, Chafizadeh M. Absorption of bile acids from the large bowel in man. J Clin Invest. 1968;47:2070–8.
65. Metcalf AM, Phillips SF, Zinsmeister AR, MacCarty RL, Beart RW, Wolff BG. Simplified assessment of segmental colonic transit. Gastroenterology. 1987;92:40–7.
66. von der Ohe, Thomforde GM, Camilleri M. Differential regional effects of octreotide on human gastrointestinal motor function. Gastroenterology. 1994;106:A585(abstr.).
67. Thornton JR, Heaton KW. Do colonic bacteria contribute to cholesterol gallstone formation? Effects of lactulose on bile. BMJ. 1981;282:1018–20.
68. Ruppin DC, Murphy GM, Dowling RH and the British Gallstone Study Group. Gall stone disease without gall stones – bile acid and bile lipid metabolism after complete gall stone dissolution. Gut. 1986;27:559–66.
69. Pereira SP, Hussaini SH, Kennedy C, Dowling RH. Gallbladder stone (GBS) recurrence after medical dissolution: do GBS recur true to type? Gut. 1994;35(Suppl. 2):S57(abstr.).
70. Gollish SH, Burnstein MJ, Ilson RG, Petrunka CN, Strasberg SM. Nucleation of cholesterol monohydrate crystals from hepatic and gall-bladder bile of patients with cholesterol gall stones. Gut. 1983;24:836–44.
71. Groen AK, Noordam C, Drapers JAG, Egbers P, Jansen PLM, Tytgat GNJ. Isolation of a potent cholesterol nucleation-promoting activity from human gallbladder bile: role in the pathogenesis of gallstone disease. Hepatology. 1990;11:525–33.
72. Jungst D, Lang T, von Ritter C, Pratschke E, Paumgartner G. Cholesterol nucleation time in gallbladder bile of patients with solitary or multiple cholesterol gallstones. Hepatology. 1992;15:804–8.
73. Ponchon T, Barkun AN, Bertrand P et al. Gallstone disappearance after extracorporeal lithotripsy and oral bile acid dissolution. Gastroenterology. 1989;97:457–63.
74. Ell C, Kerzel W, Schneider HT et al. Piezoelectric lithotripsy: stone disintegration and follow-up results in patients with symptomatic gallbladder stones. Gastroenterology. 1990;99:1439–44.
75. Mok HYI, Bell GD, Dowling RH. Effect of different doses of chenodeoxycholic acid on bile-lipid composition and on frequency of side-effects in patients with gallstones. Lancet. 1974;2:253–7.
76. Thistle JL, Yu PYS, Hofmann AF, Ott BJ. Prompt return of bile to supersaturated state followed by gallstone recurrence after discontinuance of chenodeoxycholic acid therapy. Gastroenterology. 1974;66:789(abstr.).
77. Iser JH, Murphy GM, Dowling RH. Speed of change in biliary lipids and bile acids with chenodeoxycholic acid – is intermittent therapy feasible? Gut. 1977;18:7–15.
78. Reuben A, Maton PN, Murphy GM, Dowling RH. Bile lipid secretion in obese and non-obese individuals with and without gallstones. Clin Sci. 1985;69:71–9.
79. Carey MC, Cohen DE. Biliary transport of cholesterol in vesicles, micelles and liquid crystals. In: Paumgartner G, Stiehl A, Gerok W, editors. Bile acids and the liver. Lancaster: MTP Press; 1987:287–300.
80. Petroni ML, Jazrawi RP, Ahmed H, Finch PJ, Dormandy J, Northfield TC. Cholesterol nucleation time measurement in nasobiliary or nasoduodenal bile. Comparison with surgical bile. Scand J Gastroenterol. 1993;28:803–8.
81. Hussaini SH, Pereira SP, Kennedy C, Murphy GM, Dowling RH. Bile physical chemistry and cholesterol (CH) crystal nucleation time (NTs) – the missing links in gallbladder stone (GBS) recurrence. Gut. 1993;34(Suppl. 1):S51.
82. Iser JH, Maton PN, Murphy GM, Dowling RH. Resistance to chenodeoxycholic acid (CDCA) treatment in obese patients with gall stones. BMJ. 1978;1:1509–12.
83. Gleeson D, Scrivens N, Murphy GM, Dowling RH. Resistance and acquired tolerance to ursodeoxycholic acid (UDCA): a possible cause of treatment failure. Clin Sci. 1986;70:A26(abstr.).
84. Marks JW, Lan S-P, the Steering Committee and the National Cooperative Gallstone Study Group. Low-dose chenodiol to prevent gallstone recurrence after dissolution therapy. Ann Intern Med. 1984;100:376–81.
85. Ruppin DC, Murphy GM, Dowling RH et al. Effect of low-dose ursodeoxycholic acid,

placebo and diet on bile acid and bile lipid metabolism after gallstone dissolution: a national multi-centre post-dissolution trial. In: Paumgartner G, Stiehl A, Gerok W, editors. Bile acids and cholesterol in health and disease. Lancaster: MTP Press; 1982:257–65.

86. Shiffman ML, Vickers FF, Stefler LTP. A multicenter double-blind, placebo-controlled trial of ursodeoxycholic acid (urso) for prevention of gallstone (GS) formation in obese patients during very low calorie diet (VLCD) induced weight reduction. Gastroenterology. 1994;106:A982(abstr.).

87. Jungst D, Brenner G, Pratschke E, Paumgartner G. Low-dose ursodeoxycholic acid prolongs cholesterol nucleation time in gallbladder bile of patients with cholesterol gallstones. J Hepatol. 1989;8:1–6.

88. Tazuma S, Sasaki H, Mizuno S et al. Effect of ursodeoxycholic acid administration on nucleation time in human gallbladder bile. Gastroenterology. 1989;97:173–8.

89. Spengler U, Sackmann M, Sauerbruch T, Holl J, Paumgartner G. Gallbladder motility before and after extracorporeal shock-wave lithotripsy. Gastroenterology. 1989;96:860–3.

90. Rhodes M, Allen A, Lennard TWJ. Mucus glycoprotein biosynthesis in the human gallbladder: inhibition by aspirin. Gut. 1992;33:1109–12.

91. Rhodes M, Allen A, Dowling RH, Murphy GM, Lennard TWJ. Inhibition of human gall bladder mucus synthesis in patients undergoing cholecystectomy. Gut. 1992;33:1113–17.

92. Lee SP, Carey MC, LaMont TJ. Aspirin prevention of cholesterol gallstone formation in prairie dogs. Science. 1981;211:1429–30.

93. LaMont TJ, Turner BS, DiBenedetto D, Handin R, Schafrer AI. Arachidonic acid stimulates mucin secretion in prairie dog gallbladder. Am J Physiol. 1983;245:G92–8.

94. Broomfield PH, Chopra R, Sheinbaum RC et al. Effects of ursodeoxycholic acid and aspirin on the formation of lithogenic bile and gallstones during loss of weight. N Engl J Med. 1988;319:1567–72.

95. Hood K, Gleeson D, Ruppin DC, Dowling RH and the British/Belgian Gallstone Study Group. Prevention of gallstone recurrence by non-steroidal anti-inflammatory drugs. Lancet. 1988;2:1223–5.

96. Levy PF, Smith BF, LaMont JT. Human gallbladder mucin accelerates nucleation of cholesterol in artificial bile. Gastroenterology. 1984;87:270–5.

97. O'Donnell LJD, Wilson P, Guest P et al. Indomethacin and postprandial gallbladder emptying. Lancet. 1992;339:269–71.

98. LaMorte WW, Booker ML, Scott EE, Williams LF Jr. Increases in gallbladder prostaglandin synthesis before the formation of cholesterol gallstones. Surgery. 1985;98:445–51.

36
Ultrasonographic study of gallbladder and gastric dynamics in obese people after oral cholestyramine

P. PORTINCASA, A. DI CIAULA, V. PALMIERI,
G. P. VAN BERGE HENEGOUWEN and G. PALASCIANO

INTRODUCTION

We have recently shown that acute ingestion of the bile acid sequestrant cholestyramine (CH) alone or with a test meal markedly enhances gallbladder emptying in healthy subjects[1]. This effect of CH might be of clinical relevance since the gallbladder motility defect is thought to play a key role in the multifactorial pathogenesis of cholesterol gallstones[2]. In 1992 we reported for the first time that oral CH was able to improve gallbladder hypomotility in gallstone patients[3]. Gallbladder stasis might also represent a risk factor for cholesterol gallstone formation in obesity[4,5] and therapeutic tools able to reverse the gallbladder motility defect in obese people might prevent cholesterol crystal formation and further aggregation to gallstones. Indeed, restoring gallbladder emptying with a limited amount of dietary fat during low-calorie dieting has been reported to prevent gallstone formation in obese subjects[6], while cholecystokinin (CCK)-induced frequent gallbladder contraction prevented gallstone formation in patients on total parenteral nutrition[7].

In this study we used ultrasonography to test whether, and to what extent, gallbladder dynamics in obese subjects is influenced by oral CH. A group of healthy volunteers served as controls. Since several studies point to a physiological role for CCK in the inhibition of gastric emptying[8,9], we also assessed antral emptying by sonography.

METHODS

We studied 12 obese (2 male, 10 female, mean age 37 ± 5 SEM years) and 15 lean healthy volunteers (4 male, 11 female, age 31 ± 3 years). Body mass

Table 1 Indices of gallbladder and gastric antral emptying in lean and obese subjects after test meal or test meal plus cholestyramine (CH)

	Lean (n = 15)		Obese (n = 12)	
	Test meal	*Test meal + CH*	*Test meal*	*Test meal + CH*
Gallbladder emptying				
Fasting volume (ml)	21.6 ± 1.7	19.4 ± 1.4	39.4 ± 6.9^b	39.8 ± 4.6^b
Residual volume				
Percentage	18.6 ± 2.4	2.8 ± 0.9^a	36.9 ± 6.1^b	15.6 ± 3.8^a
ml	4.0 ± 0.5	0.6 ± 0.2^a	12.3 ± 1.8^b	5.0 ± 0.7^a
AUC	7504 ± 332	9106 ± 276^a	4807 ± 606^b	7103 ± 533^a
Gastric emptying				
Maximum antral area (cm^2)	15.0 ± 2.0	12.0 ± 0.9	12.6 ± 1.2	11.7 ± 0.8
AUC	7908 ± 491	4083 ± 968^a	5521 ± 578^b	4395 ± 963

Data are mean $\pm$ SEM; AUC = area under emptying curve (% $\times$ 120 min); maximum antral area = measured immediately after ingestion of the liquid test meal; [a]$p < 0.05$ versus prior test meal; [b]$p < 0.05$ vs lean subjects

index was 39 ± 3 and $21 \pm 0.8 \, kg/m^2$ in obese and lean subjects, respectively. Gastric and gallbladder emptying was simultaneously evaluated using *real-time* ultrasound equipment with a 3.5 MHz convex probe. Measurements were taken in the fasting state (after an overnight fast), immediately after the ingestion of a liquid test meal, and at 5–15-min intervals until 2 h postprandially. Gallbladder volume was calculated by the ellipsoid formula[1] and indices of gallbladder emptying were fasting gallbladder volume, residual gallbladder volume (the minimum volume reached at the completion of emptying) and area under emptying curve (AUC). For the study of gastric emptying the probe was positioned at the epigastrium to measure gastric antral area in a single longitudinal section. Indices of gastric emptying were fasting and maximal postprandial antral area, percentage residual antral areas (calculated at each time point[10]) and AUC. On two different days subjects were randomized to receive a test meal (two egg yolks in 200 ml water, 120 kcal) or test meal plus CH (4 g dissolved in water).

RESULTS

Data on gallbladder and antral emptying in response to test meal alone or with CH are depicted in Table 1. Fasting gallbladder volume of obese patients was significantly larger than that of lean controls ($p < 0.05$). Gallbladder emptying in response to a standard meal was impaired in obese patients (increased residual volume both in percentage and ml), as compared to controls. During the whole study period of 120 min gallbladder volumes of obese subjects were significantly larger than those of controls (resulting in a 36% decrease of AUC). Fasting antral areas were 5.0 ± 0.3 and $5.6 \pm 0.6 \, cm^2$ in lean and obese subjects, respectively. After meal ingestion antral areas increased to the same extent in both groups (Table 1). However, antral emptying was deranged in obese patients, who showed greater antral areas than lean individuals throughout the study period, up to 75 min

($p < 0.05$) and a 30% decrease of AUC. Although time to reach the smallest postprandial area was longer in obese subjects than controls, difference did not reach statistical significance (93 ± 8 versus 85 ± 7 min).

The addition of CH to the test meal significantly enhanced gallbladder emptying in both obese subjects and controls. Residual gallbladder volume showed a 85% and a 59% decrease in lean and obese subjects, respectively, compared to values obtained with the test meal alone (Table 1). However, we noticed a delay of gastric emptying when CH was given to lean subjects, with a two-fold decrease of AUC as compared to the test meal alone. In obese subjects the ingestion of CH did not change the gastric emptying pattern seen with the test meal alone.

None of the subjects reported side-effects following the ingestion of cholestyramine.

DISCUSSION

Greater fasting and residual gallbladder volume may be a crucial factor to cholesterol crystal growth and gallstone formation in obese people, who already have a supersaturated bile with cholesterol[11]. Our preliminary observations suggest that in obese patients a low dose of oral CH significantly enhances postprandial gallbladder emptying and markedly reduces gallbladder residual volumes in the absence of side-effects. This finding may have clinical relevance for the correction of the obesity-related gallbladder stasis. It is likely that CH affects gallbladder dynamics mostly by interrupting the negative feedback mechanism between intraluminal bile acids and CCK release, since studies in animals[12,13] and humans[12,14] have shown that endogenous CCK increases following ingestion or intraduodenal infusion of CH, which remains unadsorbed in the intestinal lumen.

Furthermore, we[1] and others[12] have found that CCK-receptor antagonists greatly inhibit the effect of CH on the gallbladder as well as on the pancreas[12,13]. Both gallbladder and gastric emptying were impaired in obese subjects; this suggests that multiple motility defects of the gut may exist in these patients. Decreased oesophageal and gastric emptying, for example, have been previously described in obese subjects[15,16]. In this study, acute ingestion of CH inhibited gastric emptying in lean subjects, most likely through a CCK-dependent mechanism[17,18]. Interestingly, gastric emptying after acute CH did not further deteriorate in obese people. It is possible that the already manifest defect of stomach emptying masked the effect of CH, or that obesity is associated with CCK resistance in some organs[19]. Effects that may both retard and accelerate gastric emptying following administration of CCK have also been recently described[20].

CONCLUSIONS

Acute administration of a low dose of cholestyramine enhances postprandial gallbladder emptying in obese patients as well as in lean subjects. In lean subjects, but not in obese patients, acute cholestyramine delays the gastric emptying of a standard liquid meal.

It is conceivable that in obese subjects with gallbladder stasis, cholestyramine may have a potential role in the prevention and non-surgical therapy of gallstones. We are currently extending our work to evaluate whether a chronic trial with cholestyramine is able to produce a sustained effect on gallbladder and antral emptying in obese subjects.

Further studies are also needed to clarify the prokinetic properties of cholestyramine in clinical conditions presenting with gallbladder stasis.

References

1. Palasciano G, Portincasa P, Belfiore A, Baldassarre G, Albano O. Opposite effect of cholestyramine and loxiglumide on gallbladder dynamics in humans. Gastroenterology. 1992;102:2071–6.
2. LaMorte WW. Biliary motility and abnormalities associated with cholesterol cholelithiasis. Curr Opin Gastroenterol. 1993;9:810–16.
3. Portincasa P, Di Ciaula A, Baldassarre G, Palmieri V, Velardi A, Palasciano G. Cholestyramine improves gallbladder motor function in gallstone patients. Gastroenterology. 1992;102:329A.
4. Marzio L, Capone F, Neri M, Mezzetti A, De Angelis C, Cuccurullo F. Gallbladder kinetics in obese patients: effect of a regular meal and a low calorie meal. Dig Dis Sci. 1988;33:4–9.
5. Palasciano G, Portincasa P, Belfiore A et al. Gallbladder volume and emptying in diabetics: the role of neuropathy and obesity. J Intern Med. 1992;231:123–7.
6. Stone BG, Ansel HJ, Peterson FJ, Gebhard RL. Gallbladder emptying stimuli in obese and normal-weight subjects. Hepatology. 1992;15:795–8.
7. Sitzman JV, Pitt HA, Steinborn PA, Pasha ZR, Sanders RC. Cholecystokinin prevents parenteral nutrition induced biliary sludge in humans. Surg Gynecol Obstet. 1990;170: 25–31.
8. Liddle RA, Morita ET, Conrad CK, Williams JA. Regulation of gastric emptying in humans by cholecystokinin. J Clin Invest. 1986;77:992–6.
9. Kleibeuker JH, Beekhuis H, Jansen JBMJ, Piers DA, Lamers CBHW. Cholecystokinin is a physiologic hormonal mediator of fat-induced inhibition of gastric emptying. Eur J Clin Invest. 1988;18:173–7.
10. Wedmann B, Schmidt G, Wegener M, Coenen C, Ricken D, Althoff J. Effects of age and gender on fat-induced gallbladder contraction and gastric emptying of a caloric liquid meal: a sonographic study. Am J Gastroenterol. 1991;86:1765–70.
11. Angelin B, Einarsson K, Ewerth S, Leijd B. Biliary lipid composition in obesity. Scand J Gastroenterol. 1981;16:1015–19.
12. Gomez G, Upp J, Lluis F et al. Regulation of the release of cholecystokinin by bile salts in dogs and humans. Gastroenterology. 1988;94:1036–46.
13. Koop I, Lindenthal M, Schade M, Traytmann M, Adler G, Arnold R. Role of cholecystokinin in cholestyramine-induced changes of the exocrine pancreas. Pancreas. 1991;6:564–70.
14. Koop I, Dorn S, Koop H et al. Dissociation of cholecystokinin and pancreaticobiliary response to intraduodenal bile acids and cholestyramine in humans. Dig Dis Sci. 1991: 1625–32.
15. Maddox A, Horowitz M, Wishart J, Collins P. Gastric and oesophageal emptying in obesity. Scand J Gastroenterol. 1989;24:593–8.
16. Mercer CD, Rue C, Hanelin L, Hill LD. Effect of obesity on oesophageal transit. Am J Surg. 1985;49:177–81.
17. Fried M, Erlacher U, Schwizer W et al. Role of cholecystokinin in the regulation of gastric emptying and pancreatic enzyme secretion in humans. Studies with the cholecystokinin-receptor antagonist loxiglumide. Gastroenterology. 1991;101:503–11.
18. Allescher HD, Tougas G, Vergara P, Lu S, Daniel EE. Nitric oxide as a putative nonadrenergic noncholinergic inhibitory transmitter in the canine pylorus in vivo. Am J Physiol.

1992;3:G695–702.
19. McLaughlin CL, Baile CA. Decreased sensitivity of Zucker obese rats to putative satiety agent cholecystokinin. Physiol Behav. 1980;25:543–8.
20. Fraser R, Fone D, Horowitz M, Dent J. Cholecystokinin octapeptide stimulates phasic and tonic pyloric motility in healthy humans. Gut. 1993;34:33–7.

37
Gallbladder and bile duct stones: endoscopic treatment

P. B. COTTON

INTRODUCTION

Endoscopy literally includes laparoscopy, but this presentation is restricted to the use of flexible instruments. Cannulation of the bile duct (and pancreatic duct) under direct vision using an endoscope passed through the mouth was first performed more than 25 years ago. Endoscopic retrograde cholangiopancreatography (ERCP) is now a routine procedure with many diagnostic and therapeutic applications. ERCP-based endoscopic sphincterotomy has become the primary method for removing bile duct stones[1]. Initially introduced for management of retained or recurrent duct stones in elderly and frail patients who had undergone cholecystectomy, its success led to widespread use in good-risk patients also, and before cholecystectomy in certain clinical contexts (e.g. jaundice, acute cholangitis and gallstone pancreatitis). Laparoscopic cholecystectomy (LC) has added a new dimension recently, since few laparoscopists yet attempt to explore the bile duct. The relationship between ERCP and LC is a matter of considerable debate.

ERCP AND SPHINCTEROTOMY – RESULTS AND RISKS

Experts in ERCP can achieve biliary cannulation in at least 95% of attempts[1,2]. More important are the results in routine practice – especially since LC is essentially a community procedure. Preliminary data from one community-based study show that similar high rates of success can be achieved by practitioners with a lifetime experience of less than 200 ERCP procedures[3]. Failures of cannulation and sphincterotomy are often due to anatomical problems, such as previous Billroth II gastrectomy and large diverticula. The success rate for removing stones is dependent upon the expertise and persistence of the endoscopist, the patient selection, and the definitions used[1,4]. Virtually all extrahepatic stones less than 10 mm in diameter should be removable[5]. Stones greater than 15 mm pose significant

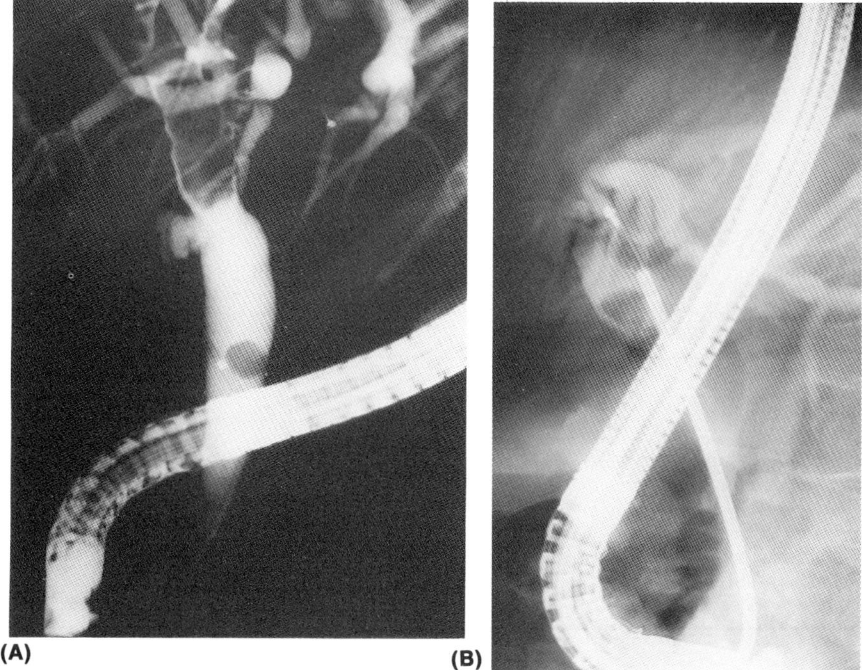

Fig. 1 A: 'Piston' stone in the common hepatic duct. **B**: Use of the Olympus BML mechanical lithotripter; the stone has fragmented

problems, especially when there is a duct stricture or distal narrowing[6]. The recent development of an effective through-the-scope mechanical lithotripter has made it possible to remove approximately 80% of large and 'difficult' stones (Fig. 1)[7-9]. There are now very few indications for other adjuvant techniques such as intraductal lithotripsy (with electrohydraulic or laser probes), extracorporeal shock lithotripsy, and chemical dissolution[10-14]. Biliary stents can provide good temporary drainage when stones prove difficult to remove; long-term stenting has been advocated, but is not always satisfactory[15].

Intrahepatic stones pose problems of a different magnitude. Some can be removed after ERCP sphincterotomy with skilful use of guidewires, balloons and baskets, but the success rate is low, especially in the presence of strictures or multiple segmental involvement[16]. Percutaneous and surgical techniques are often necessary.

The overall complication rate for endoscopic sphincterotomy and stone management is usually quoted at around 10%, with a mortality of 1%[1]. These blanket figures cover considerable variations, depending upon precise definitions, expertise, patient selection and methods for data collection[17]. Seven US centres with endoscopy databases have collected data on complications prospectively for periods of 1–5 years, using agreed criteria[18]. Among 1921 sphincterotomies (for stone), there were a total of 112 complications

Table 1 Complications of sphincterotomy for stone: prospective study in seven US centres

Total sphincterotomies	1921
Complications	112 (5.8%)
Mild	70 (3.6%)
Moderate	26 (1.3%)
Severe	12 (0.5%)
Fatal	4 (0.2%)

Standardized definitions according to Cotton et al.[17]. Data published in abstract form (ref. 18)

Table 2 Complications of sphincterotomy for stones: 440 consecutive cases at Duke University Medical Center (1989–93)

	Totals	Mild	Moderate	Severe	Fatal
All complications	23 (5.9%)	12	6	4	1
Pancreatitis	6	4	2		
Immediate bleeding	1	1			
Delayed bleeding	5	2	3		
Chest problems	2	1	1		
Infection/cholangitis	3	1		1	1
Endoscopic perforation	1			1	
Sphincterotomy perforation	2	1		1	
Other complications	3	2		1	

(5.8%). Seventy (3.6%) were mild, 26 (1.3%) moderate, 12 (0.6%) severe, and four (0.2%) were fatal (Table 1). The fatalities occurred in patients with serious co-morbidities. Pancreatitis remains the commonest direct procedure-related complication[17,19]; other feared complications such as perforation and bleeding are now seen comparatively rarely (Table 2). Preliminary data from a multi-centre community-based study suggest that the risks are not significantly higher in non-expert hands[3].

The widespread use of laparoscopic cholecystectomy has resulted in more young patients with normal-sized ducts being referred for endoscopic stone management, which has focused greater attention on short- and long-term risks. Some studies suggest that the direct risks of sphincterotomy are higher in patients with smaller ducts[20]. Paradoxically, however, the risks appeared to be lower in the prospective multi-centre US study[18]. Among 238 sphincterotomies for stone in patients aged less than 60, with bile ducts less than 9 mm in diameter, there were only two moderate complications, one severe, and no fatalities.

Long-term consequences of sphincterotomy are a legitimate concern[21,22]. The largest study so far reported that 10% of patients who had previously undergone sphincterotomy for stones had further biliary problems in a follow-up period of 6–11 years (all were post-cholecystectomy)[23]. Problems included sphincterotomy stenosis, new stones and non-obstructive cholangitis. All patients were treated conservatively. This cohort was derived in the 1970s, among older patients with larger ducts; more data are required concerning younger patients and smaller ducts. There is nothing to indicate

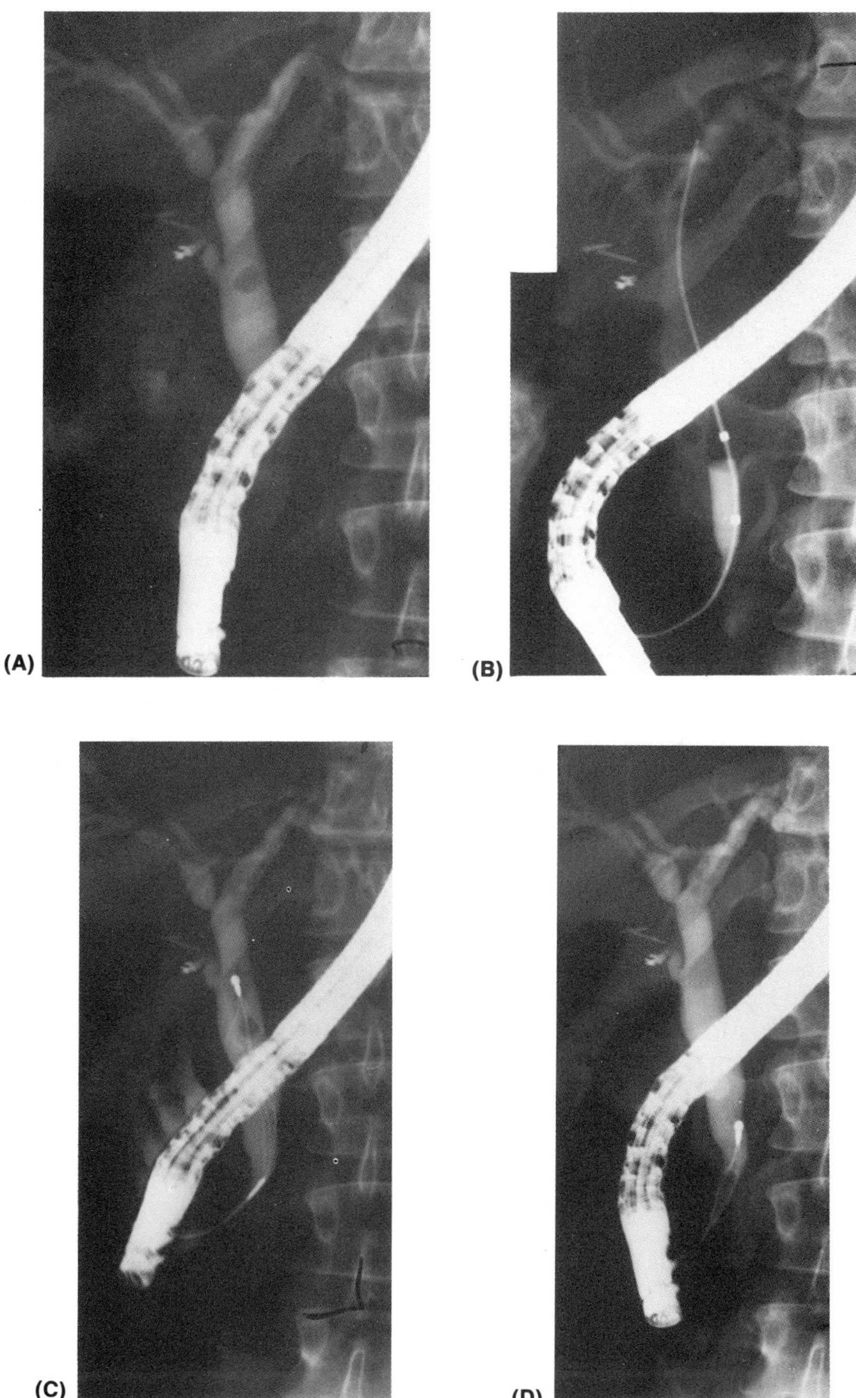

(A)

(B)

(C)

(D)

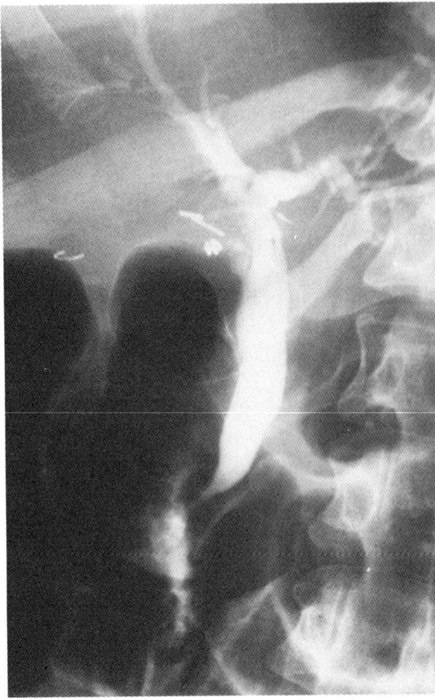

Fig. 2 **A**: An 8 mm stone retained after laparoscopic cholecystectomy. **B**: Balloon dilatation of the biliary sphincter to 8 mm. **C**: Basket entrapment of the stone. **D**: Withdrawal of the stone through the papilla. **E**: Empty bile duct with drainage

any substantial long-term hazard, but the possibility had led to renewed interest in removing stones from the bile duct at endoscopy without performing a sphincterotomy.

ENDOSCOPIC REMOVAL OF DUCT STONES WITHOUT SPHINCTEROTOMY

Relatively small stones can be pulled through the intact papilla at ERCP, with or without balloon dilatation of the sphincter (Fig. 2). This technique was originally described in 1983[24], and interest has revised recently. May and colleagues reported on 24 patients with stones less than 8 mm in diameter. All stones were removed with balloons and baskets, without performing a sphincterotomy; two patients developed mild pancreatitis[25]. An Irish group published similar encouraging results, including stones of up to 20 mm diameter[26]. There are no data on long-term follow-up of these patients, but damage to the sphincter appears unlikely. It is possible to combine this technique with other adjuvant methods such as mechanical lithotripsy and chemical dissolution.

INDICATIONS FOR ENDOSCOPIC MANAGEMENT OF DUCT STONES

ERCP is the diagnostic and therapeutic procedure of choice in any patient suspected of harbouring recurrent or retained stones after cholecystectomy[1].

In the presence of a T-tube, percutaneous radiological intervention provides an excellent alternative[27]. Repeat surgery should be necessary only rarely; for example in the context of prior surgical biliary diversion, repeated stone recurrence (for operative drainage), and for multiple intrahepatic stones.

ERCP is also appropriate in many patients who have not undergone cholecystectomy. This applies particularly in the context of acute suppurative cholangitis[28,29]. The consensus among most surgeons and endoscopists has recently been reinforced by the results of a randomized controlled trial published from Hong Kong; patients treated surgically had a 30-day mortality of 32%, compared with 10% for endoscopy[30]. Urgent ERCP is used also in some patients with acute gallstone pancreatitis. Randomized studies have validated this approach in patients with a predicted poor outcome[31]. It also appears logical in patients with pancreatitis who do not settle quickly (within 24–48 h) after hospital admission, especially if there is evidence of developing biliary obstruction. In these contexts it is assumed the patient will proceed to cholecystectomy once the acute illness has subsided. However, some elderly and high operative risk patients have been followed without cholecystectomy after endoscopic duct clearance. Many series show that the need for cholecystectomy is less than 20% when patients are followed for periods of up to 5 years[32-35]. Predicting the need for surgery is a subject of considerable interest. Although a small study suggested that non-visualization of the gallbladder at the time of ERCP stone extraction was a strong predictor for early cholecystitis[36], this has not been substantiated[33]. Dynamic isotope studies of gallbladder function may have some role in this context[37]. Endoscopic approaches have been given a further boost recently by the widespread introduction of LC.

ERCP AND LC

Approximately 10% of patients undergoing cholecystectomy for gallbladder stones also harbour stones in the bile duct[38-40]. Somewhat lower figures are being noted in recent LC series, possibly because patients are presenting for surgery earlier than before[21,41]. Some experts can explore the bile duct at laparoscopy and remove stones through the papilla or cystic duct[42,43] but these techniques are not yet widely available – and are unlikely to be so for some years. This means that most patients with duct stones must undergo open surgical exploration or ERCP/stone extraction. The merits of different approaches and combinations have been widely discussed[38,43,44]. It has been suggested (without any controlled data) that endoscopic sphincterotomy is more dangerous than open surgical duct exploration in relatively young and fit patients, and that the combination of LC and ERCP/sphincterotomy should be confined to the elderly and frail[43]. The complication data quoted earlier in this review suggest that the endoscopic approach is very safe even in the young. Furthermore, most patients are reluctant to undergo open surgery. In practice the important question is whether to perform ERCP/stone extraction before LC, or to wait and see if it is needed afterwards. Some have submitted all patients undergoing LC to a preoperative ERCP – to define ductal anatomy, and to rule out or remove stones[45]. This is clearly inappropriate, since the yield is likely to be no greater than the risks – quite apart from the additional costs. Thus, a selective approach to pre-LC/ERCP is widely accepted. Most would recommend ERCP in any patient with a very high likelihood of a duct stone (i.e. jaundice, cholangitis, stone on imaging, or non-resolving acute gallstone pancreatitis). The correct approach is less clear in patients with only moderate or low suspicion for a duct stone (e.g. some elevation of liver function tests or dilatation of the bile duct). Clinical, biochemical and radiological data can be combined to determine a percentage risk for stone; this number can be used to calculate the most cost-effective approach (e.g. by computer modelling) but, in real life, decisions are made according to local expertise and consensus[38].

An alternative to performing ERCP before LC is to do it afterwards only when LC demonstrates a stone (which cannot be removed laparoscopically). Experienced endoscopists will be successful in the vast majority of cases. Patients in whom stone extraction fails can be referred for more expert endoscopic attention, or may need open surgical intervention (albeit very rarely).

The size of any duct stone demonstrated at LC will influence the action taken. Some surgeons convert immediately to open surgery if the stone is large (greater than 10–15 mm), believing that subsequent endoscopic extraction is more likely to fail. Some recommend an expectant policy with stones less than 3 mm in diameter, assuming that most will pass without hazard[42]. More data are required to establish the safety of this approach.

There has been some discussion concerning the timing of ERCP/LC. If ERCP is performed first, LC should follow quickly, ideally on the next day; a longer delay may allow new stones to pass from the gallbladder into the duct. Equally, ERCP for management of a stone found during LC should be undertaken within very few days, to reduce the risk of impaction. ERCP and LC can be done together, under the same anaesthetic[46]. Although theoretically attractive, this approach has not found favour because of the practical difficulties involved. Laparoscopic transduodenal sphincteroplasty is even being proposed.

ENDOSCOPIC MANAGEMENT OF GALLBLADDER STONES

Recent enthusiasm for laparoscopy has overwhelmed the prior trend towards treatment of stones without removal of the gallbladder (e.g. by shock-wave lithotripsy, percutaneous cholecystostomy and percutaneous chemical dissolution). Should there be a resurgence of interest in retaining (relatively) healthy gallbladders in the future, endoscopists may be able to contribute further. It is technically possible to place a catheter through the papilla and cystic duct into the gallbladder, to permit chemical dissolution of gallbladder stones[47]. This endoscopic transcystic approach has also been used to remove gallbladder stones with a basket (Fig. 3), and to place a drain for management of acute cholecystitis[48,49].

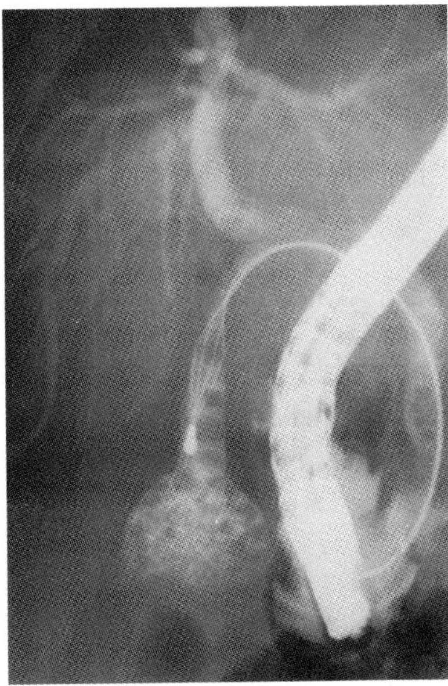

Fig. 3 ERCP extraction of a stone from the gallbladder using a basket passed through the cystic duct

PERCUTANEOUS CHOLANGIOSCOPY

Small flexible endoscopes can be passed through established T-tube and percutaneous transhepatic tracks. Stone extraction can be achieved with baskets, with or without direct vision laser or electrohydraulic lithotripsy[50]. Descending sphincterotomy has also been described. These techniques have been used primarily in the Orient for patients with multiple intrahepatic duct stones[51].

CONCLUSION

Laparoscopic cholecystectomy is now used in 80–90% of patients with gallbladder stones; 5–10% of these patients have concomitant stones in the bile duct, most of which are treated by ERCP/sphincterotomy before or after LC. Precise indications for different approaches continue to evolve. Each surgical/endoscopic team needs to develop and test algorithms which suit their interests and expertise, and provide most cost-effective management. The most important remaining questions are:

1. Can we improve preoperative methods for predicting and detecting duct stones (e.g. intravenous cholangiography revisited, other forms of scanning)?
2. How will laparoscopic duct exploration develop in the community?
3. Will endoscopic treatment of duct stones without sphincterotomy become widespread?
4. Can laparoscopic and ERCP techniques be taught more effectively, so

as to maximize their effectiveness and minimize the risks?
5. In which patients should gallbladder stones be treated without cholecystectomy?

References

1. Cotton PB. Endoscopic management of bile duct stones (apples and oranges). Gut. 1984;25:587–97.
2. Sivak MV. Endoscopic management of bile duct stones. Am J Surg. 1989;158:228–38.
3. Davis WZ, Onken J, Cotton PB. ERCP and laparoscopic cholecystectomy; academic and community practice patterns. Am J Gastroenterol. 1994 (In press).
4. Lambert ME, Betts CD, Hill J, Faragher EB, Martin DF, Tweedle DEF. Endoscopic sphincterotomy: the whole truth. Br J Surg. 1991;78:473–6.
5. Lauri A, Horton RC, Davidson BR, Burroughs AK, Dooley JS. Endoscopic extraction of the bile duct stones: management related to stone size. Gut. 1993;34:1718–21.
6. Classen M, Hagenmuler F, Knyrim K et al. Giant bile duct stones – nonsurgical treatment. Endoscopy. 1988;20:21–6.
7. Chung SCS, Leung JWC, Leong HT, Li AKC. Mechanical lithotripsy of large common bile duct stones using a basket. Br J Surg. 1991;78:1448–50.
8. Mavrogiannis C, Romanos A, Mavratzotis D et al. Mechanical, through-the-scope, lithotripsy for common bile duct (CBD) stones. Endoscopy. 1992;24:633A.
9. Shaw MJ, Vennes JA. Results of a multicenter trial using a mechanical lithotripter for the treatment of large bile duct stones. Am J Gastroenterol. 1993;83:730–3.
10. Cotton PB, Kozarek RA, Shapiro RH et al. Endoscopic laser lithotripsy of large bile duct stones. Gastroenterology. 1990;99:1128–33.
11. Leung JWC, Chung SSC. Electrohydraulic lithotripsy with peroral choledochoscopy. Br J Surg. 1989;399:595–8.
12. Ponchon T, Martin X, Barkun A et al. Extracorporeal lithotripsy of bile duct stones using ultrasonography for stone localization. Gastroenterology. 1990;98:726–32.
13. Neoptolemos JP, Hoffman AF, Moosa AR. Chemical treatment of stones in the biliary tree. Br J Surg. 1986;73:515–24.
14. Palmer KR, Hoffman AF. Intraductal mono-octonoin for the direct dissolution of bile duct stones. Experiences in 343 patients. Gut. 1986;27:196–202.
15. Cotton PB, Forbes A, Leung JWC et al. Endoscopic stenting for long-term treatment of large bile duct stones: 205 year follow-up. Gastrointest Endosc. 1987;33:411–13.
16. Libby ED, Edwards P, Leung JWC, Cotton PB. Endoscopic treatment of intrahepatic duct stones. Gastroenterology. 1993;104:A569.
17. Cotton PB, Lehman G, Vennes J et al. Endoscopic sphincterotomy, complications and their management. An attempt at consensus. Gastrointest Endosc. 1991;37:383–93.
18. Cotton PB, Geenen J, Sherman S et al. Sphincterotomy for stone is safer than advertised, even in young patients with small ducts. A multicenter prospective study. Gastrointest Endosc. 1994;40(In press).
19. Sherman S, Lehman GA. ERCP and endoscopic sphincterotomy-induced pancreatitis. Pancreas. 1991;6:350–67.
20. Sherman S, Ruffolo TA, Hawes RH, Lehman GA. Complications of endoscopic sphincterotomy. A prospective series with emphasis on the increased risk associated with sphincter of Oddi dysfunction and non-dilated ducts. Gastroenterology. 1991;101:1068–75.
21. Cetta F. Common duct stones in the era of laparoscopic cholecystectomy: changing treatments and new pathologic entities. J Laparoendosc Surg. 1994;4:41–2.
22. Johnston GW. Iatrogenic chymobilia – a disease of the nineties? Hepato-Pancreato-Biliary Surg. 1991;4:187–90.
23. Hawes RH, Cotton PB, Vallon AG. Follow-up at 6–11 years after duodenoscopic sphincterotomy for stones in patients with prior cholecystectomy. Gastroenterology. 1990;98:1008–12.
24. Staritz M, Ewe K, Meyer zum Buschenfelde K-H. Endoscopic papillary balloon dilation (EPD) for the treatment of common bile duct stones and papillary stenosis. Endoscopy. 1983;15:197–8.

25. May GR, Cotton PB, Edmunds SEJ, Chong W. Removal of stones from the bile duct at ERCP without sphincterotomy. Gastrointest Endosc. 1993;39:749–53.
26. MacMathuna P, White P, Clarke E, Lennon J, Crowe J. Endoscopic sphincteroplasty: a novel and safe alternative to papillotomy in the management of bile duct stones. Gut. 1994;35:127–9.
27. Nussinson E, Cairns SR, Vaira D, Dowsett JF, Mason RR. A 10 year single centre experience of percutaneous and endoscopic extraction of bile duct stones with T tube *in situ*. Gut. 1991;32:1040–3.
28. Leese T, Neoptolemos JP, Baker AR, Carr-Locke DL. Management of acute cholangitis and the impact of endoscopic sphincterotomy. Br J Surg. 1986;73:988–92.
29. Leung JWC, Chung SCS, Sung JJY, Banez VP, Li AKC. Urgent endoscopic drainage for acute suppurative cholangitis. Lancet. 1989;1:1307–9.
30. Lai ECS, Mok FPT, Tan ESY, Lo C-M, Fan S-T, You K-T, Wong J. Endoscopic biliary drainage for severe acute cholangitis. N Engl J Med. 1992;326:1582–6.
31. Williamson RCN. Endoscopic sphincterotomy in the early treatment of acute pancreatitis. N Engl J Med. 1993;328:279–80.
32. Cotton PB, Vallon AG. Duodenoscopic sphincterotomy for removal of bile duct stones in patients with gallbladders. Surgery. 1982;91:628–30.
33. Davidson BR, Neoptolemos JP, Carr-Locke DL. Endoscopic sphincterotomy for common bile duct calculi in patients with gallbladders in situ considered unfit for surgery. Gut. 1988;29:114–20.
34. Martin DF, Tweedle DEF. Endoscopic management of common duct stones without cholecystectomy. Br J Surg. 1987;74:209–11.
35. Hill J, Martin DF, Tweedle DEF. Risks of leaving the gallbladder in situ after endoscopic sphincterotomy for bile duct stones. Br J Surg. 1991;78:554–7.
36. Worthley CS, Toouli J. Gallbladder non-filling: an indication for cholecystectomy after endoscopic sphincterotomy. Br J Surg. 1988;75:796–8.
37. Holbrook RF, Jacobson FL, Pezzuti RT, Howell DA. Biliary patency imaging after endoscopic retrograde sphincterotomy with gallbladder in situ. Arch Surg. 1991;126:738–42.
38. Cotton PB. Endoscopic retrograde cholangiopancreatography and laparoscopic cholecystectomy. Am J Surg. 1993;165:474–8.
39. Pitt HA. Role of open choledochotomy in the treatment of choledocholithiasis. Am J Surg. 1993;165:483–6.
40. Johnson A, Hosking S. Appraisal of the management of bile duct stones. Br J Surg. 1987;74:555–60.
41. The Southern Surgeons Club. Prospective analysis of 2528 laparoscopic cholecystectomies. N Engl J Med. 1991;324:1073–8.
42. Carroll B, Phillips E. Laparoscopic removal of common duct stones. Gastrointest Endosc Clin N Am. 1993;3:239–48.
43. Fletcher DR. Laparoscopic cholecystectomy. Gastrointest Endosc Clin N Am. 1993;3:249–58.
44. Cotton P, Baillie J, Pappas T *et al.* Laparoscopic cholecystectomy and the biliary endoscopist. Gastroenterol Endosc. 1991;37:94–7.
45. Heuhaus H, Feussner H, Ungeheuer A, Hoffmann W, Siewert JR, Classen M. Prospective evaluation of the use of endoscopic retrograde cholangiography prior to laparoscopic cholecystectomy. Endoscopy. 1992;24:745–9.
46. Deslandres E, Gagner M, Pomp A *et al.* Intraoperative endoscopic sphincterotomy for common bile duct stones during laparoscopic cholecystectomy. Gastrointest Endosc. 1993;39:54–8.
47. Soehendra NH, Schulz V, Nam C *et al.* ESWL and gallstone dissolution with MTBE via a nasovesicular catheter. Endoscopy. 1990;22:176–9.
48. Tamada K, Seki H, Sato K *et al.* Efficacy of endoscopic retrograde cholecystoendoprosthesis (ERCCE) for cholecystitis. Endoscopy. 1991;23:2–3.
49. Johlin FC, Neil GA. Drainage of the gallbladder in patients with acute acalculous cholecystitis by transpapillary endoscopic cholecystotomy. Gastrointest Endosc. 1993;39:645–51.
50. Geisinger MA. Percutaneous biliary stone extraction. Radiologic and combined radiologic–endoscopic techniques. Gastrointest Endosc Clin N Am. 1991;1:105–24.
51. Han JK, Choi BI, Park JH, Han MC. Percutaneous removal of retained intrahepatic stones with a pre-shaped angulated catheter: review of 96 patients. Br J Radiol. 1992;65:9–13.

38
Extracorporeal shock-wave treatment of gallbladder and bile duct stones

G. PAUMGARTNER

INTRODUCTION

Gallstones represent a considerable health problem in the general population. Their prevalence in the adult population is about 10%[1]. Symptomatic gallbladder stones and bile duct stones require active treatment[2].

GALLBLADDER STONES

The various treatments for gallbladder stones are listed in Table 1 according to increasing invasiveness; oral bile acid dissolution therapy being the least invasive, open cholecystectomy the most invasive procedure.

Surgeons and medical physicians agree that cholecystectomy – either by laparotomy or by laparoscopy – is the standard treatment for symptomatic gallbladder stones. It can be performed irrespective of the type, number and size of the stones[3]. However, many patients are reluctant to undergo surgery or general anaesthesia despite the low risks of morbidity and mortality. Frequently, the patient insists on the least invasive treatment that would eliminate stones and symptoms.

Oral bile acid dissolution therapy is not invasive, but it is effective only in patients with very small radiolucent stones[4]. To overcome this limitation of oral bile acid dissolution therapy we have developed extracorporeal shock-wave lithotripsy of gallstones, which is also non-invasive, and we have

Table 1 Treatments for cholecystolithiasis listed according to increasing invasiveness

1.	Oral bile acid dissolution therapy
2.	Extracorporeal shock-wave lithotripsy
3.	Topical dissolution therapy
4.	Laparoscopic cholecystectomy
5.	Open cholecystectomy

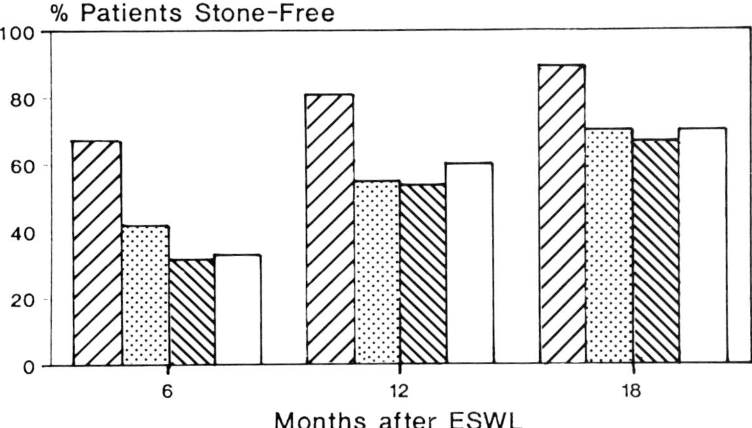

Fig. 1 Percentage of patients free of stones at various time points after extracorporeal shock-wave lithotripsy (ESWL) and adjuvant bile acid therapy calculated by actuarial analysis. ▨, Patients with a single stone ≤20 mm in diameter; ▤, patients with a single stone 21–30 mm in diameter; ▧, patients with two or three stones with a cumulative diameter ≤30 mm; ☐, patients with a single stone exhibiting a thin (<3 mm) calcified rim. Total number of patients = 931

combined fragmentation with medical dissolution[5].

Extracorporeal shock waves can be generated by electrohydraulic, piezoelectric or electromagnetic means[6]. Our group uses an electrohydraulic lithotripter which employs underwater spark discharge for shock-wave generation and an ellipsoidal reflector for focusing[5,7]. Monotherapy with ursodeoxycholic acid or combination therapy with ursodeoxycholic acid plus chenodeoxycholic acid is used for dissolution of stone fragments[7]. A prospective randomized trial from our group has shown that the two regimens do not differ with regard to efficacy. We now prefer monotherapy with ursodeoxycholic acid because it causes diarrhoea in only 5% of patients, whereas combination therapy causes diarrhoea in 18%[8].

The patients selected for extracorporeal shock-wave lithotripsy by our group had symptomatic, uncomplicated cholecystolithiasis; one to three radiolucent stones, diameter 5–30 mm, no calcifications or only a thin radiopaque rim (<3 mm) in a gallbladder that opacified on an oral cholecystogram[7,9]. For evaluation of efficacy the patients were then classified according to the number, diameter and radiolucency of the stones. The results of high-energy lithotripsy combined with adjuvant bile acid therapy in 931 patients treated by our group are given for the various subgroups of patients in Figure 1[10]. The highest success rate was obtained in the group of patients with a single radiolucent stone 20 mm or less in diameter. Of these patients about 70% cleared their fragments within 6 months, 80% within 12 months and about 90% within 18 months. The stone-free rate decreased with increases in the size and number of stones, and with the presence of a calcified rim. In Table 2 the results of our group[7] obtained in patients with radiolucent solitary gallbladder stones 20 mm or less in diameter, are compared with those of others[11–16]. Six months after lithotripsy the stone-free rate ranged

Table 2 Efficacy of extracorporeal shock-wave lithotripsy combined with adjuvant bile acid therapy in patients with a single radiolucent gallbladder stone up to 20 mm in diameter*

				Percentage of patients stone-free	
Author/reference	Year	No. of patients	Device†	6 months	12 months
Benninger et al.[11]	1992	98	PE	60	76
Elewaut et al.[12]	1993	169	PE	61	84
Greiner et al.[13]	1990	231	EH	41	68
McSherry et al.[14]	1991	175	PE	47	68
Pelletier et al.[15]	1991	147	PE	46	69
Sackmann et al.[17]	1991	122	EH	68	84
Wehrmann et al.[16]	1993	79	EM	68	80

*Only studies comprising more than 50 patients with solitary stones up to 20 mm in diameter, followed for at least 12 months, have been included
†PE, piezoelectric lithotripter; EH, electrohydraulic lithotripter; EM, electromagnetic lithotripter

between 41% and 68%; 12 months after lithotripsy it was between 68% and 84%.

An important factor for the success of lithotripsy is gallbladder emptying. When we measured gallbladder emptying during cholecystokinin infusion in patients who had cleared their gallbladder of all fragments within 18 months after lithotripsy, and compared it to gallbladder emptying in patients matched for gallstone volume, sex and age, who had not cleared the gallbladder within 18 months after lithotripsy, there was a significant difference[17]. The patients who had cleared their gallbladder of all fragments within 18 months ejected nearly twice as much of the fasting gallbladder volume (59%) as patients who did not become stone-free within this time period (32%). In a prospective study[18], patients with an ejection fraction of 60% or more became free of stones much faster, and at significantly higher rate, than patients with an ejection fraction of less than 60%. This underlines the importance of gallbladder emptying for fragment clearance.

Side-effects directly related to shock-wave lithotripsy have been minimal. Most adverse effects and complications were related to the passage of fragments after lithotripsy, pancreatitis in 2%, cholestasis in 1% and cholecystitis in 1%. Endoscopic sphincterotomy was required in 1%. Less than 5% of all patients underwent cholecystectomy within 24 months of follow-up[3,7]. Biliary pain, probably caused by the passage of fragments, occurred in about one third of patients, mainly during the first 2–3 months after lithotripsy[7]. In published trials on several thousands of patients, no fatalities attributable to lithotripsy have been reported.

Patients who had successfully undergone a gallbladder-preserving treatment are at the risk of stone recurrence. The cumulative stone recurrence rate at 4 years after successful bile acid dissolution therapy is much lower (about 12%) in patients who initially had a single stone than in patients who initially had multiple stones (about 45%)[19]. In our group of patients treated by shock-wave lithotripsy and bile acids, 90% have had a single stone. The recurrence rate in this group of patients was only 20% after 4 years[20]. Besides initial stone number, incomplete gallbladder emptying and increased

Table 3 Characteristics of the optimal candidate for extracorporeal shock-wave lithotripsy of gallbladder stones

1. Symptomatic, uncomplicated cholecystolithiasis
2. Solitary, radiolucent stone
3. Stone diameter 5–20 mm
4. No calcifications
5. Gallbladder emptying > 60%

Table 4 Efficacy of extracorporeal shock-wave lithotripsy of bile duct stones

Author/reference	Year	No. of patients	Device*	Percentage of patients stone-free
Greiner et al.[23]	1992	229	EM	90
Lee et al.[24]	1990	70	EM	61
Moody et al.[25]	1989	56	EH	79
Toom et al.[26]	1991	49	EM	86
Sauerbruch et al.[22]	1992	103	EM	88

*Abbreviations as in Table 2

conversion of cholic acid to deoxycholic acid appear to be risk factors for gallstone recurrence[21].

Based on our results on efficacy and recurrence, the optimal candidate for shock-wave lithotripsy has the characteristics listed in Table 3.

BILE DUCT STONES

For treatment of bile duct stones open or laparoscopic choledochotomy, endoscopic procedures and extracorporeal shock-wave lithotripsy are available. The mainstay of therapy of bile duct stones, especially in cholecystectomized and in high-risk patients, is endoscopic procedures. In experienced hands endoscopic sphincterotomy and stone extraction are successful in over 90% of patients with extrahepatic bile duct stones. Shock-wave lithotripsy is indicated when routine endoscopic procedures including mechanical lithotripsy fail, provided that access to the bile duct has been established by nasobiliary tube and the orifice of the common bile duct in the intestine is large enough for spontaneous passage or extraction of fragments[4].

The reasons for failure of endoscopic procedures in 103 patients who underwent shock-wave lithotripsy in our institution were impaction of stone(s) in 47%, inaccessible or very large stones in 44%, and bile duct stenosis in 9%[22]. 52% of the patients had multiple stones, 48% a single stone and 14% had intrahepatic stones. The mean size of the stones was 20 mm; 66% of the patients became stone-free after the first lithotripsy session and 88% after the second or third lithotripsy session.

In Table 4 the results obtained by our group[22] are compared with those of other studies[23-26], including 50 or more patients. In the majority of these studies the bile ducts could be cleared of all stones in about 80–90% of the patients. Repeat sessions were often required, and endoscopic extraction of fragments was necessary in the majority of patients, because fragment size is usually larger than after lithotripsy of gallbladder stones. Extracorporeal shock-wave lithotripsy was relatively safe, despite the fact that mainly elderly, high-risk patients were treated. The most important adverse effect during shock-wave treatment was cardiac arrhythmia; after treatment it was sepsis originating from the biliary tree[22]. We therefore advise antibiotic prophylaxis. Mild and transient haemobilia was observed in less than 10%. Haematoma of the liver and mild attacks of biliary pancreatitis were rare complications. The 30-day mortality rate was about 1%[22].

References

1. Paumgartner G, Sauerbruch T. Gallstones: pathogenesis. Lancet. 1991;338:1117–24.
2. Paumgartner G, Carr-Locke DL, Dubois F, Roda E, Thistle JL. Strategies in the treatment of gallstone disease. Gastroenterol Int. 1993;6:65–75.
3. Sauerbruch T, Paumgartner G. Gallbladder stones: management. Lancet. 1991;338:1121–4.
4. Paumgartner G. Nonoperative management of gallstone disease. In: Sleisenger MH, Fordtran JS, editors. Gastrointestinal disease. Philadelphia: Saunders; 1993:1844–57.
5. Sauerbruch T, Delius M, Paumgartner G et al. Fragmentation of gallstones by extracorporeal shock waves. N Engl J Med. 1986;314:818–22.
6. Paumgartner G, Sauerbruch T. Extracorporeal shock wave lithotripsy of gallstones. In: Zakim D, Boyer TD, editors. Hepatology: a textbook of liver disease. Philadelphia: Saunders; 1991:1561–8.
7. Sackmann M, Pauletzki J, Sauerbruch T, Holl J, Schelling G, Paumgartner G. The Munich gallbladder lithotripsy study: results of the first 5 years with 711 patients. Ann Intern Med. 1991;114:290–6.
8. Sackmann M, Pauletzki J, Aydemir U et al. Efficacy and safety of ursodeoxycholic acid for dissolution of gallstone fragments: comparison with a combination of ursodeoxycholic acid and chenodeoxycholic acid. Hepatology. 1991;14:1136–41.
9. Sackmann M, Pauletzki J, Delius M, Holl J, Sauerbruch T, Paumgartner G. Noninvasive therapy of gallbladder calculi with a radiopaque rim. Gastroenterology. 1992;102:988–93.
10. Paumgartner G, Pauletzki J, Sackmann M. Ursodeoxycholic acid treatment of cholesterol gallstone disease. Scand J Gastroenterol. Supplement 1994 (in press).
11. Benninger J, Schneider HT, Hahn EG, Ell C. A clinical comparison of an electrohydraulic and a piezoelectric shockwave lithotripter in gallstone therapy. Am J Gastroenterol. 1993;88:58–63.
12. Elewaut A, Crape A, Afschrift M, Pauwels W, De Vos M, Barbier F. Results of extracorporeal shock wave lithotripsy of gall bladder stones in 693 patients: a plea for restriction to solitary radiolucent stones. Gut. 1993;34:274–8.
13. Greiner L, Jakobeit C. Biliary shock-wave lithotripsy: experience of the first 3 years in 612 patients. In: Swobodnik W, Ditschuneit H, Soloway RD, editors. Gallstone disease. Berlin: Springer; 1990:177–93.
14. McSherry CK, EDAP Investigators Group: the results of the EDAP multicenter trial of biliary lithotripsy in the United States. Surgery. 1991;173:461–4.
15. Pelletier G, Delmont J, Capdeville R et al. Treatment of gallstones with piezoelectric lithotripsy and oral bile acids. A multicenter study. J Hepatol. 1991;12:327–31.
16. Wehrmann T, Hurst A, Lembcke B, Jung M, Caspary W. Biliary lithotripsy with a new electromagnetic shock wave source. A 2-year clinical experience. Dig Dis Sci. 1993;38:2113–20.
17. Sackmann M, Eder H, Spengler U et al. Gallbladder emptying is an important factor in fragment disappearance after shock-wave lithotripsy. J Hepatol. 1993;17:62–6.
18. Pauletzki J, Sailer C, Klüppelberg U et al. Gallbladder emptying is a determinant of gallstone clearance after lithotripsy. Gastroenterology. 1993;104:A375.
19. Villanova N, Bazzoli F, Taroni F et al. Gallstone recurrence after successful oral bile acid

treatment. A 12-year follow-up study and evaluation of long-term postdissolution treatment. Gastroenterology. 1989;97:726–31.

20. Sackmann M, Niller H, Klueppelberg U *et al.* Gallstone recurrence after shock wave therapy. Gastroenterology. 1994;106:225–30.

21. Berr F, Mayer M, Sackmann M, Sauerbruch T, Holl J, Paumgartner G. Pathogenic factors in early recurrence of cholesterol gallstones. Gastroenterology. 1994;106:215–24.

22. Sauerbruch T, Holl J, Sackmann M, Paumgartner G. Fragmentation of bile duct stones by extracorporeal shock-wave lithotripsy. A five-years experience. Hepatology. 1992;15: 208–14.

23. Greiner L, Jakobeit C, Schuhmacher R. Bile duct extracorporeal shock-wave lithotripsy – seven years experience. Gastroenterology. 1992;102:A113.

24. Lee SH, Fache JS, Burhenne HJ. The value of extracorporeal shock-wave lithotripsy in the management of bile duct stones. Am J Roentgenol. 1990;155:775–9.

25. Moody FG, Amerson JR, Berci G *et al.* Lithotripsy for bile duct stones. Am J Surg. 1989;158:241–7.

26. Toom R den, Nigs HGT, Blankenstein M van, Lameris JS, Schroeder FH, Terpstra OT. Extracorporeal shock wave treatment of common bile duct stones: experience with two different lithotripters at a single institution. Br J Surg. 1991;78:809–13.

39
Implications of laparoscopic cholecystectomy

O. T. TERPSTRA

Laparoscopic cholecystectomy (LC) is associated with a shorter hospital stay, a quicker convalescence and a better cosmetic result. Drawbacks of this new approach to treating gallbladder stones are the 'learning curve', resulting in more injuries of the common bile duct, a longer operation time, and less training in the conventional procedure of removing the gallbladder at laparotomy.

Little attention is paid to other side-effect of the introduction of LC: the shift in diagnostic and therapeutic procedures in the management of the patients with symptomatic gallbladder stones. To evaluate this effect data were obtained from the Foundation on Information in Health Care (SIG) in The Netherlands during the period 1991–93. In this period the number of cholecystectomies performed in The Netherlands increased by 21.2%. This is in sharp contrast with the declining number of cholecystectomies observed in The Netherlands, and most Western countries during the past decade, before 1991. The percentage of surgical common bile duct explorations decreased in the same period by 28.3%. Endoscopic cholangiography increased by 69.5% and endoscopic papillotomy by 55.4%. In 1993 an endoprosthesis was placed in the bile ducts in 15.9% more cases than in 1991.

The introduction of laparoscopic cholecystectomy has led to a change in the management of patients with uncomplicated gallbladder stones. This resulted in an increased number of cholecystectomies and an increased use of endoscopic cholangiography and papillotomy. The added risk of these procedures in treating uncomplicated gallstones is predicted to lead to a higher incidence of late complications, and higher mortality for the population with gallbladder stone disease. The same observations are made in other countries, e.g. Australia. From the data it can be concluded that the application of a technique aimed at minimizing the surgical trauma leads to an overall increase in morbidity and mortality: the paradox of the introduction of safer technology.

Index